Pain Medicine

THE REQUISITES IN ANESTHESIOLOGY

SERIES EDITOR **Roberta L. Hines,** MD
Chair and Professor
Department of Anesthesiology
Yale University School of Medicine
New Haven, Connecticut

Pain Medicine

THE REQUISITES IN ANESTHESIOLOGY

Stephen E. Abram, MD
Professor
Department of Anesthesiology
Medical College of Wisconsin
Milwaukee, Wisconsin

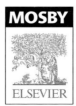

MOSBY

ELSEVIER

MOSBY
ELSEVIER

1600 John F. Kennedy Boulevard
Suite 1800
Philadelphia, PA 19103-2899

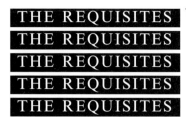

THE REQUISITES is a proprietary trademark
of Mosby, Inc.

PAIN MEDICINE: THE REQUISITES IN ANESTHESIOLOGY

ISBN-10: 0-323-02831-4
ISBN-13: 978-0-323-02831-8

Notice

Knowledge and best practice in this field are constantly changing. As new research and experience broaden our knowledge, changes in practice, treatment and drug therapy may become necessary or appropriate. Readers are advised to check the most current information provided (i) on procedures featured or (ii) by the manufacturer of each product to be administered, to verify the recommended dose or formula, the method and duration of administration, and contraindications. It is the responsibility of the practitioner, relying on his or her own experience and knowledge of the patient, to make diagnoses, to determine dosages and the best treatment for each individual patient, and to take all appropriate safety precautions. To the fullest extent of the law, neither the Publisher nor the Editor assumes any liability for any injury and/or damage to persons or property arising out or related to any use of the material contained in this book.

Library of Congress Cataloging-in-Publication Data
Pain medicine : the requisites in anesthesiology / Stephen E. Abram, editor. – 1st ed.
      p. ; cm. – (Requisites in anesthesiology series)
   ISBN-0-323-02831-4
   1. Pain medicine. I. Abram, Stephen E. II. Series.
   [DNLM: 1. Pain–drug therapy. 2. Anesthesia. WL 704 P14678 2006]
RB127.P332496 2006
616'.0472–dc22   2005053421

Acquisitions Editor: Joanne Husovski
Developmental Editor: Anne Snyder
Project Manager: David Saltzberg
Design Direction: Steven Stave
Marketing Manager: Emily McGrath-Christie

Printed in the United States of America

Last digit is the print number: 9   8   7   6   5   4   3   2   1

Working together to grow
libraries in developing countries

www.elsevier.com | www.bookaid.org | www.sabre.org

ELSEVIER   BOOK AID International   Sabre Foundation

To the Anesthesiology Residents and Pain Medicine Fellows who have worked with me in the Pain Clinic over the past 30 years. You have worked tirelessly and (mostly) without complaint to improve the lives of countless patients suffering from intractable pain. Your efforts have provided relief, comfort, and hope to our most vulnerable and underserved patients.

To Pam, for her support and encouragement throughout this project.

Stephen E. Abram, MD

Contributors

Stephen E. Abram, MD
Professor
Department of Anesthesiology
Medical College of Wisconsin
Milwaukee, Wisconsin

Caridad Bravo-Fernandez, MD
Department of Anesthesiology
Medical College of Wisconsin
Milwaukee, Wisconsin

Mikhail Fukshansky, MD
Pain Management Fellow
Assistant Professor
Department of Anesthesiology
University of Texas MD Anderson Cancer Center
Houston, Texas

Robert E. Kettler, MD
Department of Anesthesiology
Medical College of Wisconsin
Milwaukee, Wisconsin

Randa Noseir, MD
Assistant Professor
Department of Anesthesiology
Medical College of Wisconsin
Milwaukee, Wisconsin

Therese O'Connor, FFARCSI
Dip Pain Medicine
Consultant in Anesthesia and Pain Management
Sligo General Hospital
Sligo, Ireland

Phillip Phan, MD
Senior Anesthesia Resident
Baylor College of Medicine
Houston, Texas

Arun Rajagopal, MD
Interventional Spine and Pain Clinic
St. Mark's Hospital
Salt Lake City, Utah

Constantine Sarantopoulos, MD, PhD
Director
Pain Management Center
CJ Zablocki Veterans Administration Medical Center
Milwaukee, Wisconsin
Associate Professor
Department of Anesthesiology
Medical College of Wisconsin
Milwaukee, Wisconsin

Hariharan Shankar, MD
Fellow in Anesthesiology
Department of Anesthesiology
Medical College of Wisconsin
Milwaukee, Wisconsin

Mary Lou Taylor, PhD
Department of Anesthesiology
Medical College of Wisconsin
Milwaukee, Wisconsin

Jaya L. Varadarajan, MD
Attending Physician
Jane B. Pettit Pain and Palliative Care Center
Children's Hospital of Wisconsin
Milwaukee, Wisconsin
Assistant Professor
Department of Anesthesiology
Medical College of Wisconsin
Milwaukee, Wisconsin

Mark S. Wallace, MD
Department of Anesthesiology
University of California San Diego
La Jolla, California

Steven J. Weisman, MD
Jane B. Pettit Chair in Pain Management
Children's Hospital of Wisconsin
Milwaukee, Wisconsin
Professor
Departments of Anesthesiology and Pediatrics
Medical College of Wisconsin
Milwaukee, Wisconsin

Thomas J. Whalen, MD
Private Practice
Albuquerque, New Mexico

Preface

This volume of the Requisites in Anesthesiology series was created to provide Anesthesiology residents with guidelines for the treatment of many common pain problems and to serve as a study guide for the Anesthesiology board examinations. In addition, we expect that it will serve as a valuable pain management text for anesthesiologists and other specialists involved in the treatment of acute, chronic, and cancer pain. While a textbook of this scope cannot provide sufficient depth of knowledge for all painful conditions, it should impart a sound basic understanding of many of the pain problems encountered in a community practice.

Pain Medicine has been late in adopting the principles of evidence–based medicine that have been incorporated into other medical disciplines. There are many reasons for this. The problems encountered in a pain clinic are heterogeneous and include neuropathic, somatic, and visceral sources of pain, both peripheral and central pain states, and contributions from psychological issues, substance abuse, psychiatric comorbidities, and antisocial and self-destructive behaviors. We deal with long-standing refractory problems for which the accepted therapies have low success rates. The ability to successfully conduct randomized controlled trials under such circumstances is limited. Nevertheless, increasing numbers of well-conducted outcome trials and case series are leading us toward therapies with demonstrable efficacy and away from those with low chances of success. The emergence of new outcome data will necessarily lead to changes in therapies. Some of the treatment recommendations expressed in this book will be abandoned or modified; others will be confirmed.

Still other changes will come as the rapid advances in the basic science of pain perception are translated into clinical therapies. Our understanding of the mechanisms of nociception, neuropathy, and central sensitization has advanced rapidly, but few of these breakthroughs have resulted in efficacious therapies. Hopefully this will change.

As purveyors of medical technology, we are drawn to those therapies that involve technical innovation. Some of these technologies have provided substantial improvements in the lives of patients who have not benefitted from more conventional treatments. Others have not been shown to be of significant benefit. Others are effective in a small minority of patients. Unfortunately, these sophisticated and often expensive interventions are ineffective for a substantial number, possibly a majority, of patients with chronic pain. We must therefore rely on the basic tools of pain management that have evolved over the past half century: physical rehabilitation, cognitive-behavioral therapy, pharmacological intervention, and addiction medicine. These are not therapies that produce dramatic and rapid results, and reimbursement for their providers is typically poor; but they are essential to the successful treatment of most patients with long-standing pain.

It is the aim of this textbook to provide an introduction to the entire range of treatment options available for patients with intractable pain. There are few treatment algorithms or care maps presented, as few have been developed. The trainee in Pain Medicine will be dependent on the experience and expertise of faculty mentors as he or she learns how to incorporate treatment options into a coherent plan. However, even the least experienced physician can provide a valuable service to the most difficult and complex patients by listening carefully, examining thoroughly, offering to help, and providing explanations. There are two statements that patients never want to hear: "I don't know what's wrong with you," and "There is nothing I can do for you." We can always provide a logical, if not totally proven, explanation of why a patient has pain, and there is always something that can be done to help.

Contents

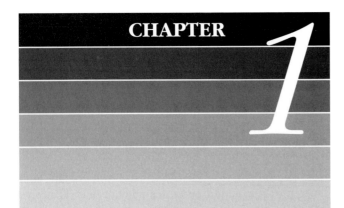

Pain Pathways and Mechanisms

CONSTANTINE SARANTOPOULOS

INTRODUCTION

The sensation of pain is the final result of a complex and interactive series of mechanisms integrated at all levels of the nervous system from the periphery through the spinal cord to the higher cerebral structures. "Pain" describes a conscious, unpleasant sensory and emotional experience that can be induced by a wide variety of events to which humans can be subjected. It can be defined as the perception of an unpleasant sensation originating from an area of the body, produced by actual or potential tissue damage, or described in terms of such damage. However, advances in our knowledge of the physiology of pain over the last years have lead to other relevant terminology.

The emphasis on the stimulus that activates the pain pathway and its immediate consequences has been recognized by the use of the word "nociception," introduced by Sherrington in the early 1900s. *Nociception* is

1

a specialized form of sensory signaling, describing the generation, transmission, and processing of information associated with the actual or potential tissue damage. At its simplest level of organization, nociception can be considered the electrical, chemical, and synaptic activity in the sensory afferent neuron. At higher levels it includes the motor reflex responses evoked by that stimulus, and at even higher levels it may describe the response evoked by such stimuli that are organized at the brainstem level into cardiovascular, hormonal, or other responses to pain. According to Sherrington, pain is a nociceptive reflex with a psychical component. "Nociceptors" are the peripheral sensory neurons that respond selectively to noxious stimuli, thus having the capacity to discriminate between painful and nonpainful sensory input.

Pain can be produced by activation of the specific nociceptors in the periphery, and in this case is characterized as "nociceptive" pain. However, it may also result from injury or alterations to sensory fibers or from disease or damage to the central nervous system (CNS) itself. This is called "neuropathic" pain. A progressive unraveling of the neuroanatomical substrate and cellular mechanisms underlying pain has been in process, and an increasing understanding of these mechanisms facilitates the development of novel strategies for more effective treatment.

In the 17th century, René Descartes described man as a *machine*: Man functioned as any other machine, differing only in sensitivity and reasoning capacity. He claimed that the nerves are connected to the sensory endings and convey the sensations to the brain. Through a nerve, an effective stimulus makes its way to the brain and produces the sensation of pain. Luigi Galvani was the first to suggest, in the late 18th century, the electrical nature of the nerve conduction, and Du Bois-Reymond measured injury currents in nerves using a galvanometer in 1840.

In the following centuries, the foundations of modern anatomy and physiology were laid. With the discovery of even more detailed knowledge, we have our present understanding of the science of pain. However, the views of Descartes have so thoroughly permeated our concepts about physiology and anatomy that it has been difficult to escape them. They have lead to a persistent search of pain fibers, pathways, and pain centers in the brain. The result was the concept of the pain as a specific projection system, which lead to ways to treat severe chronic pain with chemical, electrical, or physical "neural blockade," utilizing a multitude of different ablative or neurosurgical lesions. We know now that these procedures frequently fail and the pain tends to return, even in forms worse than those we attempt to abolish. This is explained by the dynamic, plastic properties of the neural tissue itself, something that was not conceived by the early theorists.

Modern pain theories evolved from a number of divergent views, which have been argued over the last 100 years. In the 1960s, Melzack and Wall[1] integrated the strong data of the specificity and pattern theories with the belief that the "straight-through" connection of the Cartesian model was contradicted by the more modern theories; they proposed the *Gate Control Theory*, highlighting the dynamic central nervous system mechanisms as an essential component in pain processes. According to the Gate Control Theory, large and small diameter nerve fibers project to the substantia gelatinosa and the central sensory transmission neurons. Signals of pain (high-threshold signals) are conveyed by small fibers. Large fibers convey low-threshold, normally nonpainful signals. Input from the large fibers results in activation of central control mechanisms, which subsequently project back and modify the gate control system. This theory forced biomedical sciences to accept the brain as an active system that filters, selects, and modulates inputs. The dorsal horns were also accepted as active sites at which dynamic activities (i.e., inhibition, excitation, and modulation) occurred instead of merely passive transmission stations. The cutting of nerves and pathways was gradually replaced by methods to modulate the input, such as physical therapy, transcutaneous electrical nerve stimulation (TENS), or spinal cord stimulation (SCS).

Finally, over the last few years, there has been a significant contribution to the understanding of pain from the advances in the basic sciences, such as molecular biology, electrophysiology, and basic pharmacology. Particular attention is now focused on cellular and subcellular aspects and signaling mediators as well as the development of more rationalized treatments for both acute and chronic pain.

PAIN PATHWAYS

The "pathways of pain" as classically understood, consist of a three-neuron chain that transmits pain signals from the periphery to the cerebral cortex. Starting from the periphery, the first order (or primary afferent) neuron has its cell body in the dorsal root ganglion and two axons. The peripheral axon projects distally to the tissue it innervates. The proximal axon extends centrally to the dorsal horn of the spinal cord. In the dorsal horn, this axon synapses with the second-order neuron, the axon of which crosses the spinal cord through the anterior white commissure and ascends in the spinothalamic tracts to the thalamus. At that site, it synapses with the third order neuron, which projects through the internal capsule and the corona radiata to the postcentral gyrus of the cerebral cortex, where information is somatotopically organized and perceived (Fig. 1-1).

Peripheral Pathways

The spinal nerves are formed by the junction of the anterior (ventral) and posterior (dorsal) spinal roots

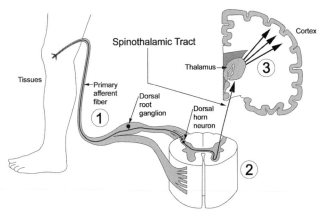

Figure 1-1 Basic organization of pathways of pain transmission from the periphery to the brain. (Copyright 2004 Catherine Twomey/Medical Center Graphics, Milwaukee, Wisconsin.)

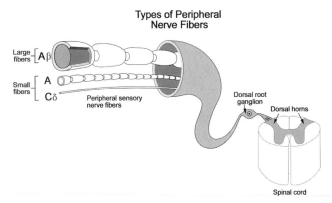

Figure 1-2 Types of nerve fibers involved in sensory transmission. (Copyright 2004 Catherine Twomey/Medical Center Graphics, Milwaukee, Wisconsin.)

(see Fig. 1-1). Motor and autonomic efferent fibers exit through the ventral spinal roots, while input of sensory afferent fibers is through the dorsal roots. After a limited course, the spinal nerves divide into anterior and posterior primary rami. Thus, sensory and motor fibers are distributed to both primary rami. The posterior rami innervate the posterior (dorsal) spinal and somatic muscular and cutaneous structures (such as the muscles and skin of the back), while the anterior rami form the various neural plexuses and peripheral nerves of the body.

The peripheral nerves are composed of axons from somatic and visceral (autonomic) systems, with sensory (afferent) and motor (efferent) components in each system. Somatic sensory fibers from several spinal nerves often fuse to form peripheral nerves. However, each spinal nerve still conveys cutaneus sensory input from a conceptually discrete area of skin. These discrete areas are called *dermatomes* and provide a clinically useful sensory map of the body surface (but there is some overlap and nonuniformity in their distribution). The cutaneous somatic input retains a radicular organization, as do the bone (sclerotomes) and the muscles (myotomes) afferents.

The nerve fibers are characterized by their degree of myelination, diameter, and velocity of electrical signal conduction. The A fibers are large, myelinated, and of rapid conduction. The Aα subtype convey motor signals to the muscles. The Aβ fibers convey sensory such as touch, pressure, and proprioception, and the Aγ innervate muscle spindles. The Aδ fibers convey signals of touch, heat, and pain faster than the C fibers, which also convey similar modalities that are non-myelinated, smaller, and slower. Aδ and C fibers are referred to as *small fibers*, while the Aβ are called *large fibers* (Fig. 1-2). The B fibers are small myelinated fibers, which convey preganglionic sympathetic signals. Pain signals are conveyed by a subpopulation of the small fibers.

The visceral afferents convey sensory information (including pain) from the viscera. They are pure sensory fibers, but follow the nerves of the autonomic nervous system and are divided into those that accompany the sympathetic nerves and those that follow the parasympathetic nerves. Nociceptive information from the abdominal and thoracic viscera is transmitted by sensory fibers, which follow the sympathetic pathways. The visceral afferents that accompany the sympathetic nerves traverse the prevertebral ganglia (e.g., the ganglia in the celiac plexus) without synapsing, reach the paravertebral sympathetic chain via the splanchnic nerves, and then reach the segmental nerves (T1 to L2) via the white rami communicantes (or sometimes the grey), and finally their cell bodies in the dorsal root ganglia (Figs. 1-3 and 1-4). From there, both the somatic and the visceral information follow a similar course toward the cerebral cortex.

Most visceral afferents from the sigmoid colon, rectum, neck of the bladder, prostate, and cervix of the uterus accompany the parasympathetic efferent fibers entering the cord in the dorsal roots of S2 to S4. The visceral afferents of the vagus nerve have their cell bodies in the nodose ganglion and transmit information such as bloating, distention, and nausea-like sensations, but not pain, except perhaps from those innervating the hypopharynx and the upper respiratory tract. They can, however, modify the responsiveness of the nociceptive dorsal horn neurons.

PRIMARY AFFERENT FIBERS

Any tissue noxious alterations that involve extreme mechanical distortion, thermal stimulation, or changes in the chemical milieu at the peripheral sensory terminals will evoke the verbal report of pain in humans and efforts to escape in animals as well as more complex responses. The circuitry that serves the transduction and encoding of this information, starts with the activation of

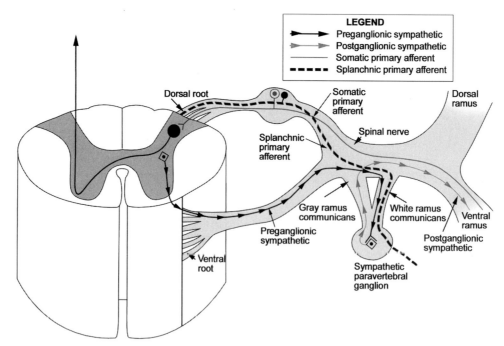

Figure 1-3   Transmission of pain signals from visceral organs via the sympathetic chain and spinal nerves. (Copyright 2004 Catherine Twomey/Medical Center Graphics, Milwaukee, Wisconsin.)

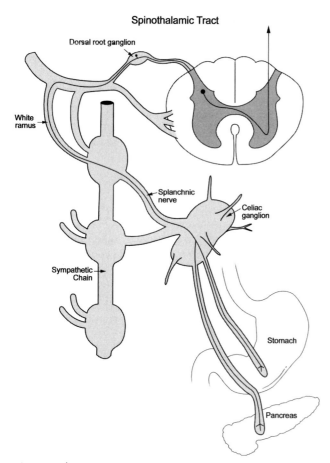

Figure 1-4   Transmission of pain signals from upper abdominal viscera. Celiac plexus. (Copyright 2004 Catherine Twomey/Medical Center Graphics, Milwaukee, Wisconsin.)

the nociceptors, the subsequent depolarization of the primary afferent axons, the transmission of the information to the bodies of the neurons in the dorsal root ganglia, and finally to the synapses with the dorsal horn cells (see Figs. 1-1, 1-2, and 1-3).

Cell Bodies

The cell bodies of the primary afferent somatic fibers are located in the dorsal root ganglia (DRG). The cell bodies of the primary afferent visceral fibers are also located in the DRG, but some of these visceral afferents may have cell bodies in the sympathetic ganglia or organs of origin.

Nociceptors

The primary afferent fibers encode and convey different modalities of sensation. They are classified as *nociceptors* (if they respond to high-threshold noxious stimuli), *mechanoreceptors* (if they encode and convey mechanical information), *thermoreceptors* (responsible for thermal information), *chemoreceptors* (for chemical information), and so forth.

Nociceptors belong either to the Aδ or the C type of sensory fibers (see Fig. 1-2) but not all Aδ and C fibers are nociceptive fibers. Most Aδ and C fibers have free nerve endings without any specialized structures (such as the Meissner's and Pacinian corpuscles or the proprioceptive endings). About 75% of the Aδ, and a variable number of C, respond to low-threshold mechanical, chemical, and thermal stimuli, and the remainder are pure nociceptors. Stimulation of the cutaneous Aδ nociceptors leads to localized, sharp, pricking pain of fast perception, whereas stimulation of the C receptors results in burning or dull, poorly localized pain of a more delayed perception. This has more to do with the signaling of tissue inflammation and the modification of the behavior toward withdrawal, immobility, and rest. When we touch a hot object, the initial acute, sharp painful sensation (first pain sensation) is conveyed by Aδ fibers, followed by a delayed, more dull, and ongoing painful burning feeling, transmitted via the C fibers.

With the exception of pathologic conditions, two criteria are necessary to define a nociceptor: The first is a response threshold higher than that of low-threshold mechanoreceptors and thermoreceptors. For example, frankly noxious stimuli capable of causing skin damage can activate only certain cutaneous nociceptors and be perceived as painful by humans. The second criterion is an ability to encode the intensity of nociceptive stimuli in terms of increasing firing frequency of action potentials. When these two criteria are considered, the nociceptors have the capacity to distinguish clearly between noxious and innocuous events in the signals they send to the CNS.

It is very difficult to provide an absolute taxonomy of nociceptors, but functionally they can be classified as follows (although their characterization is complicated by several factors such as terminological inconsistencies, species differences, contrasting properties, and methods of detection):

1. **High-Threshold Mechanical Nociceptors (HTM).** They are Aδ mostly, which according to other classification systems are classified as A-fiber Mechano-Heat nociceptors Type I (type I AMH). They are high-threshold, rapidly conducting mechanonociceptors, but they respond weakly to high intensity thermal stimuli. Although they have very high heat thresholds, when a heat stimulus of sufficient intensity and duration is delivered, they are sensitized and may respond to heat. They are particularly prevalent in the glabrous skin (but the major part for the nociceptive innervation of the skin comes from the C polymodal receptors).

2. **Myelinated Mechano-Thermal Nociceptors (MMTN).** They are also Aδ fibers, which respond in a graded fashion to progressively intense stimuli. They are also classified as Type II A Mechano-Heat Nociceptors (type II AMH) and are distinguished by a substantially lower threshold for activation. They have a lower threshold to noxious heat and respond more rapidly. These nociceptors are the first to signal pain sensation.

3. **C-fiber Mechano-Heat Nociceptors (CMH).** They have a heat threshold between 38°C and 50°C and encode for the intensity of pain induced by noxious heat stimuli. They typically show fatigue or habituation as well as sensitization.

4. **Pure Thermal Receptors.** They respond to heat alone, showing an all or none response.

5. **C Polymodal Receptors (CPN).** They make up 95% of the human C sensory fibers and respond to a variety of noxious stimuli: intense heat, intense mechanical force, and chemical stimuli. A significant percentage (probably most) of these receptors are *silent* or *sleeping* nociceptors under normal conditions; they are inactive and unresponsive and do not participate in any sensory input of nociception. However, inflammation or tissue injury can cause the sensitization of these nerves fibers, after which they "awaken." After sensitization, these fibers can be stimulated and may easily develop evoked or spontaneous discharges. This sensitization depends on the activation of second-messenger systems by the action of mediators such as bradykinin, prostaglandins, serotonin, and histamine. The phenomenon of *primary hyperalgesia* (enhanced pain and reduced threshold at the site of the injury) is believed to be a consequence of the sensitization of these nociceptors during the process of inflammation.

Distribution of Nociceptors

Most of these nociceptors have been described in the skin of primates and humans. (In the skin there is 70% C and 10% Aδ fibers as well as 20% Aβ fibers, but the ratio can vary.) Nociceptive input from noncutaneous tissues is different and has distinctive characteristics.

Muscle pain seems to be C-fiber mediated. A separate nomenclature was proposed by Lloyd[2] in 1943 regarding the nerves supply skeletal muscles; group I and II are thickly myelinated, fast conducting fibers that innervate muscle spindles and tendon organs, and Ruffini and Pacinian corpuscles, respectively. Group III (thinly myelinated, equivalent to Aδ fibers) and IV (unmyelinated, equivalent to C) fibers are predominantly free nerve endings, which are considered to be nociceptors.

Electrophysiologic and psychophysical studies have focused on three issues relevant to muscle pain:

1. The most relevant stimuli for exciting muscle nociceptors are mechanical and chemical stimuli.

2. Regardless of the type of the nociceptor excited, only one quality of pain sensation arises from the skeletal muscles; that of deep, highly unpleasant, cramping, and poorly localized pain.

3. The duration of the muscle pain and the temporal summation contributes to diffuse localization associated with the rapid expansion of the area of the perceived pain shortly after the pain onset.

The joints have both myelinated and nonmyelinated nociceptors, which transmit pain at the extreme range of motion, with any motion when sensitized by inflammation. Bone and teeth have both Aδ and C innervation, and the teeth have Aβ as well. The periosteum is supplied by a dense plexus of Aδ and C fibers and has the lowest pain threshold of all the deep tissues. The cancellous bone is also well-supplied, but cortex and marrow have little nociceptive supply.

Cerebral blood vessels are surrounded by a dense plexus of sensory nerves, and this network constitutes a homogeneous population of C polymodal receptors.

Although less well-characterized than nociceptors in the skin, there is evidence for the existence of polymodal C and Aδ fibers in internal organs, such as the heart and the gut. As mentioned before, nociceptive information from the viscera of the thorax (heart, lower esophagus) and upper abdomen (stomach, biliary tract, upper gut, pancreas) reaches the dorsal horns of the spinal cord via sensory fibers that travel with the splanchnic nerves and pass through the sympathetic chains (with the exception of the upper respiratory tract). Nociceptive information from the lower gut and bladder reaches the cord via sensory fibers that accompany the sacral parasympathetic nerves. There is also a small possibility that both sympathetic and vagal afferents may contribute to cardiac pain, although stimulation of the vagal afferents doesn't result in conscious painful sensation. In the visceral nerves, the ratio of Aδ to C fibers is 1 to 10. Only 10% of the dorsal horn fibers are visceral afferents, but 75% of the dorsal horn cells receive input of visceral sensory information. The density of visceral afferents is generally low compared to the skin, and the visceral nociceptive units have large, weakly defined, and multiple receptive fields. These factors contribute to the poor localization of the visceral pain, and explain why spatial summation is needed in order to elicit pain.

Proprioceptive information from the face and oropharynx are conveyed through primary afferents of the trigeminal nerve to cell bodies in the trigeminal mesencephalic nucleus (a unique example of peripheral sensory nerves with cell bodies inside the central nervous system). Other primary afferents have cell bodies in the gasserian ganglion, like the DRG afferents, with projections through the sensory trigeminal root to the brain stem, terminating in the main sensory nucleus and spinal trigeminal nucleus. The spinal nucleus, in particular, receives the input of nociceptive information from the trigeminal system.

Dorsal Root Ganglia and Dorsal Roots

Between 60% and 70% of DRG cell bodies are connected to small diameter Aδ or C fibers. The number of fibers projecting centrally exceeds the number of ganglion cell bodies by 43%. According to the classical views, primary afferents pass into the spinal cord through the dorsal roots. As the dorsal roots approach, the spinal cord divides into many rootlets (12 to 15) and follows a differential distribution pattern (Fig. 1-5). Close to the dorsal root entry zone, the small nociceptive fibers (Aδ and C) migrate to the lateral side, while the large fibers (Aβ) are positioned more medially. Because small pain fibers move laterally before entering the spinal cord, a selective posterior rhizotomy has been developed in the past, attempting to ablate the lateral dorsal rootlets while sparing the more medially located large fibers. However, it has a high rate of failure. This is explained by the accumulating evidence of the presence of pain fibers in the ventral roots, and the possibility that some primary afferents may pass into the cord from ventral roots as well.

Entry to Spinal Cord—Lissauer's Tract

Upon entering the spinal cord, the central processes of the primary afferents are distributed in three ways:

1. At the entrance to the spinal cord, the afferents may send a main branch directly to the dorsal horn of the segment of entry, or may send branching collateral fibers rostrally and caudally up to several segments beyond the segment of entry. Then, upon the final penetration of the collaterals into the dorsal horn parenchyma, the terminal fields also ramify rostrally and caudally for several segments.

2. The route of these ascending and descending collaterals, as far as the large fibers are concerned, is located in the dorsal (posterior) columns of the spinal cord, which are located more medially (see Fig. 1-5). However, the small fibers enter the spinal cord from the most lateral divisions of the dorsal roots, and their branching collaterals ascend or descend in sites lateral to the dorsal columns. Thus,

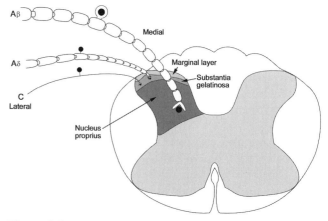

Figure 1-5   Structure of dorsal roots at the level of entry to the dorsal horns of the spinal cord. (Copyright 2004 Catherine Twomey/Medical Center Graphics, Milwaukee, Wisconsin.)

they contribute to the formation of the Lissauer's tract, which also includes small fibers originating from cells of the substantia gelatinosa in the dorsal horns (which also provide ascending or descending fibers by one or two segments) (Fig. 1-6).

3. The primary afferent endings are finally distributed and synapse in the dorsal horns of the spinal cord, but this distribution is determined from the fiber size (small or large) and type (visceral or somatic). The small fibers end in the more superficial laminae of the dorsal horns (marginal layer and substantia gelatinosa), while the large fibers end deeper in the nucleus proprius (Fig. 1-7). However, this organization can change dynamically under conditions of injury of the peripheral nerve.

DORSAL HORNS OF THE SPINAL CORD

The central pathways that further process nociceptive information begin at the level of the spinal cord dorsal horns. Interneuronal networks in the dorsal horn are responsible not only for transmission of the nociceptive information to neurons that project to the brain, but also modulate that information and pass it on to other spinal cord neurons, including flexor motoneurons and nociceptive projection neurons. Certain processes lead to enhanced reflex actions, sensitization of projection neurons, and increased nociceptive transmission. Other inputs result in inhibition of the synaptic transmission and projection neurons.

The spinal grey matter can be best viewed as a system of layers or zones that are continuous in all segments. In 1952, Rexed[3] described that at any level the spinal cord is organized into several laminae, which are continuous and homologous from the sacral up to the cervical lev-

els. He divided the spinal cord into 10 laminae, based on type, density, and myelinization of the cells.

Lamina I or the *marginal layer* is a thin band "capping" the grey matter (see Fig. 1-7). In lamina I, different types of cells can be found. Populations of these neurons respond to intense cutaneous and visceral stimulation. Most of these cells project to the brain via contralateral ascending tracts. Lamina II is also called substantia gelatinosa (SG), and is subdivided into an outer (IIo) and an inner part (IIi). It contains a large, densely packed concentration of small neurons and has an absence of myelinated axons. Substantia gelatinosa is a key station for integration and modulation of the nociceptive information. A significant proportion of the SG neurons receive input from Aδ and C fibers and are excited by thermal or mechanical stimulation, but many of the SG cells are interneurons, projecting to other SG neurons (see Fig. 1-7). In many ways, Lamina III is considered a transition between II and IV, but sometimes is included, together with the laminae IV and V, into the *nucleus proprius*. Cells in the nucleus proprius may be classified as those that respond almost uniquely to innocuous, low-threshold (Aβ) input, and those that respond to Aβ, Aδ, and C input. Lamina X surrounds the central canal, and some of its cells can convey nociceptive information (see Fig. 1-7).

As mentioned above, the distribution of the primary afferents into the dorsal horns of the spinal cord depends on their size and function. The large myelinated fibers enter into the dorsal columns. After having sent branches to the dorsal horn at the segment of entry or collaterals to nearby segments, they terminate at synapses in the nuclei gracilis and cuneatus (in the higher spinal segments). Collateral branches from the large fibers synapse mainly to the nucleus proprius (laminae III, IV, and V). Some fibers synapse into the

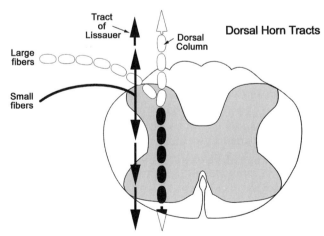

Figure 1-6 The tract of Lissauer and dorsal columns. (Copyright 2004 Catherine Twomey/Medical Center Graphics, Milwaukee, Wisconsin.)

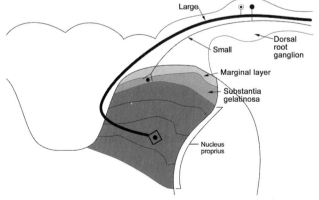

Figure 1-7 Differential distribution of large and small afferent fibers into the laminae of the dorsal horns. (Copyright 2004 Catherine Twomey/Medical Center Graphics, Milwaukee, Wisconsin.)

motor neurons of the ventral horns, where they feed monosynaptic reflexes (see Figs. 1-6 and 1-7). The C fibers end in the lamina I, and mainly in the SG (particularly in the IIo) (see Figs. 1-6 and 1-7). They also end in laminae V and X (central canal). The Aδ fibers share common features of both the large Aβ and the C fibers, regarding their pattern of termination. Some (especially the non-nociceptive fibers) pass medially and enter into laminae III and IV, while others pass directly to I, IIo, V, and X. Visceral afferents synapse with cells in laminae I and V, where somatic afferents also terminate; these cells are called viscerosomatic dorsal horn neurons. This dual innervation is known as *convergence*, and may be a mechanism of the phenomenon of the referred pain.

Neurons of the Dorsal Horns

Primary afferents relay sensory information to different populations of neurons upon entering the spinal cord. These neurons can be classified by different systems. In the simplest formulation, there are three categories of dorsal horn neurons:

1. *Projection neurons*, which send axons out of the spinal cord, to terminate in supraspinal centers. They are responsible for the rostral transmission of sensory information.
2. *Propriospinal neurons*, which send axons that extend over several spinal segments. They participate in hetero-segmental reflexes and interactions among stimuli administered to separate loci.
3. *Interneurons*, with axons terminating in the vicinity of the parent cell body. They are small cells, which serve as relays, and participate in local processing and integration of information. They can be either excitatory or inhibitory. These interneurons are more prevalent in the substantia gelatinosa (SG), which is a very important station of processing and control of the nociceptive information. These interneurons project to other neurons, form a network, and then can modify the activity of other neurons, not only in the II lamina, but in the marginal layer and the nucleus proprius as well. The outer IIo SG cells receive mostly high-threshold mechanical and thermal input of nociceptive nature from the small fibers, while the inner IIi SG cells receive low-threshold mechanical information. Descending inhibitory axons from higher centers in the brain also end up in IIo. The cells that receive the nociceptive input from the small fibers are inhibited by the low-threshold input from the large fibers, and vice versa. Thus, many lamina II cells can increase or decrease the firing threshold of other cells.

In many cases the response of these cells depends on the function of the afferent input (low-threshold versus high-threshold afferent input). In other situations, the net response of the cell is determined by the complex excitatory/inhibitory milieu in which the cell is subjected in the dorsal horn, and complex activity patterns may arise.

The following functional classification can be proposed according to an activity-dependent categorization:

Class 1: *Low-Threshold (LT) Cells*
These are neurons that respond selectively to non-nociceptive signaling. They are most prevalent in lamina IV, and the majority of their input is conveyed by large myelinated Aβ fibers. They respond maximally to light touch, pressure, hair movement, and/or vibration. Stimulation of their receptive fields within the noxious range produces no increase in firing frequency.

Class 2: *Multireceptive Cells or Wide Dynamic Range (WDR) Cells*
Their name implies the fact that their dynamic response is determined by the intensity of the incoming stimulus. The intensity of the stimulation from the periphery is thus encoded by this response. The WDR cells receive both low-threshold (non-nociceptive) and high-threshold (nociceptive) input via the convergence of afferent input from both large diameter myelinated Aβ, and small diameter lightly myelinated Aδ and unmyelinated C fibers. Their output differentially encodes for the intensity of the stimulus. They respond to both non-nociceptive and nociceptive information by changing their firing frequency (they fire at a higher frequency as afferent stimulus intensity increases, over a range from the innocuous to noxious levels). The highest concentrations of WDR cells are centered around lamina V, with smaller populations in laminae I and X. Other properties of these cells include:

- **Large receptive fields.** These fields have centers responding to a range of both noxious and innocuous stimulation, and a less sensitive surrounding area activated only by noxious stimulation. There is an even larger surrounding inhibitory peripheral field. The excitatory fields enlarge, and the inhibitory disappear in the *spinalized* state.
- **Low frequency (>0.33 Hz).** Repetitive stimulation incoming from C fibers only (but not from A) produces a gradual increase in their firing frequency, until the WDR neuron reaches a state of virtually continuous discharge. This is known as the *wind-up* phenomenon.
- **Convergence.** The same WDR cell can be excited by cutaneous or deep (muscle, joint, viscera) input, providing a substrate of musculo-somatic or viscero-somatic convergence, which explains the phenomenon of the referred pain.

Class 3: *Nociceptive Specific (NS) Cells or High-Threshold (HT) Cells*

They respond exclusively to stimuli within the noxious range. Class 3A cells are principally excited by Aδ nociceptors and respond almost exclusively to noxious mechanical stimulation. Class 3B cells that receive input from both Aδ and C fibers respond to both noxious heat and noxious mechanical input. Both are more concentrated in lamina I, with lower numbers in laminae V and X. They have small receptive fields (but larger than those of the primary afferents) and many have convergent fields from muscle and skin. NS cells produce activity graded in proportion to the stimulus intensity, and they also code for both stimulus location and magnitude.

Class 4: *Deep Cells*

Deep cells respond maximally to stimulation of subcutaneous structure, such as muscles or joints, and often they have convergent cutaneous or visceral input.

Neurochemistry of Primary Afferents

Nociceptive primary afferents synthesize a diversity of substances potentially involved in the synaptic transmission and modulation of the nociceptive information. These include the glutamate and other excitatory amino acids (EAA), neuropeptides, such as the tachykinin substance P (sP) and calcitonin gene related peptide (CGRP), adenosine triphosphate (ATP), nitric oxide (NO), prostaglandins (PG), and neurotrophins (growth factors). These potential transmitters, a variety of other neuropeptides, various enzymes, and several other molecules display a complex pattern of colocalization, comodulation, and corelease in primary afferent fibers. Actually, each specific, functional type of primary afferents possesses a characteristic complement of markers, but this has yet to be fully demonstrated by research. In any case, the neurochemical composition of the primary afferents varies qualitatively and quantitatively as a function of several factors, and differences are apparent amongst various tissues, between normal state versus peripheral tissue inflammation or nerve injury, and amongst various fiber classes. The neurochemical characterization of specific classes of primary afferents is far from complete and remains the topic of intensive research.

A substantial population of the small fibers is sensitive to capsaicin, which is an ingredient of the hot peppers. A subpopulation of the capsaicin-sensitive neurons contains neurotransmitter such as the sP and CGRP, while a second contains the lectin IB-4. Substance P (sP) is more prominent in C fibers originating from the muscles and deep tissues, than in C fibers innervating the skin. Cutaneous Aδ fibers contain little or no sP, while their major transmitters are excitatory amino acids (e.g., glutamate, aspartate). Excitatory amino acids, tachykinins (sP), and CGRP are colocalized in a subset of capsaicin-sensitive, small nociceptive C fibers. The tachykinins (e.g., sP and neurokinin A) act at the neurokinin NK_1 and NK_2 receptors, respectively, while CGRP at (at least) two receptors in the dorsal horn cells.

Excitatory amino acids, such as glutamate, also act at specific membrane receptors. These include the metabotropic receptors (coupled via G proteins to second messengers), and inotropic receptors (coupled directly to cation channels that allow the influx of calcium and sodium). The major types of inotropic receptors are the α-amino-3-hydroxy-5-methyl-4-isoxazolepropionate (AMPA)/kainate and N-methyl-D-glutamine (NMDA) receptors. The above receptors show a complex pattern of localization on various postsynaptic neurons in the dorsal horns as well as presynaptically on the primary afferents. Activation by EAAs of AMPA receptors is the principal mechanism involved in the input from Aβ fibers to the dorsal horn cells.

EAA acting at the AMPA receptors also mediate the direct monosynaptic response from the acute simple nociceptive input, while EAAs, tachykinins (sP), and possibly CGRP all cooperatively and synergistically elicit postsynaptic responses from repetitive or persistent noxious stimulation, leading to temporal summation and amplification of responses in the dorsal horn cells. Release of the transmitters is reduced by the presynaptic action of agents known to be analgesics, such as opioids and α_2-agonists (clonidine). The same agents acting postsynaptically may reduce the excitability of the dorsal horn neurons. The inhibitory amino acid γ-aminobutyric acid (GABA) also may have a similar action by inhibiting the primary afferent depolarization. Glycine has inhibitory, mainly postsynaptic hyperpolarizing actions.

ASCENDING PATHWAYS

Second-order neurons, or projection neurons in the spinal cord transmit information of pain via axons that cross the midline and ascend to a number of regions of the brainstem and diencephalon, including the thalamus, periaqueductal gray (PAG), parabrachial region, and bulbar reticular formation as well as to the limbic structures in the hypothalamus, amygdaloid nucleus, and other sites. Depending on the site of projection, they are being classified as spinothalamic, spinomesencephalic, spinoreticular, and so forth. These are shown schematically in Figure 1-8. The existence of a visceral nociceptive pathway in the dorsal columns involving the postsynaptic dorsal column pathway has also been demonstrated.

Spinothalamic Tract

The anterolateral quadrant of the spinal cord contains the most important pathway for ascending nociceptive fibers. These range from the spinal cord to the thalamus, thus forming the spinothalamic tract (Fig. 1-8). Most of the cells project to the contralateral thalamus, although a small fraction ascends and projects ipsilaterally. The axons most often decussate through the ventral white commissure at a very short distance from the cell body, enter the ventral funiculus, and then shift into the lateral funiculus as they ascend. Spinothalamic axons are arranged somatotopically; at cervical levels, those representing the lower extremity and caudal body are placed more laterally, and those representing the upper extremity and rostral body more anteromedially. The spinothal-

amic tract in humans mediates the sensations of pain, cold, warmth, and touch.

Two parts of the spinothalamic tract are discerned. One part, phylogenetically newer, projects from laminae I and V to the contralateral lateral thalamus and is known as *neospinothalamic tract.* Neospinothalamic tract cells that project to the lateral thalamus have receptive fields on a restricted area of the skin, thus are well-suited to function in signaling the sensory-discriminative aspects of pain. These aspects include the detailed perception and detection of noxious stimuli, and their characteristics in terms of quality, intensity, location, duration, and temporal pattern. The other part, phylogenetically older, projects from deeper laminae to the contralateral medial thalamus, and is known as the *paleospinothalamic tract.* The cells of origin of the paleospinothalamic tract have very large receptive fields, often encompassing the entire surface of the body and face. Some cells receive input from both the skin and the viscera. The large receptive fields suggest a role in the motivational-affective aspects of pain. These aspects include the relationship between pain and mood or emotions rather than sensory discrimination, the attention to pain and memory of pain, the capacity to modify the behavior as a result of the pain, and the capacity to cope with and tolerate pain and its rationalization.

The neospinothalamic tract is part of the neospinothalamic (or lateral) system, which rapidly conveys information of more detailed and discriminative nature. The paleospinothalamic tract is part of the paleospinothalamic (or medial) system, which slowly conveys tonic information. The paleospinothalamic system sends connections to the reticular activating system, the limbic system, the PAG, and the hypothalamus. Through these connections, evoked responses alter the motivational drive, the endocrine function, the respiratory, and the cardiovascular function.

Different response patterns in the dorsal horn cells may reflect the differing roles in the processing and experience of pain. WDR cells and/or cells with smaller receptive fields may encode the intensity and location of cutaneous, noxious stimuli, providing significant input to neospinothalamic tract. In contrast, nociceptive specific cells of superficial laminae project via the paleospinothalamic tract to medial thalamus nuclei, concerned with the emotional–behavioral aspects of pain.

Nevertheless, the spinothalamic tract cells have not only excitatory but also inhibitory receptive fields. Inhibition can occur when stimuli are applied contralaterally, or to dermatomes remote from those of the excitatory receptive field, but spinothalamic tract cells can also be inhibited effectively by repetitive electrical stimulation of the peripheral nerves. The best inhibition is produced by stimulation of a peripheral nerve in the same limb as the excitatory receptive field, but some inhibition occurs when nerves in other limbs are stimulated.

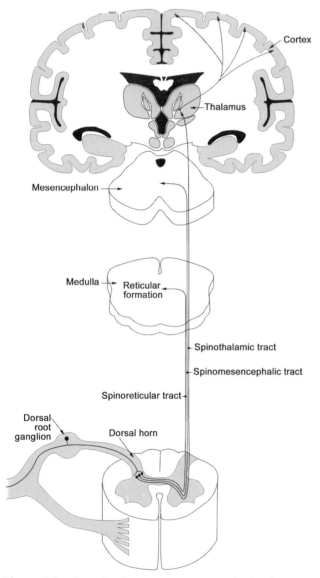

Figure 1-8   Second-order sensory neurons projecting from dorsal horns to higher CNS structures. Spinothalamic tracts project to the thalamic nuclei, while spinomesencephalic ones to mesencephalon, mediating different functions. (Copyright 2004 Catherine Twomey/Medical Center Graphics, Milwaukee, Wisconsin.)

Several other pathways accompany the spinothalamic tract in the white matter of the anterolateral quadrant of the spinal cord.

Spinomesencephalic Tract

The spinomesencephalic tract includes several projection systems that terminate in different areas of the midbrain (see Fig. 1-8). The cells of origin are located in laminae I and IV-VI (mostly V), and project to midbrain nuclei, such as the PAG and the cuneiform nucleus. Spinomesencephalic neurons have complex receptive fields on widely separated areas of the body, and respond best to noxious stimuli, but also to innocuous stimuli. There is a rough somatotopic organization. Different components of this tract have different functions:
1. Projections to the PAG contribute to aversive behavior and activate the *descending analgesia system* that arises from the PAG.
2. The projections to the cuneiform nucleus access the midbrain locomotor center and the ascending reticular activating system.
3. Projections to other nuclei may also be related with production of analgesia.

Spinoreticular Tract

Many of the cells of origin of the spinoreticular tract are located in the deep layers of the dorsal horn and in laminae VII and VIII of the ventral horns. The spinoreticular tract projects, without somatotopic organization, to several nuclei in the caudal medulla. More rostral projections go to the lateral reticular nucleus, the nucleus gigantocellularis, and the paragigantocellularis dorsalis and lateralis. Another major termination in the brainstem is in the parabrachial region. Functions of the spinoreticular tract are to signal homeostatic changes to autonomic centers in the brainstem, activate endogenous analgesia systems, and relay information that triggers motivational-affective responses.

Spinolimbic Tract

This is a multisynaptic pathway that carries information to the medial thalamus, from which it is relayed to the limbic system. A possible anatomic substrate for this pathway is the spinoreticular tract, but direct spinohypothalamic and spino-amygdalar pathways have been described. This tract is a major bilateral projection, relevant to the motivational and emotional aspects of pain.

Postsynaptic Dorsal Column Pathway

Classical view holds that the dorsal column pathways convey graphesthesia, two-point discrimination, and position sense. However, evidence has implied an additional functional role of the dorsal columns in the relay of visceral pain from the pelvis in humans. Visceral nociceptive signals from pelvic organs (including the uterus and vagina), as well as from the sacrum and perineum, is relayed via this tract to the thalamus. This pathway can be ablated via a limited midline myelotomy, in order to relieve intractable pelvic pain in patients with cancer.

SUPRASPINAL SYSTEMS CONTRIBUTING TO THE PROCESSING OF PAIN

Reticular Activating System

The reticular activating system has connections with the thalamus, hypothalamus, cortex, and PAG, and nociception is among its most effective inputs. The extensive interconnections of the reticular activating system with other supraspinal sites may also explain the multiple influences on suffering from pain.

Thalamus

The thalamus relays signals from the ascending afferents to the cortex (see Fig. 1-8), contributing to the awareness of the pain. Two parts can be identified:
1. The *neothalamus (lateral thalamus)* is located laterally and ventrobasally, is highly organized on a somatotopic basis, receives input from the neospinothalamic tract, and sends projections to the sensory SI cortex for localization and discrimination of pain. The neothalamus includes the ventroposterolateral nucleus (VPL) and the ventroposteromedial nucleus (VPM). In both nuclei, a small number of cells are nociceptive specific, and a slightly larger number are WDR cells. The proportion of thalamic neurons relevant to nociception compared with neurons activated only by innocuous stimuli is low (about 10%). The nociceptive neurons of the VPL have restricted receptive fields on the contralateral side, and most (85%) respond to both cutaneous and visceral stimuli; although the cutaneous input is somatotopic, the visceral input is not viscerotropic.
2. The *paleothalamus (medial thalamus)* includes the medial and intralaminar nuclei, is not somatotopically organized, and projects diffusely to a wide area of the cortex. Several of its neurons are nociceptive, responding as nociceptive specific (NS) or WDR, with large, usually bilateral receptive fields. This suggests that they do not contribute to sensory discrimination, but play a role in motivational-affective behavior, and possibly in memory processing.

Limbic System

Pain is quite often accompanied by affective-motivational responses, which are important to behavior. These are mediated via the limbic system. A variety of lesions to parts of the limbic system have been shown to psychophysically dissociate the reported stimulus intensity from its affective component.

The hypothalamus (part of the limbic system) incorporates nociceptive information, which may influence the integration of homeostasis via the autonomic nervous system and neuroendocrine response.

CEREBRAL CORTEX

Evidence favors the participation of both the cortex and the thalamus, not only in the sensory-discriminative aspects of pain, but also in the motivational-affective aspects. Although old views attributed little importance to the cortex in the appreciation of pain, responses have now recorded from nociceptive cortical neurons, and evidence from imaging studies reveals that the human cerebral cortex participates in nociception. Cortical areas most prominently involved include the somatosensory SI and SII cortex, the anterior insula, and the anterior cingulate gyrus. The primary somatosensory cortex (SI) has been viewed as the first level of conscious pain perception, treating the incoming information about pain as any other novel stimulus. Processes in SI are very dynamic across all somatosensory modalities and provide input for motor control and performance. However, it seems likely that the SI is not "the pain center" because it is the interaction of SI with the other pain-related areas (cortical and subcortical), rather than the activity of the SI itself, that results in the experience of the pain. So, destruction of the SI leads to altered pain perception but not to abolition of pain. Also, because of the neuroplasticity dynamics, properties of the SI nociceptive neurons are altered in subjects with chronic pain when compared to pain responses of SI neurons in subjects without chronic pain.

MODULATION OF NOCICEPTIVE INFORMATION

The anatomic tracts through which afferent information evoked by high-threshold (noxious) information travels, are traditionally known as the "pain pathways." In fact this schematic definition vastly oversimplifies and distorts the true organization. At every synapse, the transmission through the dorsal horn and brain stem is not "straight-through," but is subjected to significant modulation. In some instances, the modulation diminishes the pain message, but in others actively facilitates the transmission and amplifies the message of pain. In regards to the attenuation of the incoming nociceptive messages, it is well-known that the activation of opioid receptor, α_2 adrenoreceptors, serotonin receptors, adenosine receptors, muscarinic, GABA, and other receptors, is implicated.

The activation of afferent nociceptive input results in the subsequent activation of a number of circuits in the spinal cord and supraspinal levels. These include some interactive systems of neurons that serve to alter the afferent message, thus changing the sensory perception of the stimulus. Inhibitory modulation exists at several levels, including the level of the dorsal horns (Fig. 1-9), but there are two primary endogenous sources of these modulatory systems that can attenuate pain: (1) the descending bulbospinal pathways (serotoninergic or noradrenergic), and (2) the intrinsic interneurons in the dorsal horns (enkephalinergic and GABA-ergic or glycinergic). Both monoamines and endorphins are released in the dorsal horns by high-intensity nociceptive input. Spinal transection inhibits this effect indicating that the release is dependent on a spino-bulbo-spinal negative feedback loop.

Descending Modulatory Systems

Melzack and Wall first clearly proposed in 1962 that descending systems from supraspinal sources could modulate nociception (see Fig. 1-9). According to the Gate Control Theory, large and small diameter nerve fibers project to the substantia gelatinosa and the central sensory transmission neurons and can

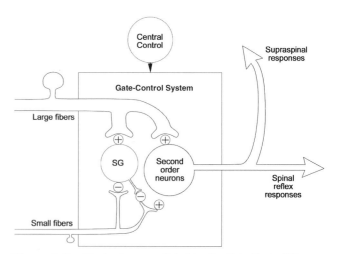

Figure 1-9 Mechanisms predicted by the Gate Control Theory. (Copyright 2004 Catherine Twomey/Medical Center Graphics, Milwaukee, Wisconsin.)

differentially modulate the further transmission of pain. Signals of pain are conveyed by small fibers. Large fibers convey low-threshold, normally nonpainful signals, which can inhibit the input from small fibers. Input from the large fibers results in activation of central control mechanisms, which subsequently project back and modify the gate control system. In 1969, Reynolds[4] performed abdominal surgery on rats, without chemical anesthesia, during stimulation of the region of the midbrain PAG. Since then, numerous investigations have been made of what became known as the *descending analgesia systems* (Fig. 1-10). These pathways utilize several neurotransmitters, including endogenous opioids, serotonin, and/or catecholamines. The anatomic structures of the brainstem that give rise to them include the PAG, the locus ceruleus, subceruleus, and Kölliker-Fuse nuclei, the nucleus raphe magnus (NRM), and several nuclei of the reticular formation. In addition, higher structures including the cerebral cortex, and various limbic structures including the hypothalamus, contribute to the analgesia pathways. Conditions of "stress" can produce opioid and non-opioid mediated analgesia; this can be a learned response, triggered also in the absence of nociception. The descending analgesia systems descend in the dorsolateral funiculus, with fibers that project to neurons in laminae I, IIo, IV, and V and have the following general properties:

1. They act presynaptically and reduce the release of neurotransmitters from the primary afferent nociceptive terminals (Aδ and C, but not from Aβ fibers).

2. They inhibit the response of the dorsal horn cells both directly, and indirectly (via the inhibition of excitatory interneurons and the activation of inhibitory interneurons), and these postsynaptic actions are probably of greater importance.

3. They preferentially inhibit the excitation of WDR cells by noxious, as compared to innocuous stimuli.

4. Monoamines are considered to be the major neurotransmitters released from these descending pathways, although several other transmitters may be colocalized and coreleased (e.g., acetylcholine, GABA, enkephalin).

5. Both endogenous opioid and nonopioid local spinal cord systems may mediate the inhibition of the response of the dorsal horn cells.

Descending pathways, however, do not exclusively exert inhibitory actions in the dorsal horns, but descending facilitatory pathways do exist. Many cerebral regions, including the cortex, may be the origin of excitatory projections to the dorsal horns. In addition, individual transmitters may exert multiple actions in the dorsal horns, depending on the type of neuron they target (inhibitory versus excitatory). There is now evidence that descending facilitatory systems can excite both the terminals of nociceptive primary afferents as well as intrinsic dorsal horn neurons. Experiments in primates showed that dorsal horn WDR cells, projecting to the thalamus, can be excited without any primary afferent input, just as a response to a conditioned stimulus previously connected with pain.

The Periaqueductal Gray

The PAG has been implicated in complex behavioral responses to stressful or to life-threatening situations. These responses tend to promote recuperative behavior after a defense reaction. These behaviors are mediated by activation of complex ascending and descending projections. PAG produces mixed aversive and analgesic effects. However, the effectiveness of the PAG to suppress both spinally and supraspinally organized responses to noxious stimuli is thought to result in large part from the inhibition of nociceptive transmission at the level of the spinal cord dorsal horns. The PAG receives direct somatotopic spinomesencephalic input deriving from laminae I and IV-VI contralaterally. Although some PAG neurons project directly to the spinal cord, most of the connections between the PAG and the spinal cord are indirect. PAG neurons project to: (1) the nucleus raphe magnus (NRM) and the adjacent reticular formation, located in the rostral ventromedial medulla, and (2) to locus ceruleus, and other nuclei in the parabrachial area (dorsolateral pons). Stimulation of the PAG causes inhibition of nociceptive dorsal horn neurons, including spinothalamic tract cells (see Fig. 1-10). This inhibition is produced

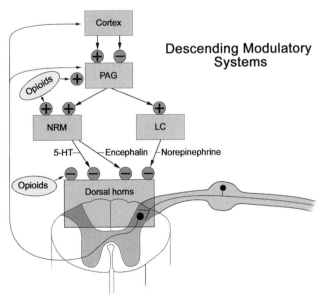

Figure 1-10 Descending systems that modulate the transmission of pain. (Copyright 2004 Catherine Twomey/Medical Center Graphics, Milwaukee, Wisconsin.)

via 5-HT$_3$ and 5-HT$_{1A}$ receptors, α_2 adrenoreceptors (norepinephrine and α_2-agonists applied directly to the spinal cord produce analgesia), GABA$_A$, and glycine receptors. The actions on the serotonin receptors are mediated by release of serotonin (5-HT) from axons projecting from the nucleus raphe magnus, and those on adrenoreceptors are mediated by norepinephrine, released from noradrenergic axons projecting from the locus ceruleus. GABA and glycine perhaps are released by inhibitory interneurons in the dorsal horns, or by other long descending axons from the medulla.

The PAG is also an important substrate for opioid analgesia, with a dense concentration of opioid peptides and receptors. Microinjection of opioids into the PAG produces a dose dependent, μ-mediated, naloxone reversible antinociception. (This is thought to be mediated by an indirect mechanism, by directly inhibiting the activity of GABA-ergic inhibitory interneurons.)

The Rostral Ventromedial Medulla

The descending inhibition resulting from activation of the PAG neurons is largely mediated through a relay in the rostral ventromedial medulla (RVM). RVM plays a significant role in the nociceptive modulation, in which serotoninergic mechanisms are clearly important, yet insufficiently understood. RVM is also an important substrate for opioid antinociception, and it is believed to contribute to the antinociceptive action of systemically administered opioids. These seem to act via a complex mechanism including both direct and indirect, excitatory and inhibitory actions on neurons that project and modulate the spinal nociceptive transmission ("on" and "off" cells).

The exact action of the analgesia from systemically administered opioids most likely reflects their ability to simultaneously activate elements of an interconnected opioidergic network whose elements span the whole neuraxis, from the forebrain to the spinal cord (see Fig. 1-10). The PAG-RVM axis appears to be linked with opioid-sensitive sites in the forebrain, including the amygdala and the nucleus accumbens, which form a part of an opioid dependent mesolimbic loop. In addition, the interaction of the axis with the spinal sites seems to be of synergistic nature (concurrent spinal and supraspinal administration leads to prominent synergy).

Locus Ceruleus, Subceruleus, and Parabrachial Area

Noradrenergic projections to all regions of the spinal cord arise from these areas, which are known as the dorsolateral pontine catecholamine cell groups A$_5$, A$_6$, and A$_7$. Their stimulation produces inhibition of nociceptive neurons in the deep dorsal horns. Noradrenergic terminals have been shown to make direct contact with dorsal horn neurons, including spinothalamic cells. The analgesic effect is mediated by α_2-adrenoceptors.

Intrinsic Interneuron Systems in the Dorsal Horns

These intrinsic interneurons play an integrative role within the cord in facilitating communication between various segments and various cells. In addition, they play a critical role in processing nociceptive afferent input, participate in excitatory circuits implicated in dorsal horn processes of neuronal sensitization and referred pain, and also in mediating the actions of the descending analgesia systems.

Spinothalamic neurons may be directly activated by primary afferents, but also indirectly via excitatory interneurons (particularly cells in deeper laminae, which are activated by C fibers via intervening interneurons in IIo). Excitatory amino acids may be the primary transmitters.

Inhibitory interneurons, by contrast, limit the flow of nociceptive input. Most inhibitory interneurons reduce nociception by directly targeting nociceptive specific or WDR cells and/or presynaptic primary afferent terminals.

The descending axons of the serotoninergic and noradrenergic neurons may contact the dendrites of the spinothalamic tract neurons (this is the case particularly regarding the noradrenergic axons), but they may also contact local inhibitory (enkephalinergic, glycinergic, or GABA-ergic) interneurons in the superficial dorsal horn. They may also exert presynaptic influences to the primary afferent endings. Thus, the descending inhibition of the nociceptive input is likely to be mediated in part by the activation of these interneurons in the dorsal horns. A population of these interneurons release endogenous opioids (i.e., enkephalin, dynorphin). The opioids (endogenous or exogenous) reduce the nociceptive transmission in the dorsal horns by a combination of presynaptic (on the primary afferents) and postsynaptic (on the dorsal horn cells) actions. They reduce the primary afferent action potential duration and transmitter release via decreasing the calcium channel conductance, and hyperpolarize the dorsal horn neurons by enhancing the potassium channel conductance. Other interneurons release GABA or glycine, likewise altering the release of transmitters or the postsynaptic excitability. GABA$_A$ receptor mediated inhibition occurs through largely postsynaptic mechanisms, while GABA$_B$ mechanisms preferentially suppress presynaptic transmitter release. Although baclofen, a GABA$_B$ agonist, has antinociceptive action in vitro, it is of limited use in chronic pain because of the increased excitability of the postsynaptic dorsal horn neuron disproportionately to the amount of the transmitter released. GABA-ergic and glycinergic interneurons have a high level of tonic or evoked activity, and loss of their function results into a spinal processing system in which low-threshold afferent input is handled as if noxious. Cholinergic inhibitory interneurons have been described, which act via multiple muscarinic and probably nicotinic receptors localized on primary afferent terminals and dorsal horn neurons. Intrathecal administration of muscarinergic substances, such as neostigmine, produces analgesia.

Nociceptive neurons can be inhibited also by activation of the large, primary afferent fibers, or their collaterals in the dorsal columns. Such activation initiates local spinal circuits of interneurons in the substantia gelatinosa, which subsequently produce presynaptic inhibition of the C fibers in the same segments. Release of inhibitory transmitters, such as the GABA, from the interneurons is implicated. Natural activation of large myelinated fibers by vibratory stimuli and electrical stimulation of the dorsal columns are known to reduce chronic pain. This is relevant to the Gate Theory, which predicates that sensory input from the large fibers inhibits the nociceptive input from the small fibers. Stimulation of nociceptive afferents can also lead to inhibition of dorsal horn neurons, through both spinal and supraspinal components. A large population (92%) of the WDR cells (versus 10% of the NS cells) has distant, large inhibitory receptive fields (even in the contralateral body); high-threshold stimulation of their fields can inhibit their nociceptive evoked activity. Viscerosomatic neurons are also inhibited from stimulation of distant sites.

MECHANISMS OF PAIN

The transmission of pain from peripheral tissues through the spinal cord to the higher centers of the brain is not a passive, simple process using exclusive *straight-through* pathways. The spinal and supraspinal circuits have the potential to alter dynamically the relationship between the stimulus and the perception and response to pain. Altered perception regarding the localization of the painful input underlies the phenomenon of "referred pain." *Plasticity* is the inducible capacity of the nociceptive transmission systems that mediate pain for change. In other words, plasticity is the ability of the nervous system to modify the output/input relationship. The interplay between excitatory and inhibitory systems will determine the intensity of the messages delivered to the higher levels of the CNS and sensed. The incoming messages may be attenuated or enhanced, depending on particular circumstances. The latter state can result from the condition of *central sensitization*.

Referred Pain and Visceral Pain Phenomena

Referred pain is the pain that is localized in a different site than the site of its origin. In general, pain originating from visceral organs, like the heart or the abdominal viscera, is primary referred and perceived to an overlying or adjacent somatic area. It can be accompanied by other phenomena, such as cutaneous (secondary) hyperalgesia, reflex muscle spasm, deep tenderness, and intense autonomic hyperactivity. Visceral or deep nociception, in particular, can produce secondary hyperalgesia and muscular spasm proportional to the intensity of the original stimulus. Persistent and intense nociception can lead to prolonged excitability in the dorsal horn neurons, with expansion of their receptive fields and reduction of their depolarization thresholds. These phenomena can also spread beyond the initially involved segments, with further extension of the spasm. Autonomic reflexes can also produce many different viscero-visceral, vascular, and neuroendocrine responses, which together with the muscular spasm lead to a new nociceptive source that may outlast the original.

The mechanistic substrate of the referred pain is related to the convergence of cutaneous, deep somatic, and visceral input on to certain populations of dorsal horn neurons, so that spinothalamic tract neurons receive convergent input from visceral and overlying somatic structures. Convergence can occur also in supraspinal levels. The ratio of Aδ to C fibers in the viscera is 1/10 versus 1/2 in the skin, and the visceral afferents innervate larger areas with extensively overlapping receptive fields. The above factors explain why visceral pain is poorly localized, dull and aching versus the localized sharp ectodermal pain.

MECHANISMS AND HYPOTHESES EXPLAINING THE DIFFERENT PHASES OF PAIN

Different states or types of pain, reflecting a large range of sensory experiences exist, can be viewed as the expression of different neurophysiological mechanisms, not necessarily of absolute teleological significance. Under normal conditions, a physiologic state exists in which there is a close correlation between the noxious stimulus and the perception of a painful response. However, changes induced by the nociceptive input or by the coexisting conditions can result in variations in the quality and intensity of the perception of the pain produced by a certain noxious stimulus. These changes tend to be temporary, as homeostatic mechanisms tend to restore the system to the normal interrelationships between stimulus and pain. Nonetheless, very intense or prolonged nociceptive input, or disruption or loss of the normal input, distort the nociceptive system to such an extent that the correlation between stimulation and pain is lost. A contribution to the understanding of these mechanisms, made by Cervero and Laird,[5] proposed that pain can be viewed in three states, or *phases* ranging from a more normal, adaptive, to an abnormal, nonproductive end of a spectrum. These phases are not exclusive; at any given time, several of the underlying mechanisms may coexist in the same individual. The three phases of pain are:

1. The input, processing, and perception of a brief or transient noxious stimulus, corresponding to what we perceive as a brief, transient, acute painful sensation.
2. The consequences of a prolonged noxious stimulation and nociceptive input resulting from tissue damage and peripheral inflammation. These comprise the substrate of the chronic, nociceptive pain states.
3. The consequences of damage or injury to the neural tissue itself, including the peripheral neuropathies and central neuropathic states. This correlates with the various neuropathic pain states.

Phase 1: Brief, Transient Acute Pain

Under normal conditions, the nociceptive primary afferent fibers do not display any spontaneous activity. Nonetheless, the brief application of a mechanical or thermal noxious stimulus will cause discharges of these small fibers. This is proportional to the intensity of the stimulus, and results into subsequent reports of sensation of pain in humans and escape behavior in animals. There is a close correlation between the intensity of the stimulus, the discharges in the primary afferents, and the subjective expression of pain. Information is propagated predominantly by the Aδ fibers. The underlying synaptic events from this acute response to a noxious stimulus are mediated predominantly by glutamate acting at the AMPA/kainate receptors (Fig. 1-11), but only to a minimal degree by neurokinins (substance P) acting at NK$_1$ receptors. The consequence is a phasic response of a discrete population of the dorsal horn neurons, leading to a brief discharge of action potentials and activation of discriminative-sensory pathways. This phase corresponds to the adaptive, warning role of acute, localized, and transient exposure to (particularly cutaneous) noxious stimulation.

Phase 2: Chronic Nociceptive Pain

Conditions of tissue damage and persisting inflammation lead to very intense and prolonged noxious stimula-

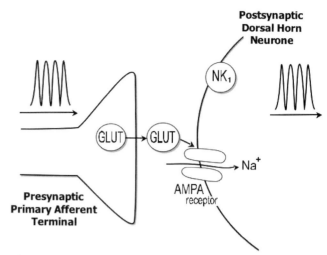

Figure 1-11   Synaptic transmission of brief, acute pain.

tion. There is a significantly increased afferent traffic to the nociceptive pathways, such that the response properties of their components and mechanisms may change. Not only is there an increased afferent input to the CNS from the injured area, but in addition, nociceptive spinal cord neurons modify their responses, moving to more excitable state. In this phase of pain, the subject experiences spontaneous pain, painful sensations evoked from stimulation of the injured area as well as pain from stimulation of the undamaged surrounding area. The curve which describes the relationship between the intensity of the pain and that of the stimulus shows a leftward shift (Fig. 1-12). The relevant clinical phenomena are: (a) hyperalgesia, which is an increased response (increased pain) to a stimulus which is normally painful, but much less; and (b) allodynia, which is pain evoked by a stimulus that does not normally produce pain. This enhancement of the response of the nociceptive pathways after prolonged input of stimuli of certain intensity is called *sensitization*, and constitutes an elementary form of neural "memory"

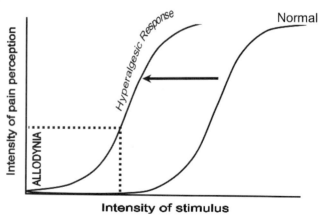

Figure 1-12   Increased responsiveness with allodynia and hyperalgesia in chronic pain states.

and "learning." Both peripheral and central mechanisms contribute so that sensitization can occur at any point from nociceptors in the peripheral tissues to the spinal cord and to the brain. A similar phenomenon, known as *long-term potentiation,* is seen in the hippocampus and is associated with memory and learning. Ultimately, a pathologic state of chronic pain may develop that involves more or less permanent changes in the CNS, persisting long after the original injury has healed.

Peripheral Mechanisms of Sensitization

Surgical or traumatic mechanical insults, chemical irritation, heat injury, or disease leading to cutaneous tissue damage or inflammation is associated with two zones of pain:

1. The first is called the area of *primary hyperalgesia* and is located over the area of the original tissue damage itself. It is characterized by spontaneous pain and increased sensitivity to mechanical, thermal, and chemical stimuli.
2. The second zone, *secondary hyperalgesia,* displays an increased sensitivity to mechanical stimuli, but not to thermal stimuli in an undamaged area surrounding the first zone.

Increased sensitivity implies: (a) a decrease in the stimulus threshold required to elicit painful response and (b) an exaggerated response to a suprathreshold stimulus. Primary hyperalgesia is produced mainly by events and mechanisms occurring in the periphery, at the level of the primary afferent nociceptive fibers. In contrast, secondary hyperalgesia is mediated by predominantly central mechanisms.

The primary hyperalgesia can be explained by changes in the transduction sensitivity, responsiveness, and activity of peripheral nociceptors as well as by the recruitment of silent nociceptors. Specific mechanisms are very complex and include:

1. Direct stimulation of nociceptive primary afferents. This can be mediated by a large variety of substances, which can act independently or synergistically to activate the nociceptor. Algogenic substances include:
    *   Kinins, such as bradykinin and kallidin, produced from activation of plasma and tissue kallikreins. Action is mediated via two types of receptors (B_1 and B_2), which can excite polymodal and mechanosensitive C as well as high-threshold $A\delta$ fibers, producing pain.
    *   Prostaglandins and leukotrienes. Prostaglandins may be derived from virtually all tissues, but, under conditions of tissue inflammation and tissue injury, immunocompetent cells and terminals of sympathetic efferent fibers become predominant sources. Mediators, such as the nitric oxide and certain cytokines (e.g., IL-1, TNF), induce the inducible enzyme cyclooxygenase (COX)-2 syn-

thase, which is the main source. The constitutive COX-1 enzyme may also play a certain role. The COX-2 form is essentially absent from healthy tissues, but gets rapidly induced under conditions of inflammation, and parallels the production of prostaglandins. Inflammation results in *de novo* synthesis of COX-2 enzyme. The COX-1 enzyme is constitutively expressed in most tissues, producing prostaglandins as part of normal healthy tissue function.

*   ATP, which can elicit pain by stimulating rapidly desensitizing, cation permeable, inotropic receptors of the P_{2X} family. Particular sources include tumor cells, endothelial cells, and/or platelets and sympathetic nerve endings.
*   Protons and vanilloids (capsaicin). Hydrogen (H^+) protons are algogenic agents. Protons depolarize nociceptors by triggering a transient Na^+ ion channel, or by opening poorly selective channels permeable to Na^+, K^+, and Ca^{++}. Capsaicin, a substance of pepper, provokes pain by opening cation-permeable ion channels with several similarities to the protons. By this activation capsaicin causes the release of sP, but prolonged application eventually leads to ultimate sP depletion from the afferent terminals, thereby inactivating the nociceptive function. Some nociceptors respond to either protons or capsaicin, but a significant overlap suggests a common site of action.
*   Serotonin (5-HT). This can be derived from many sources, and excites nociceptors via $5-HT_3$ receptors by directly gating ion channels, or sensitizes them via endocellular messenger systems.
*   Norepinephrine, derived from sympathetic efferent terminals. This does not directly excite, but enhances the sensitivity of the nociceptors via α_2 and α_1 adrenoreceptors present on the neuronal membrane. The hyperalgesia produced by norepinephrine has been shown only in the presence of tissue injury or inflammation. An excitatory effect of norepinephrine on both intact and damaged sensory neurons develops after nerve injury. Sensory neurons express α_2 receptors, and this expression is upregulated after nerve injury. It is likely that these adrenoreceptors may mediate an effect by modulating ion channel activity via G protein interactions.
*   Histamine, excitatory amino acids, tachykinins (sP), and CGRP all have sensitizing effects in the periphery.

2. Antidromic activation of nociceptive primary afferents and *neurogenic inflammation.* Classically, algogenic substances depolarize the nociceptor leading to an orthodromic transmission of impulses, from the periphery to the dorsal horns. However,

concurrently, antidromic impulses may be triggered in collateral fibers, propagating from the more proximal parts to the periphery, where they provoke the peripheral release of excitatory amino acids, sP, and other mediators. These further enhance the activity of the nociceptors by a positive feedback mechanism and elicit vascular effects, such as increased permeability and other processes. Peripherally released sP evokes the release of algogenic substances, sensitizes nociceptors, and augments the stimulation of nearby axons, thus spreading the response. CGRP leads to vasodilation and increased permeability, and the excitatory amino acids produce various feedback actions.

3. Synergistic actions and sensitization of nociceptors by the engagement of intracellular transduction systems. These events include the activation of adenyl-cyclase and phospholipase C as well as an increase in neuronal Ca^{++}. Thus, the likelihood, intensity, and duration of further discharges are enhanced. Of significance is the effect of prostaglandins and bradykinin. Previously "silent" nociceptors are recruited by this mechanism.

4. Modulatory events involving a complex pattern of reciprocal interactions amongst primary afferents, glial cells, immunocompetent cells, sympathetic terminals, etc.

5. Altered phenotype of primary afferents. Changes in the activity and properties of nociceptors in inflamed tissues may reflect modification of gene expression and altered phenotype. This may account for the increase in primary afferent levels of sP, CGRP, nitric oxide and glutamate, and other changes.

Central Sensitization

The concept of increased responsiveness of the central pathways as a consequence of intense afferent traffic was first introduced by Woolf[6] in 1983, where he described the "enhancement of the withdrawal reflex in rats after high frequency stimulation of the C fibers." Central sensitization refers to the increased responsiveness of the spinal cord, an important cause of enhanced responses of pain after prolonged, intense nociceptive input. This increased responsiveness includes the dorsal horn neurons, interneurons, and ventral horn neurons. The thalamus, cortex, and other brain areas also develop relevant changes. As a consequence of the central sensitization, low intensity or normal input of stimuli can produce an inappropriately greater response. This sensitization is mainly produced from massive and prolonged nociceptive afferent barrage mainly through the C-fibers and is associated with extensive changes in the dorsal horn cells, resulting in expansion of their receptive fields and encoding of the innocuous stimuli as painful.

Effective neural blockade with local anesthetics prior to initiation of the noxious stimulation, or appropriate preemptive suppression of the impending nociceptive signaling, may, theoretically, have the capacity to prevent these changes. This is the background of the *preemptive analgesia,* which, clinically, consists of an attempt to reduce postoperative pain or analgesic requirements by preemptively administering analgesic agents (local or general anesthetics, opioids) prior to the surgical stimulus. Nevertheless, a considerable discrepancy exists between laboratory evidence and clinical practice, and most available clinical studies have failed to show any significant benefits or are equivocal.

Mechanisms of Central Sensitization

The increased neuronal excitability and responsiveness, as a consequence of prolonged, intense nociceptive traffic, displays three general electrophysiological characteristics at the cellular level:

• A stimulus provokes a response of greater duration and intensity, involving a greater number of generated action potentials (hyperalgesia).

• Receptive fields expand so that responses can be evoked from a larger area, previously ineffective in eliciting firing (area of secondary hyperalgesia).

• The threshold for firing is reduced so that neurons can be now activated by normally subnoxious stimulus intensities. There is also appearance of novel responses to Aβ fibers (allodynia).

Two relevant events are recognized:

1. The knowledge that the prolonged nociceptive input can sensitize the neurons in the CNS is not new. In 1966, Mendell[7] showed that repetitive stimulation of primary afferent C fibers at rates ≥0.33 Hz, at constant intensity, can elicit a progressive increase in the number of the action potentials generated by dorsal horn cells and motoneurons. This phenomenon is called *wind-up* and constitutes a simple, cellular model of pain sensitization at the CNS level.

2. *Heterosynaptic facilitation* refers to the process whereby a progressive increase in neuronal excitability leads to an increased responsiveness to other inputs, specifically Aβ fibers.

Nevertheless, the processes of central sensitization are not only suggested by the above electrophysiological phenomena, but by psychophysical or behavioral studies as well. One model of spinal sensitization is the *formalin test.* Subcutaneous injection of an inflammatory substance, formalin, in the hindfoot of a rodent, results in an acute period (3 to 5 min.) of high C fibers afferent barrage activity, followed by low or minimal afferent activity. However, the recording of the parallel electrical discharge activity of the dorsal horn WDR cells in anesthetized animals as well as of the number of flinches or licking of the foot in awake animals (an indication of pain behavior), displays two distinct phases: An acute initial phase of high activity, lasting 3 to 5 minutes, followed—after a period of inactivity—by a second phase of an inappropriately intense activity, with regard to both recordings. This second phase of the resumed WDR discharge activity and the pain behavior, in spite of the minimal afferent nociceptive input, is indicative of the spinal sensitization. Pretreatment of the animals with intrathecal administration of MK801, a selective NMDA antagonist, has little effect on the initial phase, but can markedly attenuate the second phase phenomena. If the drug is given after the injection, it has no effect.

This observation underlies the significance of the excitatory amino acids acting on the NMDA receptors for the development of the spinal sensitization, but the underlying processes are of considerable complexity.

The Role of Excitatory Amino Acids and Tachykinins in the Sensitization of Dorsal Horn Neurons

The influence of transmitters, released by the primary afferent, on the activity of the dorsal horn neurons is mediated via:

1. A direct alteration in ion flux at cation-permeable channels.
2. Interactions with intracellular transduction mechanisms leading to subsequent ionic current modifications (e.g., via receptor phosphorylation).
3. Long-term effects involving processes like receptor regulation or recycling and changes in gene transcription of receptors, transmitters, and other molecules.

Brief noxious mechanical or heat stimuli produce rapid depolarization and action potential discharges in nociceptive specific and WDR dorsal horn cells. The acute response to noxious stimulation or injury is encoded peripherally as electrical discharge predominantly in Aδ, and to a much lesser degree in C fibers, subsequently the electrical discharge propagates toward the central presynaptic endings, where it evokes the release of neurotransmitters. The major transmitters in Aδ fibers are excitatory amino acids (glutamate). The acute pain is further mediated mainly by the glutamate acting at the AMPA/kainate receptors, and to a smaller extent, by substance P (from C fibers) acting at NK$_1$ receptors. Activation of the AMPA/kainate receptor elicits brief excitatory postsynaptic potentials with no cumulative response from low-frequency stimulation. The consequences are brief depolarizations of the dorsal horn neurons and activation of the central pathways.

However, under conditions of persisting inflammation, more and more C fibers become sensitized and might fire either sporadically, at a lower threshold, or as a response to previously innocuous stimuli, consequently providing a more sustained input to the dorsal

horns. In addition, silent C fibers become active during inflammation, which further increases the already enhanced afferent input. In addition to the release of excitatory amino acids, activation of C fibers results in the release of tachykinins (sP and neurokinin A). In the same dorsal horn cells previously briefly activated by the Aδ fibers, now C fiber activation can produce longer lasting excitatory postsynaptic potentials that give rise to cumulative depolarization and firing of action potentials upon repetitive stimulation. What makes the difference between the Aδ and the C fiber elicited postsynaptic response is the neuropeptide (sP and neurokinin A) content of the latter. While Aδ fiber stimulation activates mostly the non-NMDA (AMPA/kainate) receptor, input from the C fibers leads to a synergistic activation of both the AMPA/kainate and the neurokinin receptor, which with sufficient magnitude and duration can subsequently excite the NMDA receptor (Fig. 1-13). Therefore, it is suggested that NMDA receptors are modulated by activation of the neurokinin receptors.

NMDA receptors are linked to special inotropic channels, permeable to Ca^{++} (see Fig. 1-13). The sensitizing nociceptive mechanisms converge to reinforce transmission via the NMDA receptors, resulting in a pronounced, sustained elevation in Ca^{++} influx and intracellular Ca^{++} levels. However, under normal conditions NMDA receptors are quiescent, secondary to an intra-channel block by a Mg^{++} plug.

Activation of the neurokinin receptors, leads to increased activity of second messenger cascade leading to activation of protein kinase C, which phosphorylates the NMDA receptor, counteracts the Mg^{++} block, and allows NMDA receptor to operate at more negative, hyperpolarized potentials. The activation of the NMDA receptors results in increased intracellular Ca^{++} levels

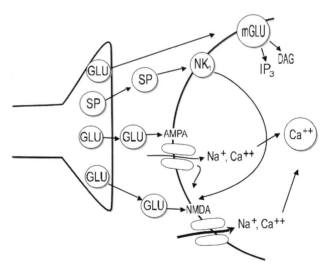

Figure 1-13   Complexity of synaptic transmission in chronic pain states.

and can elicit burst-like patterns of firing in the dorsal horn neurons. Furthermore, it may set up reverbatory, hyperexcitable circuits and reinforce the rostral transmission of the nociceptive information.

Activation of NMDA receptors and increases in intracellular Ca^{++} level play a particularly important role in triggering and maintaining neuronal sensitization in the dorsal horns, a process underlying the development of hyperalgesic and allodynic states. Key factors in an interrelated cascade of events at the cellular level include:

1. Activation of the phospholipase A_2 and production of prostaglandins, which augment the hyperalgesic state.
2. Activation of second messenger systems and production of mediators, such as inositol triphosphate and diacylglycerol, which further enhances the cascade via intracellular Ca^{++} release and activation of the protein kinase C, respectively (Fig. 1-14).
3. Increases in intracellular calcium and protein kinase C, which further enhance NMDA receptor excitation. They also increase the expression of proto-oncogenes, such as *c-fos* and *c-jun*, which act as third messengers that control transcription of "target" genes that encode various peptides or proteins, receptors, or enzymes capable of modulating responses to nociception.
4. Another mechanism involves the production of intracellular NO, which rapidly diffuses inside and outside the cell, further enhancing the nociception-driven spinal sensitization. However, it may exert a multiplicity of even contradictory actions in different cells.
5. NMDA-mediated central events, and activation of the protein kinase C, have been also associated with reduced sensitivity to opioids, so that dose escalation is required to overcome it, but clinically, this is complicated by side effects. In contrast, NMDA receptor antagonists (ketamine) potentiate the analgesic effect of opioids and may play a role in preventing central hypersensitive states.
6. A negative feedback mechanism is related to the release of adenosine after activation of the NMDA receptor. Adenosine acts on A_1 receptors on the membrane of dorsal horn neurons and has an antinociceptive effect. Adenosine, administered systemically or intrathecally, can produce analgesia.

Another way by which information of noxious stimulation can propagate centrally is associated with the relatively slower transport of chemical substances. These are called neurotrophins and can modify the metabolism of the dorsal root ganglion cells as well as the properties of the cytoplasm and the membrane of the cell body and presynaptic endings.

Finally, it is recognized that a (at least) transient, functional reduction of the tonic GABA-ergic and glycinergic inhibitory interneuronal activity can mimic and accentuate processes of dorsal horn sensitization, contributing to the allodynia and hyperalgesia. The exact mechanisms

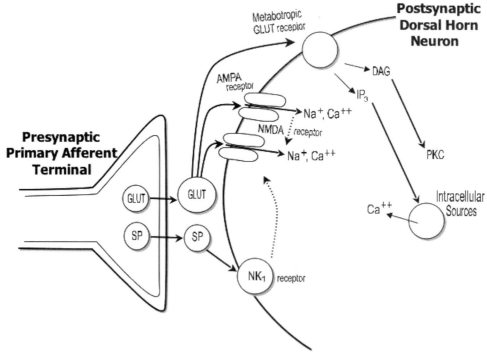

Figure 1-14   Central role of activation of NMDA receptor, calcium influx, and intracellular signaling in chronic pain states.

remain unclear, but a destruction of a subpopulation of inhibitory interneurons might be attributed to NMDA-receptor excitotoxic mechanisms. Additionally, in accordance with the Gate Theory, stimulation of Aβ fibers provides an analgesic effect, mediated via inhibitory interneurons, to the dorsal horns (this explains the pain relieving effect of manipulations, such as rubbing the painful site). Consequently, any reduction of Aβ fiber mediated stimulation of the inhibitory interneurons might disinhibit and further sensitize nociceptive neurons in the dorsal horns.

Phase 3: Neuropathic Pain

Phase 3 pains are abnormal (pathological) pain states, which develop as the consequence of disease or damage to peripheral nerves or to the CNS itself. They comprise the neuropathic pain states, which are characterized by a lack of correlation between injury and pain. In clinical terms, the Phase 1 and 2 pains are symptoms of peripheral tissue injury, but the neuropathic (Phase 3) pain is a symptom of neurological diseases that include lesions of peripheral nerves or damage to any portion of the somatosensory system within the CNS.

Neuropathic pain can be spontaneous or evoked, triggered by innocuous stimuli or associated with exaggerated responses to minor noxious stimuli. Pathophysiologically, neuropathic pain originates as an expression of substantial alterations in the normal nociceptive system induced by peripheral or central damage. However, the particular combination of mechanisms responsible for each one of the various neuropathic pain states is unique to the individual disease, or to particular patient subpopulation (patients with seemingly identical damage to their central nervous system may or may not complain of pain). Thus, it is believed that the development of neuropathic pain may involve genetic, cognitive, or emotional factors.

Damage to the sensory pathways of the nervous system may result in loss of sensory function as well as in pain and abnormal sensory symptoms (e.g., allodynia, hyperalgesia, dysesthesia). Two groups of mechanisms probably account for the latter symptoms:
1. Pathological changes in the damaged neurons; and
2. Reactive changes in response to nociceptive input, and to the loss of portions of the normal afferent input.

Characteristic sensory experiences of the neuropathic pain include:
1. Spontaneous pain with burning quality or intermittent, sharp stabbing, or lancinating pain.
2. Thermal hyperalgesia, to both cold and hot stimuli.
3. Mechanical allodynia, elicited by touch or brushing. This is a very common neuropathic manifestation, considered a hallmark of the neuropathic pain.

While the pathological changes in damaged neurons are unique to neuropathic pain states, some of the reactive changes to the nociceptive input are the expression of the pathophysiological mechanisms also seen in the chronic pain states of non-neuropathic nature. These include the mechanisms of central sensitization, as described in the previous section. In neuropathic pain states, the activation of these mechanisms may be abnormally prolonged or intense, due to ongoing abnormal input from damaged neurons. Sometimes healing never occurs, but even if successful regeneration develops, the properties of the regenerated afferents may not be completely normal. The role of supraspinal or descending mechanisms may also be significant, although not adequately clarified.

Other painful conditions, described as *Complex Regional Pain Syndrome* (or *Reflex Sympathetic Dystrophy*) can be also considered types of neuropathic pain because of the predominant role of the changes in the nervous system. The syndrome is the likely result of both peripheral and central sensitization mechanisms, in addition to dysregulation of the autonomic function. Another type of neuropathic pain, the phantom pain in amputees, may also be explained by central mechanisms, involving the dorsal horns or probably higher centers.

Pathophysiologic Mechanisms of Neuropathic Pain

Both peripheral and central changes have been identified and may play a role, of different significance amongst the different types of the neuropathic pain. However, it is not clear which of the described changes are causative mechanisms determining the pathogenesis of neuropathic pain and which are bystander events or act as correlates with indirect significance.

The peripheral mechanisms illustrate the complexity of the peripheral events involved in the generation and maintenance of pain provoked by primary afferent nerve injury. Injury to the primary afferents results in an initial, intense electrical discharge, followed by the generation of abnormal ectopic impulses, which is involved in the initiation and maintenance of the neuropathic state. Peripheral events contribute mostly to spontaneous pain and hyperalgesic responses, while allodynia-like phenomena are best explained by central mechanisms.

Neuropathic Pain: Peripheral Mechanisms
Peripheral mechanisms implicated in neuropathic pain include:
1. Alterations in afferent function after nerve injury. Acute injury to the nerve leads to an "afferent barrage." This includes the rapid, intense central discharge of both Aβ and C fibers for a period of minutes, and even several days for some fibers. Suppressing this initial barrage by applying local

anesthetics to the nerve before the injury can prevent the development of subsequent hyperalgesic manifestations.

2. The injured axons begin to sprout, and the sprouted terminals display a characteristic "confused" growth cone (neuroma) characterized by transduction properties not possessed by the original, normal axon. These include hyperexcitability to a range of various applied stimuli, and increased sensitivity to humoral (e.g., cytokines, prostaglandins, catecholamines) and mechanical factors (i.e., pressure, touch). Those stimuli and factors may enhance ongoing firing, or elicit firing in previously silent afferents. Spontaneous ectopic firing and ectopic mechanosensitivity have been shown to originate at the same sites, and many injured axons show both changes, although mechanosensitivity can occur without spontaneous firing, and spontaneous firing without mechanosensitivity. It has been shown that mechanosensitive "hotspots" develop in the neuromas, on the surface of the injured nerves, or on regenerating nerves. Clinically, their presence is responsible for the Tinel sign in carpal tunnel syndrome.

3. After the acute injury, persistent spontaneous firing also originates after an interval of days to weeks from small afferent fibers at the site of the lesion (neuroma) to the DRG and neurons in the ipsilateral dorsal horn. Again, suppression with local anesthetics appears to reduce facilitated responses. It should be noted that the DRGs contribute significantly to the ectopic neuropathic barrage and the mechanosensitivity in traumatized nerves, and when neuropathic symptoms and pain persist despite peripheral nerve blocks, ectopic sources in the DRG should be considered. During everyday movements and after manipulations, such as straight-leg lifting, the nerve roots and DRG are subjected to significant mechanical stress, with no effect normally. However, if there is mechanosensitivity due to radiculopathy, these stresses elicit ectopic impulse discharge and pain. The increases in the spontaneous excitability and responsiveness of the injured axons are mediated by changes in the expression and function of multiple ion channel subtypes localized in the DRG and neuroma: various classes of Ca^{++}, K^+, and particularly Na^+ channels are involved. Regenerating nerves show increased production, transport and concentration of aberrant sodium channels at the lesioned terminals. These regenerated channels differ significantly from those of the normal axon. This is a target for sodium-channel blocking drugs, such as mexiletine or lidocaine, which can suppress ectopic firing at concentrations not adequate to suppress normal neural conduction. Expression and increased concentration of novel adrenoreceptors has also been demonstrated.

4. Activation of damaged and adjacent intact fibers by inflammatory mediators. These include pro-inflammatory mediators (sP, CGRP, 5-HT, ATP, NO, leukotrienes, prostaglandins, nerve growth factor, cytokines, etc. They may exert direct and indirect actions on damaged and intact fibers contributing to an increase in afferent traffic.

5. Abnormal patterns of inter-neuronal communication in the DRG and/or neuroma. The apposition of the membranes of adjacent axons can lead to the direct current transfer from one to another, causing "ephaptic" excitatory cross-talk between the fibers (Fig. 1-15). Thus, sympathetic fibers or low-threshold Aβ fibers can activate high-threshold C fibers, contributing to mechanical allodynia. "Crossed-after-discharge" communication involves the depolarization of neurons as a result of the repetitive firing of their neighbors, probably mediated by diffusible mediators (ATP or K^+).

6. Increased sympathetic innervation and excitation of the DRG and/or the neuromas of the primary afferents. Following injury, primary afferent responsiveness to sympathetic stimulation is markedly augmented. After nerve damage, sympathetic terminals extend into the neuroma of the sprouting afferent axon (Fig. 1-16), with a time course parallel to the appearance of mechanical allodynia. Postganglionic sympathetic terminals also sprout and form basket-like projections around DRG cell bodies, particularly the large somata corresponding to Aβ fibers (see Fig. 1-16). Smaller fibers may also be affected. This novel sympathetic innervation has been shown to exert an excitatory drive on both the neuroma, and, independently, on DRG neurons. This is consistent with the observations that chemical sympathetic blockade, bretylium, guanethidine, and

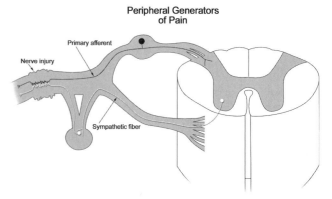

Figure 1-15   Excitatory "cross-talk" between injured peripheral fibers. (Copyright 2004 Catherine Twomey/Medical Center Graphics, Milwaukee, Wisconsin.)

Nerve Sprouting Postinjury

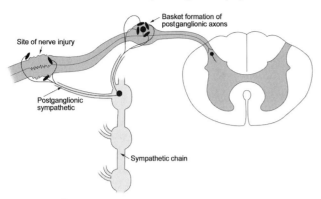

Figure 1-16 Sympathetic efferent fiber sprouting after peripheral nerve injury. (Copyright 2004 Catherine Twomey/Medical Center Graphics, Milwaukee, Wisconsin.)

adrenergic antagonists can alleviate mechanical allodynia and other manifestations of sympathetically maintained painful states. The predominant mechanism of excitation is direct action of released norepinephrine at upregulated and/or oversensitive α adrenoreceptors on the damaged primary afferents. Data favor a principal role of α_2, rather than the α_1 type (but this is confounded by the antinociceptive actions of the α_2 agonists at the central α_2 receptors). It is known that many intact DRG neurons express α adrenoreceptors, and an upregulation following axonal injury seems likely, or the receptors normally expressed may produce exaggerated responses. The sympathetic terminals themselves also express α_2 receptors, which can mediate release of prostaglandins from these terminals. Other sympathetic mechanisms include changes in vascular permeability and blood flow, edema and pressure on pressure-sensitive nociceptors, vasoconstriction, and ischemia.

Finally, it should be noted that neuropathic, painful states are not invariably sympathetic dependent. Clinically, "sympathetically maintained" and "non-sympathetic dependent" states of pain can be differentiated, based on the fact that in some patients neuropathic pain can be relieved by sympathetic blocks. Furthermore, surgical sympathectomy can itself trigger a painful syndrome in some patients.

7. With regards to the edema and trophic changes in skin, nails, and bone that characterize the longstanding cases of reflex sympathetic dystrophy, it seems that these changes are mediated by the release of various vasoactive peptides (such as sP), triggered by the antidromic impulses in C fibers. Sustained ectopic firing can travel both toward the CNS as well as antidromically to the periphery.

8. Altered phenotype of damaged fibers. The levels of many neuropeptides and receptors change in small and large afferent fibers following their injury.

Despite a decrease of sP and CGRP levels, at least at some time periods, in damaged C fibers, nociceptive transmission is maintained as a result of the residual stores of transmitters at upregulated NK_1 and CGRP receptors on sensitized dorsal horn cells. Other transmitters, such as vasoactive intestinal polypeptide (VIP) and neuropeptide Y (NPY), assume excitatory and antinociceptive roles, respectively. A reduction in the DRG cells access to nerve growth factor seems to mediate the decrease of the sP. Simultaneously to the loss of sP in the C fibers, sP actually appear in axotomized, large Aβ fibers upon their injury. The consequences of this induction of sP synthesis in the Aβ fibers are compounded by their release of glutamate, their concurrent sprouting into more superficial dorsal horn laminae (where they make inappropriate contacts with nociceptive neurons), and the upregulation of the NK_1 receptors. The Aβ fibers also increase their levels of VIP and NO, further contributing to a pronociceptive role.

9. Aberrant patterns of peripheral regeneration of damaged peripheral afferents, and alterations in their functional properties. Sprouting of intact, collateral primary afferents occurs into areas of denervated peripheral tissue while regenerating injured primary afferent fibers do not regain their original distribution in the peripheral tissues. These alterations are associated with reorganization of receptive fields of the dorsal horn neurons, with subsequent reconstruction of cortical somatosensory maps. Intact peripheral C fibers sprout to reinnervate denervated cutaneous areas after nerve injury, and these collaterals may play a role in the "extraterritorial" allodynia and hyperalgesia.

10. Surgical or traumatic interruption of primary afferent input to dorsal horns via lesions proximal to DRG produces spontaneous pain and increased responsiveness of dorsal horn neurons. Mechanisms involved are the sensitization of the dorsal horn cells by the intense transient primary afferent discharge upon the injury, a reduction of inhibitory tone, enhanced or attenuated supraspinal mechanisms of facilitation or inhibition, respectively, and a novel afferent input to denervated dorsal horns from collateral sprouting.

Neuropathic Pain: Central Mechanisms

1. There is evidence that stimulation of Aβ fibers mediates the mechanical allodynia in neuropathic pain, and that central mechanisms are required for its expression. However, the role of C fibers in the induction or maintenance of central sensitization in the neuropathic pain should not be underestimated.

It is the afferent barrage from the C fibers that triggers the WDR sensitization in the dorsal horns, and a persistent, low level of C afferent input may be necessary for maintaining central mechanisms underlying certain neuropathic states. Thus, C fiber input to dorsal horns may facilitate Aβ fiber mediated allodynia by inducing and accentuating central sensitization. Excitatory C and Aβ fibers may even synergize upon the WDR neurons.

2. Afferent sprouting of the large afferents to more superficial dorsal horn laminae involved in nociception. After primary afferent injury, there is increased sprouting and reorientation of the Aβ fiber terminals into more superficial laminae (Fig. 1-17). In particular, migration from the deeper, non-nociceptive laminae III, IV, and V into lamina IIo, a region involved in the reception, processing, and transmission of nociceptive information. In lamina IIo, Aβ fiber sprouts may interact synaptically (or otherwise) with nociceptive-specific or WDR neurons, which they would not normally access. Thus, their stimulation will be misinterpreted as noxious. This is compounded by their phenotypic switch to produce sP and VIP as well as by the upregulation of the NK_1 receptors. C fibers and descending pathways may also invade inappropriate regions of dorsal horns: regenerating damaged C fibers expand into deeper laminae contacting NS or WDR cells, producing abnormal signaling.

3. Reduction of Aβ fiber input to inhibitory interneurons. Following primary afferent injury, there is evidence of reduction of the action of the inhibitory interneurons at the small fibers and projection neurons. This is attributed to the reduction of the Aβ fiber-mediated stimulation of the inhibitory interneurons.

4. Functional reduction in the activity or physical degeneration of inhibitory interneurons. Inhibitory interneurons normally suppress the propagation of nociceptive information via inhibitory actions at the projection neurons, excitatory interneurons, and primary afferent terminals. After peripheral nerve injury, dark-staining neurons appear in the ipsilateral dorsal horn (particularly in I and II laminae). These are dying or degenerating inhibitory interneurons, and loss of their tone can induce a hyperexcitable allodynic state. As a result of peripheral nerve injury, activation of NMDA receptor by C fibers triggers the sensitization of WDR cells in dorsal horns. On this basis, it seems possible that primary afferent injury can elicit a transient massive release of glutamate. This, subsequently, via activation of NMDA receptors on to small, vulnerable interneurons, may lead to an excessive intracellular accumulation of Ca^{++}, and the induction of mechanisms provoking their excitotoxic degeneration.

5. Other central mechanisms, including the mechanisms of sensitization and increased excitability of dorsal horn neurons and possible changes in descending mechanisms of inhibition and facilitation.

6. Adaptive changes in the thalamus, cortex, and other higher centers responsible for the discriminative-sensory and affective-cognitive dimension of pain. These include alterations in the neuronal responsiveness together with a reorganization of patterns of synaptic connectivity. Higher centers (e.g., cortex, thalamus) do not behave as passive recipients or relayers of information, but are also themselves actively involved in further integration processes. Additionally, pain can be provoked by damage to CNS itself (central pain), as a result of a stroke, multiple sclerosis, malignancy, etc. However, more work is needed at the cerebral level for an improved understanding of supraspinal mechanisms of both chronic and neuropathic pain, but initial analyses at the cellular level of these mechanisms have suggested striking many similarities to events occurring at the dorsal horns.

The predominant pathophysiological abnormality that particularly characterizes neuropathic pain is that the injured sensory neurons become electrically hyperexcitable and generate ectopic firing discharge. Sympathetic stimulation activates a high proportion of ectopic discharge sites, but in each case of neuropathy the ectopic firing is sustained by a different kind of "idiosyncrasy" of precipitating factors. Only if sensitivity to sympathetic stimulation is the major factor, for example, sympathetic blockade will produce improvement. Nevertheless, suppression of the sodium channel-dependent electrical activity seems to provide more consistency since it constitutes the basis of the generator current. Finally, heredity may play a significant role in the

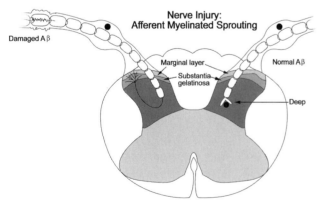

Figure 1-17 Altered large fiber distribution in dorsal horns after peripheral nerve injury. (Copyright 2004 Catherine Twomey/Medical Center Graphics, Milwaukee, Wisconsin.)

genesis and maintenance of the neuropathic pain through details that remain unknown.

CONCLUSION

To summarize, it is reasonable to distinguish several pathways and mechanisms fulfilling contrasting and complementary roles in the detection, processing, and appreciation of pain. Different systems or "phases" of pain may play different teleologic roles. The brief, transient acute pain immediately after a noxious stimulus or injury is processed mainly by systems fitted for gauging the intensity and determining the location. This sensory-discriminative component is of adaptive value in triggering evasive action to a threat, in the comparative absence of modulation by emotional or cognitive factors. On the other hand, other circuits are more involved in the affective dimension of pain and influence or are influenced by emotional-cognitive factors (Fig. 1-18). Rather than detecting stimuli, they serve the ability to rationalize and cope with pain, in particular long-term clinical pain of diverse origins. These systems are associated with mood changes reflecting and modifying pain.

Both of these systems should be regarded as complementary and operating reciprocally and interactively. Regarding the higher levels, it seems that specific "pain centers" do not exist. Rather, a "neuromatrix" of cerebral structures and multiple, interactive thalamo-cortico-limbic networks synergistically contribute to the global experience of pain. The lack of discrete, circumscribed CNS regions underlying pain sensation, is related to, and complicated by, the extensive redundancy of circuits and mechanisms transmitting nociceptive information, and the extensive pattern of reciprocal interactions amongst them. There exists a multiplicity of anatomical structures and ascending and descending pathways, neurotransmitters, inflammatory mediators, mecha-

nisms triggering abnormal patterns of firing and cascades of intracellular signals. A fundamental process underlying prolonged painful states is the sensitization of peripheral and central neurons involved in the processing of pain, and this is elicited by sustained and repetitive stimulation. Isolated selective inactivation of delineated regions of the CNS, or blockade of the actions of specific pronociceptive mechanisms, is unlikely to offer a generalized solution for counteracting the experience of pain. Many discrete therapeutic manipulations in clinical practice, including surgical procedures, sympathectomies, blocks or pharmacologic antagonisms may have limited efficacy. Nevertheless, rational strategies appropriate to the effective control of specific and defined painful conditions remain as the only realistic approaches, and advances in basic sciences provide an improved understanding of mechanisms underlying pain for the discovery of novel analgesic agents and interventions. Relevant to this, is a growing realization that a characterization of the molecular bases of the mechanisms generating rather than inhibiting nociception may provide more fertile ground for this purpose.

REFERENCES

1. Melzack R, Wall PD: Pain mechanisms: a new theory. Science 150:971-979, 1965.

2. Lloyd DPC: Neuron patterns controlling transmission of ipsilateral hind limb reflexes in cat. J Neurophysiol 6:293-315, 1943.

3. Rexed B: The cytoarchitectonic organization of the spinal cord in the cat. J Comp Neurol 96:414-495, 1952.

4. Reynolds DV. Surgery in the rat during electrical analgesia induced by focal brain stimulation. Science 164:444-445, 1969.

5. Cervero F, Laird JMA: From acute to chronic pain: mechanisms and hypotheses. Prog Brain Res 110:3, 1996.

6. Woolf CJ: Evidence for a central component of post-injury pain hypersensitivity. Nature 306:686-688, 1983.

7. Mendell LM. Physiological properties of unmyelinated fiber projection to the spinal cord. Exp Neurol 16:316-332, 1966.

SUGGESTED READING

Abram SE: Pharmacology of pain control. In Brown DL (ed): Regional Anesthesia and Analgesia. Philadelphia, W.B. Saunders, 1996, p 671.

Abram S: Preemptive analgesia. Seminars in Anesthesia 16:263, 1997.

Besson, JM, Chaouch A: Peripheral and spinal mechanisms of nociception. Physiological Reviews 67:67, 1987.

Dickenson A: Spinal cord pharmacology of pain. Br J Anaesth 75:193, 1995.

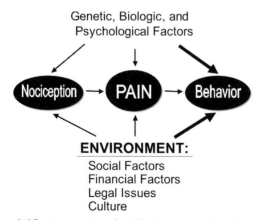

Figure 1-18 Interacting physiologic, emotional, and environmental factors in the behavioral expression of pain.

Dickenson A: Mechanisms of central hypersensitivity: excitatory amino acid mechanisms and their control. In Dickenson A, Besson JM (eds): The Pharmacology of Pain. Berlin, Springer, 1997, p 167.

Dray A: Peripheral mediators of pain. In Dickenson A, Besson JM (eds): The Pharmacology of Pain, Springer, 1997, p 21.

Fine PG, Rosenberg J: Functional neuroanatomy. In Brown DL (ed): Regional Anesthesia and Analgesia. Philadelphia, W.B. Saunders, 1996, p 25.

Harris JA: Using c fos as a neural marker of pain. Brain Research Bulletin 45:1, 1998.

Hogan Q: Reexamination of anatomy in regional anesthesia. In Brown DL (ed): Regional Anesthesia and Analgesia. Philadelphia, W.B. Saunders, 1996, p 50.

Hogan Q: Back pain: beguiling physiology (and politics), Editorial. Regional Anesthesia 22:395, 1997.

Hogan Q, Abram SE: Diagnostic and prognostic neural blockade. In Cousins M, Bridenbaugh PO (eds): Neural Blockade in Clinical Anesthesia and Management of Pain. Philadelphia, Lippincott Williams & Wilkins, 1998, p 837.

Hudspith MJ: Glutamate: a role in normal brain function, anesthesia, analgesia and CNS injury. Br J Anaesth 78:731, 1997.

Kingrey WS: A critical review of controlled clinical trials for peripheral neuropathic pain and complex regional pain syndromes. Pain 73:123, 1997.

Koltzenburg M: The sympathetic nervous system and pain. In Dickenson A, Besson JM (eds): The Pharmacology of Pain. Berlin, Springer, 1997, p 61.

Krames ES: Mechanisms of action of spinal cord stimulation. In Waldman SD, Winnie AP (eds): Interventional Pain Management. Philadelphia, W.B. Saunders, 1996, p 407.

Millan MJ: The induction of pain: an integrative review. Progress in Neurobiology 57:1, 1999.

Munglani R, Hunt SP: Molecular biology of pain. Br J Anaesth 75:186, 1995.

Myers, RR: Morphology of the peripheral nervous system and its relationship to neuropathic pain. In Yaksh TL, et al (eds): Anesthesia: Biologic Foundations. Lippincott Williams & Wilkins, 1998, p 43.

Raja SN, et al: Transduction properties of the sensory afferent fibers. In Yaksh TL, et al (eds): Anesthesia: Biologic Foundations. Lippincott Williams & Wilkins, 1998, p 515.

Sorkin LS, Carlton SM: Spinal anatomy and pharmacology of afferent processing. In Yaksh TL, et al (eds): Anesthesia: Biologic Foundations. Lippincott Williams & Wilkins, 1998, p 577.

Willis WD, Westlund KN: Neuroanatomy of the pain system and of the pathways that modulate pain. J Clin Neurophysiol 14:2, 1997.

Xu, XJ: Novel modulators in nociception. In Dickenson A, Besson JM (eds): The Pharmacology of Pain. Berlin, Springer, 1997, p 211.

Yaksh, TL: Toward a new concept of pain. In Waldman SD, Winnie AP (eds): Interventional Pain Management. Philadelphia, W.B. Saunders, 1996, p 1.

Yaksh, TL: Anatomy of the pain processing system. In Waldman SD, Winnie AP (eds): Interventional Pain Management. Philadelphia, W.B. Saunders, 1996, p 10.

CHAPTER 2

Psychological Assessment of Chronic and Cancer Pain Patients

MARY LOU TAYLOR

INTRODUCTION

Chronic pain would be so much easier to treat if it was a purely physical problem amenable to straightforward measurement. How simple it would be to say, "Ah, your pain is a 10, I will (operate right away, get your morphine drip ready, you name it)." But in truth, a patient's experience of pain is a complex combination of physical pathology, mood, affective state, coping skills, beliefs, expectations, and the patient's social and environmental milieu. It is not enough to test a patient's range of motion, strength, or sensation. Nor is it enough to look at function itself as an indicator of pain. Measures such as functional capacity evaluations and return to work have been shown to correspond poorly to actual pathology and are more heavily dependent on motivation, expectations, and the other factors cited above. Every experienced pain management specialist has seen patients with very significant spinal pathology who go to work each day as well as others with little to show on an MRI who are functionally disabled.

Pain is not simply nociception. This fact makes the psychological assessment of patients with chronic pain extremely important. Likewise, psychological assessment of cancer patients can aid in determining the most effective plans of care.

The goals of this chapter are to provide an overview of the current models of pain, discuss the purposes of psychological assessment of chronic and cancer pain patients, detail the factors most commonly assessed, and specify the most generally accepted assessment methods. This chapter will highlight the important aspects of psychological assessment. Books providing comprehensive coverage of the topic have been referenced at the end of the chapter.

CURRENT MODELS OF PAIN

"Pain is an unpleasant sensory and emotional experience associated with actual or potential tissue damage or described in terms of such damage."[1]

When the International Association for the Study of Pain (IASP) Subcommittee on Taxonomy published this definition of pain in 1986, it was an attempt to integrate an emerging body of knowledge that had expanded the concept of pain over the previous two decades. Pain is now viewed as an experience with both sensory and emotional aspects, rather than a sensory experience to which one has an emotional response. In less than 25 words, the IASP established that pain is both physical and psychological. It is by definition unpleasant, but does not require actual tissue damage to be considered "pain."

GATE CONTROL THEORY

One of the most influential concepts in the understanding of pain is the Gate Control Theory proposed by Ronald Melzack and colleagues.[2] Breaking away from the prevailing conceptualization of pain as a nociceptive phenomenon, Melzack suggested that the experience of pain has sensory-discriminative, cognitive-evaluative, and motivational-affective processes; he argued that all three dimensions must be considered to adequately treat pain. The "bottom-up" pain pathway, from periphery to brain, can be influenced (the "gate" can be opened or closed) by our emotional and cognitive processes. Factors that decrease the transmission of nociception in the dorsal horn include positive emotions, relaxation, intense concentration, and interest in life activities. Conversely, negative emotions, stress, focus on pain, and lack of distraction can "open the gate" and result in increased pain perception.

LOESER PAIN MODEL

In 1980, John Loeser further delineated pain as a multi-layered phenomenon.[3] *Nociception* is the potentially tissue-damaging stimulation that activates the firing of A-δ and C fibers in the nervous system. *Pain* is the sensation in the nervous system in response to the nociception. It is the "whole brain" experience that includes perception, evaluation, meaning, and learning. *Suffering* is a negative affective response to the overall experience of pain, and may vary widely from person to person. *Pain Behavior* is the outward expression of pain that communicates the presence of pain to others, which can vary from culture to culture as well as from person to person. Through learning, pain behavior can be maintained in the absence of physical pathology.

BIOPSYCHOSOCIAL MODEL OF PAIN

Today, pain specialists generally agree that patients' experiences of pain are determined by three factors: the biology of their bodies, their psychological makeup, and their social environment. For any patient, one of these may be more prominent at any certain time. A patient may do well with pain caused by a physical injury until other factors emerge—a recurrence of a major depression, a divorce, or loss of employment, for example. Psychological assessment of the pain patient investigates all of these spheres and looks for interactions that may help or hinder the patient's coping with chronic pain or cancer pain.

LEARNING THEORY

William Fordyce, Jr. was one of the first pain specialists to recognize and study the influence of learning on the perception of pain and the development of pain behaviors.[4] When a person is injured, the experience of pain can be reinforced and strengthened by subtle responses from the environment. If coworkers are more solicitous when a patient is limping than when he or she is walking normally, for example, the patient may unconsciously learn that limping is adaptive or productive. The reinforced limping behavior, however, may increase and prolong pain. The patient, unaware of the learning process that has taken place, may limp long after the original injury has resolved. This is an example of *operant conditioning*.

The development of chronic pain also involves *classical conditioning*, where an unconditioned response to a stimulus gets paired with another stimulus to become a conditioned response. A person who herniates a disc while gardening, for example, and immediately tightens the back muscles as an unconditioned response to the initial pain, may unconsciously tighten muscles each time he or she goes into the garden, or bends in the same way, or even thinks about being in a similar circumstance. Similarly, pain that occurs when in a negative affective state may become conditioned to that state.

Many studies have looked at the influence of these learning factors on the perception of pain. Wunsch and colleagues[5] presented volunteer subjects with non-painful and painful thermal stimuli while they were looking at pleasant, neutral, or unpleasant slides. The subjects rated both nonpainful and painful stimuli as more intense and more unpleasant when looking at the unpleasant slides than they did when viewing the pleasant or neutral slides. Subjects remained unaware that the affective associations had influenced their perception of the physical sensation. In one functional MRI study by Wager and colleagues,[6] the importance of expectation and anticipation was highlighted when actual brain activity, in response to shock, was shown to change after administration of placebo.

Learning theory strengthens the biopsychosocial model of pain by emphasizing the importance of past experience, expectations, and environmental influences on the experience of pain in the present.

PURPOSES OF PSYCHOLOGICAL ASSESSMENT IN CHRONIC PAIN

In general, there are four purposes for referring a patient for a psychological pain assessment:

1. To determine if a patient is a good candidate for a particular pain treatment. Over the years, researchers have found several psychosocial factors that correlate with good or poor outcomes to back surgery, invasive treatments such as spinal cord stimulator or morphine pump implantations, and intensive chronic pain management programs. Many insurance companies now require a psychological assessment prior to authorizing these treatments. Nelson and colleagues[7] have developed a list of exclusionary criteria for the evaluation of spinal cord stimulation candidates (Box 2-1). Though each patient must be considered individually, implantation is not generally advised for patients exhibiting "red flags."

2. To identify psychosocial factors that need to be addressed before treatment, or factors that may warrant a psychiatry or alcohol and other drug abuse (AODA) referral. Many psychological and social factors—an untreated major depression or anxiety disorder, drug or alcohol addiction, divorce proceedings, a legal battle that causes severe anger and stress—may decrease the likelihood of success for any proposed treatment. Identifying and addressing these factors prior to a treatment, whether it is a surgery or multidisciplinary treatment program, may greatly increase a patient's chances of success. Some factors identified in a psychological assessment of chronic pain, such as severe depression or psychotic disorders, may trigger referrals to psychiatry. Patients who are adequately treated for psychological disorders are much better candidates for chronic pain treatment.

3. To tailor a treatment program to a patient's individual needs. It is rare that any one treatment will adequately address chronic pain. A psychological chronic pain assessment is helpful in determining which treatments are most likely to benefit which patients, to allow the pain treatment team to use the best combination of treatments without subjecting the patient to unnecessary interventions.

4. To judge treatment progress and outcomes. Tracking progress and outcomes is useful to the patient. Data from questionnaires on functioning and coping can help identify treatment effectiveness. Likewise, they can demonstrate ineffectiveness and help guide treatment options. For example, if the goal of prescribing narcotic pain medications is to enable the patient to increase activity and improve family life, adequate assessment of these factors can help the pain specialist discuss with the patient whether continued use of the medications is helping goal attainment. Tracking outcomes furthers knowledge in the field of pain management. Many treatments work in some patients and not others. Pretreatment and post-treatment assessments help to identify which treatments are most appropriate for which patients. Finally, outcome data on the effectiveness of treatment programs is useful in working with insurance companies and third-party payers. Treatments with demonstrated ability to change the lives of patients are more readily authorized than treatments with no data.

FACTORS ASSESSED IN PSYCHOLOGICAL CHRONIC PAIN EVALUATION

In the biopsychosocial approach to chronic pain, multiple factors need to be evaluated in addition to the

---

Box 2-1   Implanted Spinal Cord Stimulation: Psychological Factors

Red flags:	Active psychosis
	Active suicidality
	Active homicidality
	Untreated or undertreated major depression
	Somatization disorder or other somatoform disorder
	Current drug or alcohol abuse
	Compensation or litigation depending on spinal cord stimulation outcome
	Inadequate social support
	Neurobehavioral cognitive deficits
Yellow flags:	Unusual pain ratings
	Nonphysiologic signs on physical exam

physical condition of the patient. Many of these factors are assessed in a psychological chronic pain evaluation. These factors include:

Mental Status

Patients with cognitive impairments, whether due to head injury, stroke, dementia, psychosis or drug effects, need special consideration in pain management treatment planning. Additionally, patients who are not cognitively capable of decision-making cannot give informed consent to treatment.

Pain History

A patient's past experience of pain and perception of what is currently wrong and why are important to elicit. Past experiences influence expectations regarding efficacy of proposed treatments. A person who has had good pain relief from surgery in the past is less likely to be willing to engage in conservative treatments in the present if given a surgical option. A person with a past history of a misdiagnosed medical disorder that was resolved by persistently changing physicians may go from doctor to doctor to find the right "cure" for chronic pain.

Learning the patient's perception of the current pain condition is also important. How did the pain begin? Patients who perceive that an injury was someone's "fault" may have a harder time managing pain. Likewise, patients whose injuries were the result of a life-threatening trauma (i.e., assault, war, severe accident) may develop symptoms of post-traumatic stress disorder or phobic anxiety that complicate treatment. One study found that chronic pain patients whose pain stemmed from specific traumatic injury reported higher pain severity, more emotional distress, and more life interference than patients whose pain onset was insidious or spontaneous.

What is causing the pain? Patients may have unclear or inaccurate ideas about pain generation that increase their fear of reinjury and affect their activity levels. What is their pain like currently, and what factors increase or decrease their pain? Patients who perceive lying down and taking medications as the only ways to decrease pain are likely to see their pain increase over time as they become more deconditioned. Patient responses to previous treatments and patient expectations are reviewed.

Family

A patient's current family situation, including relationships with ex-spouses and extended family, is important in evaluating current stress and support as well as possible reinforcers for pain behaviors. Additionally, family history may include factors important in the development or prolongation of chronic pain, such as modeling of

pain by a parent, or reinforcement of pain behaviors as a child. Family history of drug/alcohol abuse, psychological disorders, attitudes towards illness and disability, and any physical or sexual abuse the patient may have experienced are all useful information.

Education/Vocation

A complete psychological assessment includes an education and job history as well as a review of current vocational plans. It is important to know if return to work is a patient goal, and if it is reasonable. Does the patient have a job to return to, or will retraining be necessary? Are there problems with employers or coworkers? Was the patient injured on the job? Examining these goals and workplace issues helps to inform treatment: patients returning to school or to a cognitively demanding job may have difficulty if prescribed anticonvulsants or narcotics, and traumatically injured patients may experience symptoms of Post-Traumatic Stress Disorder when they return to work, for example.

Financial/Legal Status

Assessment of the extent of financial changes and stressors due to chronic pain is important. Current sources of

---

CLINICAL CAVEAT

Disincentives to Feeling Well?

- **Compensation.** The mere presence of compensation for injury is not necessarily predictive of poor treatment outcome. However, if continuance of compensation is dependent on treatment outcome, it may be a disincentive to getting well.
- **Social Support.** Patients who were previously high-functioning but overloaded with responsibility may have a disincentive to getting well if others have taken over their duties and pain reduction will mean going back to an unreasonably full schedule.
- **Learning.** Though often unconscious, patients may learn that pain behavior brings reinforcement (solicitous responses from spouse or coworkers, for example) and wellness behavior is punished.

---

compensation and current or planned litigation must be reviewed to explore the implications of reducing chronic pain and disability. Are there disincentives for getting well?

Drug and Alcohol Use

A history of alcohol use patterns, street drug or prescription drug abuse is taken, in addition to evaluating patient attitudes and compliance with currently prescribed medications. History of legal problems secondary to drug or alcohol use is addressed.

Behavior Analysis

A psychological assessment investigates the changes in activities and behaviors secondary to pain. Included is an analysis of patient-spouse and patient-family interactions and spouse/family responses to pain behaviors and wellness behaviors. Identifying reinforcers for pain behavior or punishments for wellness behavior can help formulate an effective treatment plan. Asking the patient what activities they would pursue if their pain was reduced 50% helps assess goals, values, and patient motivation. One patient, who identified staying home and watching television as his current activity level, replied that he wouldn't change at all if his pain was reduced. "I like my life the way it is." His goal was pain reduction through medication, not increased physical functioning.

Psychological History/Treatment

This includes an assessment of past history of DSM-IV diagnoses, inpatient and outpatient treatments, and the patient's responses to past psychotropic medications. Suicidal attempts and legal issues regarding psychological history are noted.

Psychological Issues Currently Affecting Chronic Pain Management

This is a broad category that assesses factors that have been shown to influence a person's response to pain and pain treatment. These include:

Optimism/Pessimism

Research has shown that a person who analyzes a negative event as personal (it's a problem within me), permanent (this happens every time), and pervasive (this happens in all circumstances) will have much more difficulty managing chronic pain. A pessimistic person whose pain level goes up after doing a certain physical therapy exercise is more likely to think, "Every time I do PT, my pain goes up. It doesn't matter what kind of exercise I do. My body just won't let me do PT," and are much more likely to drop out of treatment prematurely.

Coping Strategies

Psychological assessments investigate the patient's main coping strategies. Patients utilizing negative strategies (i.e., catastrophizing, hoping and praying, inappropriate use of health care) may benefit from therapy to learn more adaptive coping (i.e., coping self-statements, reinterpreting pain sensations, increasing activity).

Anger

Research linking anger to the development and severity of chronic pain has made advances in the past decade.

Bruehl[8] demonstrated in a 2003 study that men who are easily angered and express anger readily are more likely to display endogenous opioid dysfunction in an experimental pain challenge. Okifuji and colleagues[9] suggest that it is useful to look at anger toward specific targets as well as overall anger. Anger toward self was significantly correlated with pain levels, while anger toward the "whole world," self, significant other, insurance, and health-care providers were correlated with depression in a group of chronic pain patients. Several books postulating the link between anger and nonspecific low back pain are in publication.

Self-Efficacy

Self-efficacy is a person's belief that their actions will lead to a desired goal. Self-efficacy is closely tied to expectations and motivation and directly affects treatment compliance. Tailoring treatment to gradually increase self-efficacy can prevent treatment drop-outs.

Readiness to Change

Psychologists have studied how people change behaviors, such as stopping smoking or eating a healthy diet, and have recognized several stages in a person's journey of change. Precontemplation, contemplation, preparation, action, maintenance, and recycling have been identified as distinct phases of change. Accurately assessing a patient's readiness to change helps pain management specialists time interventions for optimal success. Starting a narcotic taper when the patient is in a precontemplation stage, for example, is likely to set up resistance and lack of compliance. Working with a patient in a precontemplation stage to move toward an action stage will take a little longer, but will be more successful.

COMPONENTS OF PSYCHOLOGICAL CHRONIC PAIN ASSESSMENT

A thorough psychological assessment for a patient with chronic pain includes four components: a clinical interview, completion of assessment tests, interviewing the spouse or significant other, and behavioral observations.

Clinical Interview

A clinical interview is an essential step in a complete chronic pain evaluation. The interviewer has the opportunity to establish a rapport with the patient and explain the goals and uses of the evaluation.

Factual information that is elicited includes the history of the pain problem, previous treatments and responses, family, social, and education/vocational history, drug and alcohol history, financial/legal status, and psychological treatment history. During the clinical interview, the psychologist asks questions to elicit information about coping strategies, affect, self-efficacy, readiness to change, and optimism. Previously undiagnosed psychological disorders that can affect chronic pain, such as obsessive-compulsive disorder, panic disorder, or major depression can be identified in a skilled clinical interview.

If the assessment is part of a multidisciplinary treatment program, the clinical interview may also be useful in beginning to provide pain management education and to establish a therapeutic relationship with the psychologist.

Assessment Tests

There is a myriad of self-report questionnaires available to assist in the evaluation of the chronic pain patient. Most pain management programs devise their own battery of tests to meet their particular needs. A routine battery may include questionnaires specific to pain and pain coping as well as more psychologically-oriented instruments. Many of these tests will be described in the following section.

Interview of Spouse or Significant Other

Interviewing the patient's closest relationship, whether it is a spouse, significant other, parent or child, can provide important additional information. When possible, it can be useful to interview the significant person both in the presence of the patient and alone. Though generally shorter than a patient clinical interview, the clinician asks questions regarding the significant person's understanding of the pain, a behavior analysis (e.g., patient's behaviors, family's responses to pain behaviors and well behaviors, patient's activity level, impact of pain on family and marital relationships), stressors (e.g., financial, social, vocational), patient's medication/drug/alcohol use, and patient's affect. Often this significant person can provide additional (and sometimes conflicting) information to broaden the psychologist's understanding of the pain patient.

Behavioral Observations

The psychologist, throughout the clinical interviews and while the patient is completing the assessment questionnaires, has the opportunity to directly observe patient behavior and the interaction between the patient and the significant other. Special attention is paid to the following questions:

1. Does the patient change behavior in the presence of others, or when aware of being observed? If the patient behavior changes when the significant other

is present, learning factors may be important in the continuance of chronic pain. If the patient is unable to sit comfortably during the interview, but sits with ease when not aware of observation, motivation is suspect.

2. What type of nonverbal pain behaviors does the patient exhibit? Limping, unusual postures, frequent postural changes, grimacing, and breath-holding are frequently observed behaviors.

CURRENT CONTROVERSY

When Do Physicians Prescribe Narcotics?

- The leading factor in whether a patient is prescribed narcotic pain medications is the patient's observed pain behaviors.
- Objective physical findings, pain severity, demographic factors, and duration of pain have been shown to have much less influence in the prescription of narcotics than pain behaviors alone.

What type of verbal pain behavior is apparent? In addition to groans, grunts, and sighs, attention should be paid to words used to describe pain or the person's situation. Words can signal extreme affective distress and a feeling of being out of control. "Torturing" and "vicious" evoke a very different frame of mind than "severe" or "penetrating."

Are there differences between what a patient says and directly observable behavior? A patient who states he or she has a sitting tolerance of 15 minutes, but who can sit through a 45-minute interview without excessive postural changes may have developed a sense of helplessness and low self-efficacy or may be overestimating disability for secondary gain. Congruence or incongruence between the patient's numeric rating scale score and their behavior is noted.

Are there behaviors that may directly contribute to chronic pain? Patients with high resting muscle tension or patients who hold their breaths and tighten up when moving have often developed secondary myofascial pain, no matter what their original injury was. Bracing and guarding against pain are behaviors that may need to be addressed in treatment, both with physical therapy and relaxation training.

PAIN/PSYCHOLOGICAL ASSESSMENT QUESTIONNAIRES

Paper and pencil instruments used in chronic pain assessment generally fall into three categories: inventories of pain/function, psychological/personality tests, and tests of pain belief and coping. Describing all of the tests developed in these areas is beyond the scope of this chapter. References at the end of the chapter will direct the interested reader to more thorough treatments of this topic.

Preparing a patient for testing is critical. Patients need to understand that they will not "pass" or "fail" the test. The purpose of the testing is to better understand the patient's experience and current condition to plan the most appropriate treatment possible.

All pencil and paper pain or psychological instruments are subjective and can be manipulated by the patient. In some circumstances, such as an evaluation for a spinal cord stimulator implant, a patient may downplay problems to appear better functioning than is actually true. In other circumstances, such as disability evaluations, patients may have incentives to exaggerate. Some tests have built-in methods for detecting "fake bad" and "fake good" response bias. However, most tests are vulnerable to manipulation. Establishing a good rapport and providing the patient with a reasonable rationale for answering honestly can help reduce this possibility.

PAIN/FUNCTION INVENTORIES

McGill Pain Questionnaire (MPQ). The MPQ, designed by Ronald Melzack in 1975,[2] includes a list of 78 words describing pain that are broken into 20 separate groups. Within each group, the words are ordered from mildest to most severe. Patients are asked to circle the one word in each group that best describes his or her pain, or to leave blank any grouping where no word applies. The descriptors fall into four main categories: sensory (shooting, burning), affective (suffocating, terrifying), evaluative (annoying, unbearable), and miscellaneous. Patients complete a pain diagram and check off adjectives describing the temporal aspects of pain. Included in the test is a Present Pain Intensity (PPI) scale, a 0 to 5 scale with the following corresponding adjectives: No Pain, Mild, Discomforting, Distressing, Horrible, and Excruciating.

The MPQ yields several scores. The Pain Rating Index (PRI) is derived from the rank values of the descriptors in each category: Sensory, Affective, Evaluative, and Miscellaneous, and a total score from all subscales. The Number of Words Chosen (NWC) is a simple count of all 20 subscales. The PPI is the number corresponding to the adjectives rating the patient's pain at the time of test administration.

The MPQ has been widely researched and shown to be a valid and reliable instrument in a wide variety of pain conditions. It is sensitive to changes in pain over time and is easily understood in a wide adult age range. It is useful in both research settings and in clinical practice, as it helps patients describe their experiences of pain and helps the clinician quantify changes over time and treatments.

Melzack published a short form of the MPQ (SF-MPQ) in 1987 that includes 15 descriptors measuring the Sensory and Affective components of pain, a Visual Analog Scale, and the PPI. Its brevity makes it useful in settings where patients are asked to fill out many questionnaires or the test is frequently administered.

Multidimensional Pain Inventory (MPI). The MPI, originally designed by Kerns, Turk, and Rudy in 1985,[10] is a 61-item questionnaire that measures a broad range of psychosocial functioning in people with chronic pain. It is divided into three sections, with each item presented on a 0 to 6 scale. Section I looks at the psychosocial effects of pain: the patient's perception of how pain interferes with work, social activities, relationships, the patient's level of suffering, negative mood, and perceived life control. Section II regards the reactions of the spouse or significant other to the patient's pain, describing solicitous, distracting, and punishing responses. The third section includes a variety of specific activities—washing dishes, riding in a car, etc.—and asks the patient to rate how frequently he or she is able to perform them.

Scoring of the MPI yields three profile categories as well as 20 subscale scores. Patients falling into the Dysfunctional profile category generally report high pain severity, life interference, and affective distress, coupled with low levels of activity and perceived life control. Patients with an Adaptive Coper profiles generally score lower on pain severity, affective distress, and interference with higher activity levels and perceived life control. Interpersonally Distressed profile patients are most notable for limited support from their significant others. In treatment programs, Interpersonally Distressed profile patients show the poorest response. Dysfunctional profile patients generally respond better when cognitive treatments are a part of their overall pain management program.

The MPI has been shown to be valid and reliable. It is sensitive to change over time and is often included in outcome research to evaluate pretreatment and posttreatment levels of functioning.

Oswestry Disability Index (ODI). The ODI is a 10-section questionnaire of functioning in areas such as personal cares, sitting, lifting, walking, social life, etc. For each section, the patient is asked to circle 1 of 6 choices that range from no disability to extreme disability.

Sickness Impact Profile (SIP). The SIP is a 136-item disability questionnaire that scores patients on 12 dimensions of functioning: ambulation, mobility, body care and movement, social interaction, communication, alertness, emotional behavior, sleep and rest, eating, work, home management, and recreation. In addition to the individual scales, the test is scored on Physical, Psychosocial, and Total Disability scales as well. The test is now available in a shortened form (SIP-68) that has been shown to be valid, reliable, and sensitive to changes in function over time.

Medical Outcomes Study 36-Item Short Form Health Survey (SF-36). This self-report questionnaire yields scores on eight scales: physical functioning, role limitations due to physical health problems, bodily pain, general health, vitality, social functioning, role limitations due to emotional problems, and mental health. It can be administered in the standard format, where most questions are answered for a time frame of the past four weeks, or an Acute format, where questions are answered for the past week. It has been used extensively in health-care quality of life research and is included in the standard batteries of many programs, though some studies have questioned its sensitivity to treatment effects.

TESTS OF PSYCHOLOGICAL FUNCTIONING

Minnesota Multiphasic Personality Inventory, Revised (MMPI-2). The MMPI-2 is considered to be the most thorough and rigorous of the general psychological questionnaires and is used in many programs in the initial assessment phase. It is a 567-item true/false test that yields 10 clinical scales and 15 content scales as well as validity scales to detect response bias or random answering. It is very useful in assessing psychological functioning and in describing behaviors based on individual profiles.

Briefly, the first three scales, Hy (Hypochondriasis), D (Depression), and Hs (Hysteria) appear to be the most telling in the evaluation of chronic pain patients. Patients with clinically elevated Hy and Hs scores (the "Conversion V"), which suggest a high somatic focus and an underreporting of emotional pain, have been shown in several studies to have poorer outcomes, especially in studies of prediction of response to surgeries. Moderately elevated Hy, D, and Hs scales, however, appear to reflect adjustment disorders secondary to pain and do not indicate poor surgical risk. Patients with many elevated scales, indicative of more significant psychopathology, generally do less well in any form of treatment.

Despite years of research, there has been limited success in identifying psychological profiles that predict the development of chronic pain (the "pain-prone personality") or that accurately predict response to many chronic pain treatments. The length of the test makes it difficult to use when outcomes are measured serially over time. Also, many chronic pain patients have difficulty completing the 567 items in one sitting. The norms of the test are based on psychiatric, rather than chronic pain populations.

Symptom Checklist-90 Revised (SCL-90-R). The SCL-90-R is a shorter test of general psychological functioning. Patients are presented with 90 physical and psychological symptoms, ranging from headaches to hearing voices, and are asked to mark how distressed they have been by each symptom within the last week. It yields nine psychological scales: Somatization, Obsessive-Compulsive, Interpersonal Sensitivity, Depression, Anxiety, Hostility, Phobic Anxiety, Paranoid Ideation, and Psychoticism. It also yields three global indices of distress. The Global Severity Index (GSI), derived from the total number of items endorsed and the intensity of perceived distress, is the most often-used indicator of current distress levels. The Positive Symptom Distress Index (PSDI) is interpreted as a measure of symptom intensity, and the Positive Symptom Total (PST) is simply the number of symptoms endorsed at any level of distress. While the SCL-90-R has the advantage of increased patient acceptance and shorter administration time, it is difficult to compare chronic pain patients with the test's normative sample of inpatient and outpatient psychiatric patients and nonpatients.

Millon Behavioral Health Inventory (MBHI). The MBHI is a measure of psychological functioning designed specifically for medical patients. The 150-item questionnaire yields scores on scales reflecting patients' basic personality and coping styles (e.g., introverted, inhibited, sociable, forceful), psychogenic attitudes (e.g., tension, pessimism, alienation), psychosomatic correlates (e.g., allergic inclination, gastro susceptibility, cardiovascular tendency), and probable responses to treatment, including outpatient pain management. The test's brevity and its focus on health improve its acceptance by patients. Also, the patient is being compared with a normative sample of medical rather than psychiatric patients. However, as with the previously discussed instruments, it

---

CURRENT CONTROVERSY

Pain Profiles

- Though the quest for accurate predictors of the development of chronic pain has spanned several decades, no "pain-prone personality" has been definitively identified.
- Many psychological factors commonly seen in chronic pain patients may be a result of the chronic pain experience, rather than a cause.
- Some research has been more successful in identifying predictors of outcome in surgery and invasive procedures, but there are no consistently accurate techniques for predicting which injured person will go on to develop chronic pain.

has not been shown to accurately predict treatment response in several studies.

Depression Scales. Two major depression scales used in chronic pain assessment are the **Beck Depression Inventory, Revised (BDI-II),** and the **Center for Epidemiologic Studies-Depression Scale (CES-D).** Both are brief (21 and 20 items, respectively) and easily scored. Both have been found to be able to accurately assess depression in a chronic pain population. The CES-D has been found to be most sensitive to changes due to treatment effects. Both include physical symptoms of depression (such as sleep disturbance, fatigue, loss of libido) that are also associated with chronic pain. For this reason, the cutoff point for diagnosing depression is higher in a chronic pain population.

Anxiety Scales. Two measures of anxiety most often used in chronic pain assessment are the **State-Trait Anxiety Inventory (STAI)** and the **Beck Anxiety Inventory (BAI).** The STAI is a 40-item self-report. Patients are asked to answer 20 items as they feel in the present, and 20 items as they generally feel. Scores are provided for trait anxiety, generally more difficult to change with brief treatment, and state anxiety, which can be more easily modified. The BAI is quite similar to the Beck Depression Inventory, in that it is a 21-item questionnaire that has patients rate each item from 0 to 3. Items include subjective, somatic or panic-related anxiety symptoms. Both tests are valid and reliable quick screens of anxiety.

TESTS OF PAIN BELIEF AND COPING

Many tests have been devised to study patient's pain beliefs and coping skills. Three of the most interesting are the **Coping Strategies Questionnaire (CSQ),** the **Survey of Pain Attitudes (SOPA),** and the **Pain Stages of Change Questionnaire (PSOCQ).**

The CSQ is a 42-item self-report that rates the patient's use of six cognitive and one behavioral coping strategy. Subscales include Diverting Attention, Reinterpreting Pain, Coping Self-Statements, Ignoring Pain, Praying and Hoping, Catastrophizing, and Increasing Activity. Two additional items that assess self-efficacy measure the patient's perceived ability to decrease pain and perceived control over pain. In studies, catastrophizing and praying and hoping have been shown to be associated with higher pain levels and disability and greater psychological distress. A goal of cognitive pain management is to increase the use of positive coping strategies.

The SOPA, first published in 1987, has undergone two revisions and is now a 57-item questionnaire that provides scores on Control, Disability, Medical Cures, Solicitude, Medication, Emotion, and Harm. It is a valid

and reliable measure of patients' attitudes regarding many aspects of pain, and has been shown to be sensitive to changes when assessing beliefs before and after conservative pain management treatment programs.

The PSOCQ more specifically assesses a patient's readiness to change to a more adaptive self-management approach to pain. Its 30 items assess four stages: Precontemplation, Contemplation, Action, and Maintenance. Studies have demonstrated that patients who place in the Precontemplation or early Contemplation stages of change are more likely to drop out of treatment that is directed toward self-management.

PSYCHOLOGICAL ASSESSMENT OF CANCER PAIN PATIENTS

Cancer patients may experience pain caused by progression of disease or as a result of treatments such as surgery, chemotherapy or radiation. While the majority of patients do not report pain at the time of diagnosis, studies indicate that 60% to 80% of patients with metastatic disease report pain. Much work has been done in the past decade to improve palliative care at the end of life, including aggressive pain management. However, as more patients survive cancer, chronic cancer pain is becoming a more prevalent and often overlooked problem.

The types of cancer pain vary widely, and include muscular, bone, neuropathic, and visceral. Likewise, the severity can range from easily controllable to extremely severe.

It is important to consider the whole person when assessing and treating cancer pain. In addition to stage of disease and etiology of specific nociception, it is useful to ascertain patients' previous levels of functioning, their goals and expectations, and the meaning they ascribe to their pain. A biopsychosocial assessment allows the clinician to address pain more completely. Just as in chronic pain, the experience of pain may be exacerbated by fear, anxiety, depression, stress, low self-efficacy, hopelessness, learning, and culture. Assessing these issues and patients' personality styles can help tailor treatment to maximize benefit.

Unlike chronic pain, cancer patients may be reticent about discussing pain, for fear of diverting attention from aggressive treatment of the cancer itself or because they don't want to "bother" the doctors who are trying to save them. Also, many patients dislike the idea of taking even more medications, while others fear that taking narcotics too soon may leave them with uncontrollable pain later on. Studies have indicated that depression and anxiety in cancer patients is higher in those who are experiencing pain and is significantly reduced when pain is adequately treated. It is important for physicians to assess pain routinely, assure patients that their pain will be adequately treated, and include a psychological assessment when appropriate.

Assessment Components

Assessment of the presence and severity of pain needs to begin at diagnosis and be frequently repeated throughout a patient's treatment. Because many patients do not experience pain until later stages of their disease/treatment, and some never have pain, a thorough psychological assessment is often performed only after pain has become problematic or chronic, or the patient has elected to undergo a difficult treatment, such as a bone marrow transplant. In general, it is better to have an initial psychological assessment earlier in the course of the disease rather than waiting until the patient is in severe pain or at the end of life.

CLINICAL CAVEAT

Cancer Pain Is Multifactorial, Too

- Cancer pain is often regarded as more unidimensional and psychological factors are often overlooked.
- Like all types of pain, cancer pain may be influenced by social, environmental, cognitive, and personality factors.
- As cancer treatments improve, more patients will shift from "cancer pain" to "chronic pain" patients.

Psychological assessment of cancer patients includes clinical interviews, self-report questionnaires, and behavioral observations.

Interview

As with chronic pain patients, it is useful to interview both the patient and the significant other or main caregiver. Information regarding prior functioning is elicited, including prior psychological diagnoses and treatment, vocation/education, family history, previous pain experience, and drug and alcohol history. Current functioning including the impact of pain on social, vocational, recreational, and self-care activities is assessed. Patients are questioned about mood, sleep, coping strategies, current stressors, and their fears and expectations regarding pain. Factors that provoke or alleviate pain and attitudes toward health-care providers and illness in general are explored. In cases where the patient is very ill, caregiver reports become more critical.

The large majority of cancer patients have no pre-existing psychiatric disorders, but a significant number may develop adjustment disorders (with depressed mood, anxiety, or both) at some point in their treatment. The

prevalence of major depression in samples of cancer patients has ranged from 13% to greater than 50%. Because a significant minority of patients with advanced cancer will experience organic brain dysfunction, a brief mental status exam is often warranted.

Questionnaires

Many of the assessments described earlier in the discussion of chronic pain assessment are also applicable to cancer pain patients.

The MPQ is valuable is identifying location, temporal aspects, and severity of pain as well as the qualitative experience of pain. The SF-MPQ can be administered quickly and can be repeated to assess treatment efficacy.

Measures of function and quality of life are important in cancer pain assessment. As described earlier, the SF-36 and its abbreviated version, the SF-12, are reliable measures of general functioning. The SIP and its shortened form, the SIP-68, cover a wide range of function but take longer to complete. The Functional Assessment of Cancer Therapy (FACT) is a quality of life index designed for patients receiving cancer treatment. Its revised version, the FACT-G, is a valid and reliable 36-item instrument that measures physical, functional, social, and emotional well-being and the patient's relationship with the physician. Other forms are available that are germane to specific cancer types.

Because the majority of cancer pain patients do not have pre-existing psychological diagnoses, the use of lengthy tests of general psychological functioning are not often used outside of research settings. Brief inventories of depression and anxiety, such as the Beck Depression Inventory and the State Trait Anxiety Inventory, may be used. Less weight is given to somatic symptoms that are common with severe illnesses or during treatments, such as sleep disturbance, weight loss, and loss of libido. The Millon Behavioral Health Inventory[11] is useful to help assess relationships with health-care providers, the patient's approach to health, and general stressors that may influence the course of treatment.

Behavioral Observations

Behavioral observation is more important for cancer pain patients who have prolonged periods of pain, pain out of proportion to their disease, or pain that is expected to be chronic though they no longer have active disease. All pain behavior is subject to operant conditioning, and the longer the patient is in pain, the more opportunities there are for reinforcement of pain behavior. During the clinical interview and while the patient is completing questionnaires, the psychologist observes behavior in a manner similar to that done with chronic pain patients.

CONCLUSION

Pain is an experience, not a sensation. The experience of pain includes cognitive and emotional components as well as sensation, and is best evaluated and treated from a biopsychosocial model rather than a purely biomedical model. A comprehensive pain management psychological assessment is useful to identify many of the factors that contribute to the etiology, exacerbation, or continuation of chronic pain conditions. Personality factors, pre-existing and current psychological disorders, financial, family, social and vocational stressors, and conditioning of pain behaviors can all seriously affect the experience of pain.

Psychological assessments are useful to determine whether the patient is a good candidate for invasive treatments such as spinal cord stimulation; to identify psychosocial factors that may need to be addressed before pain treatments, including psychiatric referrals; to tailor treatment to the patient's individual needs; and to assess treatment outcomes. An assessment includes a clinical interview, patient-completed questionnaires, behavioral observations and, where possible, interviews with significant others.

The goal of psychological assessment of pain patients is to improve understanding of the patient to maximize treatment benefit. By assessing the whole person—the history, cognitions, expectations, social system, and personality style that makes that patient unique—the most appropriate treatment options can be offered.

REFERENCES

1. International Association for the Study of Pain (IASP) Subcommittee on Taxonomy, Mersky H (ed): Classification of chronic pain syndromes and definitions of pain terms. Pain 3(suppl):S1-S226, 1986.
2. Melzack R, Wall PD: The Challenge of Pain. New York, Basic Books, 1982.
3. Loeser JD: Perspectives on pain. In Turner P (ed): Proceedings of the First World Congress on Clinical Pharmacology and Therapeutics. London, Macmillan, 1980, pp 316–326.
4. Fordyce WE: Behavioral Methods for Chronic Pain and Illness. St. Louis, CV Mosby, 1976.
5. Wunsch A, Philippot P, Plaghki L: Affective associative learning modified the sensory perception of nociceptive stimuli without participant's awareness. Pain 102:27-38, 2003.
6. Wager TD, Rilling JK, Smith EE, Sokolik A, et al: Placebo-induced changes in fMRI in the anticipation and experience of pain. Science 303:1162-1167, 2004.
7. Nelson DV, Kennington M, Novy DM, Squitieri P: Psychological selection criteria for implantable spinal cord stimulators. Pain Forum 52:93-103, 1996.
8. Bruehl S, Chung OY, Burns JW, Biridepalli S: The association between anger expression and chronic pain intensity: evidence for partial mediation by endogenous opioid dysfunction. Pain 106:317-324, 2003.
9. Okifuji A, Turk DC, Curran SL: Anger in chronic pain investigations of anger targets and intensity. J Psychosom Res 47:1-12, 1999.
10. Kerns RD, Turk DC, Rudy TE: The West Haven–Yale Multidimensional Pain Inventory (WHYMPI). Pain 23(4): 345-356, 1985.
11. Millon T, Green C, Meagher R: Millon Behavioral Health Inventory Manual, 3rd ed. Minneapolis, National Computer Systems, 1982.

SUGGESTED READING

Abram SA, Haddox D (eds): The Pain Clinic Manual. Philadelphia, Lippincott Williams & Wilkins, 2000.

Dworkin RH, Breitbart WS (eds): Psychosocial Aspects of Pain: A Handbook for Health Care Providers. Seattle, IASP Press, 2004.

Turk DC, Melzack R (eds): Handbook of Pain Assessment, 2nd ed. New York, Guilford Press, 2001.

Turk DC, Monarch ES, Williams AD: Cancer patients in pain considerations for assessing the whole person. Hematol Oncol Clin N Am 16:511-525, 2002.

Turk DC, Okifuji A: What factors affect physicians' decisions to prescribe opioids for chronic noncancer pain patients? Clin J Pain 13:330-336, 1997.

Turk DC, Okifuji A: Perception of traumatic onset, compensation status, and physical findings: impact on pain severity, emotional distress and disability in chronic pain patients. J Behav Med 19:435-453, 1996.

Nezu AM, Nezu CM, Fiedman SH, et al: Helping Cancer Patients Cope. Washington, DC, American Psychological Association, 1998.

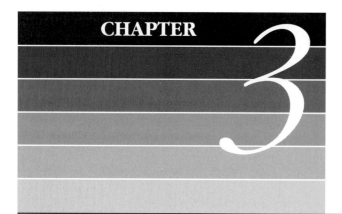

Psychological Treatment of Chronic Pain

STEPHEN E. ABRAM

INTRODUCTION

A significant portion of a chronic pain patient's disability may be acquired long after the injury or medical illness that initiated the painful condition. Some of this acquired disability is physical and is related to loss of physical condition. Inactivity leads to muscle weakness, stiffness, and pain, loss of muscular support of the spine and joints, and shortening of tendons and ligaments. Subsequent attempts at physical activity, even those involved with activities of daily living, are met with further increases in pain, and the patient's lifestyle becomes more and more sedentary, leading to more generalized pain. Weight gain is a common consequence that leads to further physical disability and to the development of other medical conditions.

A variety of learned behaviors contribute to the patient's withdrawal from a productive and rewarding lifestyle. Complaints of severe pain, groaning, and grimacing are met by solicitous behavior from family members, including offers to help with household chores and advising the patient to rest, reinforcing the sedentary lifestyle. Pain complaints allow the patient to avoid unpleasant vocational activity or social interactions, and these rewards help to perpetuate maladaptive pain behaviors.

Certain thoughts and beliefs acquired during a painful illness add to the patient's distress. Catastrophizing refers to thoughts of worst case scenarios. This type of thinking is a key predictor of a patient's pain experience and correlates with pain intensity ratings, disability, use of health-care resources, and medication use. It has three elements: a focus on threatening information: "I feel a clicking in my back whenever I move"; an overestimation of the extent of the threat: "If things get worse I will become paralyzed"; and an underestimation of internal and external resources available: "No one can do anything about my condition and I can't bear the pain any longer."

Psychological strategies are directed toward eliminating maladaptive physical and psychological responses to pain and replacing them with responses that lead to more satisfying and productive activities. The patient is taught coping strategies that provide a greater sense of control and reduction of functional disability. In many cases the resumption of a more active lifestyle will result in actual reduction of pain as the patient's physical condition improves.

COGNITIVE BEHAVIORAL THERAPY

The aim of cognitive behavioral therapy is to extinguish behaviors that lead to reduced activity, increased social isolation, and increased emotional distress, and to restore behaviors that are rewarding for the patient and for society. This involves identifying and correcting thoughts, attitudes, and beliefs that perpetuate maladaptive behaviors. The patient is taught to identify and record maladaptive thoughts and replace them with more balanced, productive ones. Thoughts and beliefs that produce anxiety or sadness and depression are replaced with positive thoughts. Evidence may be presented by the therapist that many patients with similar conditions return to normal productive lives.

Patients and family members are taught to identify environmental factors that reinforce maladaptive pain behaviors. Escaping an unpleasant or stressful work environment is a common one. Every effort should be made to keep the patient in a work environment and to modify that environment to minimize pain and stress and maximize nonpainful activity. Identification of behaviors of family and caregivers that perpetuate maladaptive behaviors is a difficult but essential part of treatment.

Stress and anger management is an important aspect of cognitive behavioral therapy. Patients are taught to identify stressors that trigger anger or anxiety. Treatment consists of assertiveness training and improvement in communication skills.

Patients are taught to work toward attaining achievable goals. Patients who try to achieve substantial improvements quickly may become frustrated and angry. If goals are broken down into smaller steps that can be accomplished more quickly and easily, the patient's belief in success is heightened and the likelihood of success increases.

Distraction techniques can be an effective tool for exerting control over pain. Rather than focusing on pain, which tends to increase pain perception, the patient's attention is focused on other thoughts and activities. Active distraction involves involvement in an activity, while passive distraction involves meditation and relaxation techniques.

Sleep deprivation can be a major impediment to achieving a more productive lifestyle. Daytime napping and loss of daytime physical activity can interfere with normal nocturnal sleep patterns. Patients should be encouraged to follow regular sleep-wake schedules. Relaxation training and other behavioral techniques can help patients to fall asleep.

A list of cognitive-behavioral techniques is shown in Box 3-1.

PATIENT EDUCATION

Misinformation and misunderstanding lead to increased anxiety, reduced motivation, and poor treatment choices by the chronic pain patient. An important aspect of education is to inform the patient about the futility of conventional surgical and interventional pain treatment

---

Box 3-1 Cognitive Behavioral Strategies

Problem Identification
   Identify thoughts, beliefs, and attitudes underlying
      maladaptive behavior
   Catastrophizing
Cognitive Restructuring
   Substitute balanced, productive thoughts for
      maladaptive ones
   Apply techniques to anxiety, depressive symptoms
Sleep Management
   Improved sleep habits
   Behavioral techniques
Extinguish Learned Behaviors
   Learned avoidance of stressful situations
   Reinforcement of maladaptive behaviors
Distraction Techniques
   Active
   Passive
Increased Self-Efficacy
   Attainable goals
Stress and Anger Management

---

techniques following multiple therapeutic failures. The patient who has undergone multiple surgical procedures despite their producing increasing pain and disability needs to learn that other options are more likely to help. They should also learn that there is a down side to many of the medications that are prescribed for chronic pain. Opioids can produce hyperalgesia, leading to increased sensitivity to pain, especially as tolerance develops and doses are escalated. They also are associated with sexual dysfunction, psychological depression, and suppression of immune function. They should also be taught to recognize signs of opioid dependence and abuse.

Patients may need to be taught that some fears about medication use may be unfounded. While some patients experience significant adverse affects of opioids, others obtain long-lasting benefit without significant dose escalation, sensory sensitization, addiction, or side effects.

Headache patients should be given information about medications that can produce rebound headaches and about environmental factors and foods that can cause or worsen headaches. They should also understand the ability of sedative and hypnotic medications used for sleep, anxiety or muscle relaxation to produce depression, dependence, memory loss, and reduced cognitive function (see Box 3-1).

Patients also need to understand the relationship between pain and stress, anger, anxiety, and depression. They also need to learn that psychological strategies can exert substantial control over pain. Explanation of descending inhibitory systems, activity-induced activation

Box 3-2   Patient Education Topics

Advisability of ongoing invasive therapies
Risks and benefits of medications for pain
   Opioid hyperalgesia
   Abuse, addiction
   Rebound phenomena
   Dispel irrational fears
Understanding acute versus chronic pain
Hurt versus harm
Interrelationship between pain, anxiety, and depression
Interrelationship between pain, stress, and autonomic
   function
Role of deconditioning in maintaining ongoing pain
   Need for exercise
   Role of physical therapy
Intrinsic pain control systems
   Exercise induced analgesia
   Descending control
Learning theory and pain behaviors

of endogenous pain control systems, aggravation of pain by stress-induced increases in muscle activity, and autonomic tone can help patients to understand how psychotherapeutic interventions can provide pain reduction as well as improved ability to cope with ongoing pain.

An important issue is the difference between hurt and harm. In the case of an acute injury, aggravation of pain during increased activity may delay healing or increase the extent of injury. This is not true of chronic pain states. As patients increase their physical activity and begin therapeutic exercises, there is bound to be some pain during the early phases of therapy. They need to understand that this pain is not a signal of tissue injury or trauma and that working through the pain is essential to their recovery (Box 3-2). They also need to be taught the value of moderation and the need to proceed in a slow, stepwise fashion. Overdoing physical activity can produce temporary setbacks that cause frustration and dissatisfaction with therapy.

Lastly, it is important that patients and their family members and caregivers understand the importance of learned behaviors and the reinforcement of pain behaviors.

While much of the patient education is carried out by the psychotherapist, it is important that the physicians and nursing personnel participate as well. If the individual who provides medication therapy or other therapeutic interventions emphasizes the need to switch to a regimen involving psychological strategies and rehabilitation along with reduction in medication use and abandonment of surgery and nerve blocks, the patient is more likely to be convinced that it is the right decision.

BIOFEEDBACK AND RELAXATION

Biofeedback and relaxation training allow the patient to exert a certain amount of control over involuntary functions such as autonomic activity and muscle tone. Relaxation techniques are relatively nonspecific but can indirectly influence the effects of anxiety and stress on muscle tone and autonomic function.

Relaxation Techniques

Progressive Muscle Relaxation
Patients are taught to systematically tense then relax individual muscle groups. The end result is the ability to selectively relax tense muscle groups.

Focused Breathing
Patients are taught to focus on their breathing and to actively control inspiration and exhalation. They may be instructed to silently repeat a soothing word or phrase with each exhalation. Short daily exercises of this sort are associated with reductions in stress, anxiety, and sympathetic tone.

Autogenic Relaxation
Patients are instructed to systematically relax specific parts of the body, providing suggestions of warmth and heaviness of the part on which they concentrate.

Guided Imagery
Once the patient achieves a relaxed state, the use of imagery can produce further beneficial effects. The relaxed state can be enhanced by imagining oneself in a pleasant, safe environment. Images of warmth, such as lying in the warm sun, can further increase skin temperature. Enhancement of coping skills can be achieved by desensitization using imagery to bring up stressful images or situations while maintaining a state of relaxation and effective coping. Images of tight muscles relaxing or unwinding can actually lead to pain reduction in some instances.

Biofeedback

Electromyogram Biofeedback
Surface electromyogram (EMG) electrodes are placed over affected muscles, such as suboccipital muscles in patients with tension headache. Increasing EMG activity produces a higher auditory tone, while lowering EMG activity produces a lower tone. Patients can be taught to selectively relax specific muscle groups using this technology.

Thermal Biofeedback
Auditory tones change in response to rising or falling skin temperature. Patients are taught to increase the tem-

perature of the hands or feet. This technique is most often used in migraine, Raynaud's phenomenon, and complex regional pain syndrome, but it can produce a state of general relaxation in a variety of pain states.

GROUP THERAPY

While one benefit of group therapy is to increase the efficiency of the psychotherapist by treating multiple patients at one time, its primary benefit is to use the dynamics of the group to benefit each of the individuals. Chronic pain patients often feel isolated and misunderstood. Interaction with other individuals who share the same problems and frustrations can provide considerable emotional support. In addition, seeing others in the group coping with the same issues encourages the individual to persevere.

Patient Selection

Patients should meet the following criteria to be considered for group therapy:
1. Have basic skills of personal interaction.
2. Have at least low-average intelligence.
3. Have no psychotic symptoms or significant personality disorder.
4. Demonstrate reasonable motivation.
5. Demonstrate compliance with psychological treatment strategies.
6. Have reliable transportation.

Group Therapy Format

Therapy usually combines a psychotherapy session and physical therapy. Group size is usually 4 to 8 patients. A typical program combines 2 hours of psychotherapy and 1 to 2 hours of physical therapy per week. Programs typically run for 5 to 8 weeks. Psychotherapy includes the entire range of cognitive behavioral therapies outlined above as well as relaxation training and education. Physical therapy generally focuses on non-specific aerobic exercise and strengthening and stretching exercises.

PSYCHIATRIC COMORBIDITY

During the course of psychological assessment and therapy, it is not uncommon for the clinical psychologist to discover that a patient has significant psychopathology that requires concomitant treatment. Recognition of significant coexisting depression and anxiety is common, and these conditions may improve as therapy for the painful condition progresses. On the other hand, severe underlying depression may be the principal rea-

son for the patient's pain complaints and referral to a psychiatrist for psychotherapy and pharmacological management may be appropriate.

Neurotic abnormal illness behaviors are occasionally encountered among patients with chronic pain complaints. Hypochondriacal reactions are characterized by health concerns that are out of proportion to the degree of pathology. There are generally three components to hypochondriacal disorders:
1. A phobic attitude toward illness.
2. A conviction that disease is present combined with lack of response to reassurance.
3. A preoccupation with bodily symptoms.

The phobic form of hypochondriasis involves feelings of anxiety combined with a focus on the physiological manifestations of anxiety. Cardiac palpitations are regarded as a sign of heart disease; headaches are due to brain tumor. Another form of hypochondriasis involves overconcern about symptoms associated with one's current condition. Hypochondriacal patients often have a history of illness or frailty as a child and were regarded as sickly by parents and teachers. There may also have been an invalid parent who exhibited illness behavior that became a behavioral model for the child. The prognosis for patients with a long history of illness and extensive utilization of healthcare resources is poor. Patients with recent onset of illness and hypochondriasis may respond fairly well to cognitive behavioral therapy, particularly when combined with a behavioral approach that discourages invalidism.

Patients with conversion disorder do not exhibit preoccupation with illness but complain of symptoms such as motor dysfunction, numbness or pain. The terms psychogenic pain and somatoform pain disorder have been used to diagnose pain complaints without an underlying source of pathology. Anxiety or depression may underlie the development of psychogenic pain.

Patients with psychoses that were formerly well-managed may decompensate with the added stress of a painful condition. Psychiatric symptoms may be a sign of underlying substance abuse or addiction. It is important to recognize severe personality disorders, as these conditions will significantly compromise the team's ability to provide satisfactory treatment. Among veterans and victims of violent crime, post-traumatic stress disorder is a common accompaniment of chronic pain. Treatment of this condition often requires long-term intervention.

SUGGESTED READING

Blackall GF: Psychological techniques in pain management. In Raj PP (ed): Practical Management of Pain, 3rd ed. St. Louis, Mosby, 2000, pp 523–528.

Fordyce WE: An operant conditioning method for managing chronic pain. Postgrad Med 53:123–138, 1973.

Kerns RD, Turk DC, Rudy TE: Comparison of cognitive-behavioral and behavioral approaches to the outpatient treatment of chronic pain. Clin J Pain 1:195–203, 1986.

Krueger RF, Tackett JL, Markon KE: Structural models of comorbidity among common mental disorders: connections to chronic pain. Advances in Psychosomatic Medicine 25:63–77, 2004.

Lipchik GL, Miles K, Covington EC: The effects of multidisciplinary pain management treatment on locus of control and pain beliefs in chronic non-terminal pain. Clin J Pain 9:49–57, 1993.

CHAPTER 4

Physical Rehabilitation of the Chronic Pain Patient

STEPHEN E. ABRAM

The goals of a physical rehabilitation program include resumption of physical exercise and improvement in exercise tolerance, reestablishment of muscle strength and flexibility, return to normal joint and spine mechanics, and decreased reliance on medications. Pain reduction is a secondary goal and, although it can never be guaranteed, it is often a welcome consequence of a successful rehabilitation program.

The major components of a physical rehabilitation program include stretching, strengthening, and exercise. A number of physical modalities are often included in a physical therapy program. These may be helpful for patients with acute injuries and can be helpful in initiating a physical therapy program in a chronically debilitated patient, but they are of minor long-term benefit. Emphasis should be on activities and exercises that promote return to normal cardiovascular, muscle, joint, and neurologic function. Another benefit of physical therapy is training in the use of assistive devices and adaptive techniques.

INTRODUCTION

Patients with chronic pain experience loss of function that is out of proportion to the extent of injury or pain they initially experienced. Reduction in normal physical activity causes reduced exercise tolerance, muscle shortening, weakness, and eventually fibrosis, joint dysfunction, and adhesions. Loss of normal patterns of neuronal afferent input can lead to functional changes in the central nervous system, such as sensitization of dorsal horn pain projection neurons, reduction in tonic descending inhibitory pathways, or activation of descending facilitation. Weight gain associated with reduced activity, emotional stress, and certain medications can greatly increase the level of disability. The deconditioning associated with pain-induced reduction in activity is often of greater consequence than the original painful condition.

PHYSICAL EXERCISE

Endurance or aerobic exercise is an essential part of the rehabilitation program. In addition to the obvious cardiovascular benefits, regular exercise will improve blood flow to skeletal muscle, activate endogenous pain suppression mechanisms, and may lead to improvements in sleep patterns and mood. Commonly used endurance exercises include walking, jogging, swimming, cycling, and stair walking. Improvement in the ability to perform these exercises will invariably improve the patient's ability to perform activities of daily living.

The eventual goal in an aerobic exercise program is to raise the heart rate to at least 70% of the individual's maximum heart rate for 20 to 30 minutes. A rough guide is: maximum heart rate = 220 minus age in years, or it can be determined more precisely using a maximal exercise treadmill test. Older patients and those with cardiac risk factors or a history of cardiovascular disease should undergo a thorough medical evaluation and receive clearance from their physician before initiating an exercise program. Patients with stable cardiovascular disease should initially aim for 50% to 60% of their maximum heart rate for 15 minutes. These patients should be monitored carefully for hypotension, chest pain, diaphoresis, or pallor during exercise. Careful monitoring and adjustment of exercise level is needed for patients with respiratory disease or peripheral vascular disease and vascular claudication.

For patients with concurrent medical illness or with far advanced disability and deconditioning, the aerobic-exercise program should be further modified. For some patients, this aspect of therapy will depend on progress in stretching and strengthening programs. However, every effort should be made to at least start this aspect of therapy. For the patient whose activity is restricted to transfers from bed to couch, dinner table or bathroom, 5 minutes of slow walking up and down the apartment hallway 3 times a day is an important first step.

STRETCHING

Stretching exercises are essential when there has been muscle shortening or contracture of tendons or joint capsules. A wide range of painful disorders are associated with muscle, ligamentous, or joint contracture, including lower back pain with hamstring and hip flexion contractures, adhesive capsulitis of the shoulder, degenerative arthritis of the knee with flexion contractures, and complex regional pain syndrome with muscle dystonias and joint contractures, to name a very few. Stretching exercises restore normal length to contracted muscles and return restricted joints to normal and often painless range of motion. Normal range of motion and muscle length should be restored before muscle-strengthening programs are started.

Passive sustained stretching involves stabilizing the bone proximal to the affected joint and slowly applying tension on the bone distal to the joint. Stretching is continued to the maximum position attainable and held for 30 seconds or more. Subsequent applications produce an increasing range of motion until the normal extent is obtained. The patient may be asked to vigorously contract then relax the muscle group to be stretched, reducing reflex muscle contraction during stretching. Sustained stretch is most effective when performed daily. Many stretching procedures can be done by the patient after adequate instruction. Once normal range of motion is achieved, active-assisted and active range of motion exercises may be added or substituted. These exercises begin to provide strength to muscles that have atrophied through disuse.

In certain conditions, such as complex regional pain syndrome (CRPS), vigorous passive range-of-motion exer-

cise can aggravate or retrigger pain and autonomic disturbances. For these patients, active or active-assisted stretching exercises, continued to an end point of relatively mild pain, may produce slow but uninterrupted improvement.

STRENGTHENING

Strength training is designed to restore muscle endurance and balance to joints and the spine. Resistive exercises, which utilize static or dynamic muscle contraction against an outside force, are used to restore muscle strength.

ISOMETRIC EXERCISE

Isometric exercise involves contraction of a muscle group against an immovable object. It involves no appreciable change in muscle length or joint movement and is useful when movement of the effective joint is painful or contraindicated. It is useful for improving or preserving muscle strength in the early postsurgical period or when there is acute, severe joint injury or inflammation. It is not very effective in restoring functional activity. It can be hazardous for patients with severe hypertension or cardiovascular disease.

ISOTONIC EXERCISE

Isotonic exercise consists of movement of a fixed, or in some cases, variable load through the entire range of motion of the joint. It can be done with free weights (e.g., barbells, dumbbells), or with variable resistance equipment, such as the Nautilus system. Progressive resistive exercise consists of a series of repetitions against

---

Box 4-1   Therapy for Complex Regional Pain Syndrome

1. Active and active-assisted stretch of affected joints
2. Strengthening of affected and disused muscles, including secondary myofascial syndrome
3. Desensitization techniques: thermal (contrast baths), mechanical
4. Initiation of endurance (aerobic) exercise training, utilizing exercise that does not aggravate extremity pain (e.g., walking, swimming)
5. Assistive devices such as splints, edema control gloves and stockings, cane, walker, crutches
6. Modalities (e.g., TENS, ultrasound)
7. Training for use of one hand or one leg for activities of daily living or vocational activities

25%, 50%, 75%, and 100% of maximum capacity. An alternative system involves the use of large elastic bands (e.g., Theraband System) that provide resistance to motion. The system offers bands with a range of resistances that are coded by color. This system is inexpensive and, following appropriate instruction, can be used regularly at home or in the workplace. The goal of isotonic exercise is to increase muscle strength and endurance. The benefits include increased circulation, improved range of motion, diminished joint stiffness, and reduced pain.

ISOKINETIC EXERCISE

Isokinetic exercise is a dynamic form of strength training using a device that controls the velocity of muscle shortening. It can provide effective strength training with less risk of injury and discomfort. It also has the advantage of identifying the extent of injury and determining when more vigorous activity is acceptable. It is often used in the early stages of rehabilitation of the chronic pain patient.

OTHER TECHNIQUES

Desensitization

Patients with CRPS and neuropathic pain who have significant problems with allodynia may benefit from tactile and cold temperature desensitization techniques.

Proprioceptive Neuromuscular Facilitation

These techniques are designed to improve proprioceptive function through the use of specific patterns of movement and other motor learning modalities.

Coordination Training

These techniques utilize repetition of specific motor activities, sensory cues, and practice aimed at increasing speed of response.

Modalities

There are a number of techniques utilized by the therapist to provide pain relief. For the most part these techniques are beneficial primarily for acute painful disorders, but some are helpful in the initial stages of chronic pain rehabilitation to facilitate stretching and strengthening programs.

Ultrasound

Ultrasound produces heating of underlying tissues by the use of high-frequency sound waves. Energy is generated at tissue interfaces, such as those between muscle and ligaments or between muscle and bone. For chronic pain patients, it can be helpful in conjunction with sustained stretching exercises, as the increased temperature may facilitate mobilization of fibrosed muscles or contracted joints and tendons. It may also provide temporary pain relief in myofascial syndromes, allowing more effective stretching of affected muscle groups. It should not be used near open epiphyses, near laminectomy sites, or on pacemaker patients.

Therapeutic Cooling

Tissue cooling is beneficial for acute sprain and muscle strain injuries. It may also be helpful for providing temporary analgesia to facilitate stretching exercises in myofascial pain. Ice massage or vapocoolant (fluoromethane) spray are applied to trigger points before initiation of stretching exercises. Both of these modalities can be used in home exercise programs, which greatly increases their benefit.

Transcutaneous Electrical Nerve Stimulation

Transcutaneous electrical nerve stimulation (TENS) can provide temporary analgesia for a variety of chronic pain disorders. Some patients experience up to several hours of reduced pain after each application and use it as a primary treatment for pain. Many patients experience pain reduction only during TENS application. For these patients, the device can be helpful for facilitating stretching or strengthening exercises. Reduction of pain during the therapy session can increase painless range of motion and accelerate progress.

Traction

Traction is occasionally helpful in certain painful cervical and lumbar spine disorders. It is mainly beneficial at reducing associated muscle spasm. The force used is inadequate to physically distract components of the spine.

CONCLUSION

Specific therapy choices are generally tailored to each patient and depend greatly on the physical examination findings. It is therefore unnecessary and often counterproductive for the referring physician to specify all of the therapeutic interventions when referring the patient to physical therapy. On the other hand, it is helpful for the physician to know which treatment options are beneficial for a given condition in order to ensure that the patient is receiving optimal care. Boxes 4-1 through 4-3 show a few commonly used therapies for several painful disorders.

Box 4-2 Therapy for Axial Low Back Pain

1. Stretching of hamstrings, hip flexors and adductors, lumbar paravertebrals
2. Abdominal strengthening
3. Aerobic exercise (e.g., walking, cycling, swimming)
4. Education: back protection and biomechanics
5. Modalities: TENS, ultrasound; cold therapy if myofascial component
6. Assistive devices: back roll when sitting; rarely use of corset or brace for certain activities

---

Box 4-3 Therapy for Lumbar Radiculopathy

1. Hamstring stretching, general flexibility exercises
2. Abdominal and gluteal strengthening
3. Endurance exercise with lumbar stabilization
4. Modalities: TENS, cold therapy if myofascial component
5. Extension (McKenzie) exercises if extension maneuvers reduce extent of radicular pain
6. Education: back protection and biomechanics
7. Assistive devices: cane if weakness or unsteady gait

Box 4-4 The Physical Therapy Prescription

Referral Diagnosis: Include any appropriate primary or secondary conditions
Examples: Lumbar radiculopathy
            Upper extremity CRPS I
            Myofascial pain involving trapezius, levator scapulae
            Cervical facet arthropathy
            Hip flexor and hamstring contracture
            Abdominal and quadriceps weakness
Precautions: Include conditions that may affect therapy or create an emergency
Examples: Seizure disorder
            Ischemic heart disease
            Neural claudication
            Diabetes
            Spinal fusion
            Osteoporosis
            Spinal cord stimulator

Therapy Goals
Examples: Reduced hip flexion contracture
            Increased quadriceps strength, knee flexibility
            Reduced mechanical and cold allodynia
            Increased aerobic exercise endurance
            Improved balance and coordination
            Reduced hand edema
            Instruction in assistive devices
            (Pain reduction is often a goal, but not a primary one)
Frequency and Duration
May depend on communication with therapist
Examples: Until effective home exercise established
            Strength training: 3 times per week for six weeks
            Stretching: daily for 2 to 3 weeks
            Endurance/aerobic training: 3 times per week for 3 weeks
Date of M.D. follow-up

The physician's physical therapy prescription should provide as much useful information as possible while leaving specific treatment options to the discretion of the therapist. Information needed in the prescription is shown in Box 4-4.

SUGGESTED READING

Bucko CC, Young JL, Cola AJ, et al: Physical therapy options for lumbar spine pain. In Cole AJ, Herring SA (eds): The Low Back Pain Handbook, 2nd ed. Philadelphia, Hanley & Belfus, 2003, pp 151–178.

Linchitz RM, Sorell PJ: Physical methods of pain management. In Raj PP (ed): Practical Management of Pain, 3rd ed. St. Louis, Mosby, 2000, pp 529–544.

Schramm-Bloodworth DM: Physical Therapy in the Pain Clinic Setting. In Abram SE, Haddox JD (eds): The Pain Clinic Manual, 2nd ed. Philadelphia, Lippincott Williams & Wilkins, 2000, pp 85–101.

Van Tulder MW, Koes BW, Bouter LM: Conservative treatment of acute and chronic nonspecific low back pain. Spine 22:2128–2156, 1997.

Willick SE, Herring SA, Press JM: Basic concepts in biomechanics and musculoskeletal rehabilitation. In Loeser JD (ed): Bonica's Management of Pain. Philadelphia, Lippincott Williams & Wilkins, 2001, pp 1815–1831.

CHAPTER 5

The Clinical Evaluation of the Patient with Chronic Pain

ROBERT E. KETTLER

INTRODUCTION

There are a number of descriptions of the components of a history and physical examination and how to elicit them.[1,2,3] The practitioner who needs to refresh the skills of a general clinical evaluation may consult those resources, or spend time with an experienced clinician. The Current Procedural Terminology (CPT) manual published by the American Medical Association (AMA) is a useful reference for the components of the history and physical examination that comprise the various levels of service.[4] This chapter will focus on matters of specific import to the evaluation of the chronic-pain patient.

AN EVIDENCE-BASED APPROACH TO CLINICAL EVALUATION

The clinician should strive to use techniques of clinical evaluation that have been shown to provide useful information. Unfortunately, many components of the history and physical examination have not undergone rigorous evaluation. The clinician should remain up-to-date with the relevant literature. Using a systematic approach to the literature can facilitate this. Asking an answerable question is the appropriate way to approach gaps in the clinician's knowledge base. The PICO technique serves as a template for the question. The P represents the Patient, Population, or Problem; the I stands for the Intervention; the C represents the Comparison or Control group; and finally, the O represents the Outcome. For example, an answerable question could be phrased as follows: What percentage of patients with lancinating symptoms improve when treated with gabapentin compared to those with burning pain but no lancinating symptoms when the pain severity is measured with a visual analog scale (VAS)?[5]

PATIENT HISTORY

Chief Complaint

The chief complaint is almost invariably the painful condition that brought the patient to the clinic in the first place. However, many patients have multiple sites of pain and often multiple painful conditions, and it may be helpful to ask the patient to address the problem that is most distressing, or the one that brought him or her to your clinic.

History of Present Illness

The necessary components of the history of present illness (HPI) can be remembered by the mnemonic

OPQRST. The O stands for Onset: the circumstances related to the beginning of the patient's pain problem. The P represents Provocative factors (those factors which exacerbate the pain) and Palliative factors (those factors which alleviate the pain). The Q prompts the clinician to ask about the Quality of the pain. It is helpful to direct the patient to describe the pain in one word: aching, burning, pounding, tearing, throbbing, etc. The anatomic distribution of the pain is represented by R (Region). The Severity (S) of the pain can be assessed by a number of techniques that will be discussed in more detail below. The T represents the Temporal factors: time of day, duration, etc. The associated symptoms (e.g., numbness, sweating) complete the HPI.

Patients often have difficulty describing the attributes of pain, so it is incumbent on the clinician to strive for clarity and quantification. The clinician can ask the patient to rate the pain on a scale of 0 to 10 or complete a VAS to quantify the severity of the pain. Another way to assess the pain's severity is to query the patient about activity changes, sleep disruption, ability to relate agreeably with family, etc. In each case the clinician should try to elicit answers that are as specific as possible.

When the patient is vague about the chronology of the pain, a technique to achieve clarity is to draw a timeline and note points that are known with certainty. The patient may be able to be more definite if provided with a reference such as this.

Bracketing may also be useful in determining the chronology of the problem or quantifying aspects of the history. In bracketing, the clinician suggests extreme boundaries for the attribute and asks the patient if the attribute falls within these boundaries. For example, if the patient says he's been in pain for years, the clinician could ask if the patient was in pain 20 years ago. If the answer is no, the clinician can ask if the pain began one year ago. By progressively narrowing the boundaries, the clinician can obtain an estimate of the duration of the pain.

Current Activity

If not elicited in the HPI it's important to document the patient's current level of activity and how it has changed since the pain problem began. It's also useful to ask the patient what level of activity is desired. This piece of information can provide a baseline to monitor progress.

Current Medications

The clinician should elicit the response of the pain problem to medications, past and current, if not done during the HPI. The list of current medications is an important piece of information about the patient's general health as well as a consideration when performing various interventional procedures.

Social History

The social history[3] provides several important pieces of information. The occupational information can indicate the effect the pain problem has on the patient's life, and the level of job satisfaction may provide prognostic information about the return to work. Asking the patient about daily activities and hobbies can also indicate the effect on the patient's life. Finally, the social history can provide information about the patient's support system. Orient suggests asking the patient about the most difficult problem faced and how it was faced as a way to assess the patient's support network.

The social history is also the component of the history where the risk of substance abuse is assessed. Unfortunately, the epidemiology of substance abuse in general and in chronic pain patients in particular is still nascent. Qualitative risk factors for substance abuse include multiple family problems, social disorganization, and psychopathology (i.e., anxiety, borderline personality disorder, depression, and sociopathy).[6] If substance abuse becomes apparent during the course of therapy, the clinician should assess the likelihood of successful intervention. If the patient sees nothing wrong with the behavior, except for the consequences of getting caught, rehabilitation is unlikely to be successful. On the other hand, if the patient views the behavior itself as wrong or harmful, rehabilitation is more likely to succeed.

Family History

The clinician should review the family history for evidence of inherited disorders and role models of chronic disease behavior.

Review of Systems

The psychiatric review is important to assess the presence of anxiety, borderline personality disorder, depression, and sociopathy.

Goldberg et al[7] have published a useful screening test for anxiety and depression. The clinician asks the patient a series of questions scoring a point for each "Yes" answer.

The screening questions for anxiety are:
1. Have you felt keyed up, on edge?
2. Have you been worrying a lot?
3. Have you been irritable?
4. Have you had any difficulty relaxing?

If the patient provides two or more "yes" answers, the clinician asks the following questions:
5. Have you been sleeping poorly?

6. Have you had headaches or neck aches?
7. Have you had any of the following: trembling, tingling, dizzy spells, sweating, urinary frequency, and diarrhea?
8. Have you been worried about your health?
9. Have you had difficulty falling asleep?

If the patient receives five points, the patient has a 50% chance of suffering from an anxiety disorder. As the score increases from five, the patients risk of anxiety increases.

The screening questions for depression are:
1. Have you had low energy?
2. Have you had loss of interests?
3. Have you lost confidence in yourself?
4. Have you felt hopeless?

If the patient provides one or more "yes" answers, the clinician should ask the following questions:
5. Have you had difficulty concentrating?
6. Have you lost weight due to poor appetite?
7. Have you been waking early?
8. Have you felt slowed up?
9. Have you tended to feel worse in the morning?

If the patient scores two, there is a 50% probability of a depressive disorder. Again the risk of the disorder increases as the score increases above the 50% threshold.

Patients with borderline personality disorder tend to have a history of unstable mood and behavior and frequently demonstrate sudden, intense, and inappropriate anger. They frequently seek care by voicing vague complaints and seem to suffer frequent crises, but they have a propensity to fail to comply with recommended therapy.[8]

Sociopathic individuals have no regard for others and act in exploitative, irresponsible ways without remorse.[8]

Laboratory Data

It is important to review pertinent laboratory information from referring physicians and facilities. Laboratory findings pertinent to painful disorders such as rheumatoid arthritis, lupus, diabetes, and HIV are essential to providing ongoing care. Neurodiagnostic tests such as electromyogram, nerve conduction studies, and tests of autonomic function should be obtained. Any radiologic imaging studies pertinent to the patient's painful condition should be reviewed. Patients should be encouraged to bring the actual films as well as dictated reports. A template for a pain-directed history is shown in Box 5-1.

PHYSICAL EXAMINATION

The physical examination serves several important functions:
1. A guide for obtaining special studies.

2. An aid to interpreting the results of special studies.
3. Facilitating the development of the physician-patient relationship.

The components of the physical examination of the chronic pain patient are the same as for all physical examinations: inspection, palpation, percussion, and auscultation. These skills require some adaptation to the chronic pain patient; those adaptations will be discussed here. The specific physical examination for a specific pain problem will be presented in the relevant chapters.

Inspection may be the most difficult of the skills to learn. DeGowin[1] states that an experienced clinician observes a prominent finding, forms an immediate diagnostic hypothesis, and begins a search for confirming or refuting evidence of that hypothesis. This process makes inspection perhaps the most productive part of the examination. Unfortunately, it is often not done in a systematic fashion, so it isn't learned easily or well. The clinician should practice and develop the power of observation on a regular basis to make use of this important part of the physical examination, particularly during the inspection of the patient's general appearance. A systematic approach to the patient's general appearance is covered below.

The skill of palpation can be improved by noting the parts of the hand most suited to each type of information that can be obtained. The fingertips are best at tactile discrimination. The back of the hand and fingers is most sensitive to temperature. The palmar surface of the metacarpophalangeal joints is most sensitive to vibratory stimuli. Finally, the grasping fingers can most readily assess position and consistency. The information obtained by palpation includes temperature, texture, moisture, crepitus, and tenderness. Palpation allows determination of the size, shape, location, consistency, tenderness, surface contour, mobility, and pulsatility of masses. Because palpation may exacerbate the patient's pain, the clinician should begin confidently with light palpation while assuring the patient that the information is necessary and gently but deliberately proceed to deep palpation. The clinician performs light palpation by placing the entire palmar surface of the palpating hand on the patient and gently probing with the approximated fingertips. As the patient adjusts to this maneuver, the clinician probes more deeply and may use the nonpalpating hand to reinforce the probing hand. Patients who are ticklish or otherwise uncomfortable with palpation may be more tolerant of the maneuver if one of the patient's hands is placed on the clinician's palpating hand.

Those components of the physical examination that have pertinence to the chronic pain patient are the general appearance and the integument, the musculoskeletal, and the neurological systems.

Box 5-1   Template for Pain-Directed History

CHIEF COMPLAINT:

HISTORY OF PRESENT ILLNESS:

Description of present pain (location, radiation, quality, intensity):
Associated symptoms (numbness, weakness, autonomic dysfunction, GI or GU dysfunction):
What relieves pain (e.g., activity, rest, position)?
When did pain start?
How did pain start (e.g., at work, in an auto accident, suddenly, as a gradual onset)?
How has the pain changed since its onset (e.g., increased, decreased, changed location)?
Previous and current medication for pain (include % relief, duration of effect, adverse effects):
Taking currently:
Not taking currently:
Other interventions (e.g., injections, TENS, PT, surgery; include dates, extent and duration of relief):

SOCIAL, VOCATIONAL HISTORY:

Married of single, other person in household:
Daily activity; what activity prevented by pain?
Employment history (e.g., current and prior employment, unemployed because of pain?, income source):
Level of education:
Use of alcohol, tobacco, street drugs:

PAST MEDICAL HISTORY:

Allergies:
Medications (not already listed; include reason for use, OTCs):
Other medical problems:

REVIEW OF SYSTEMS:

CNS:
Cardiovascular:
Respiratory:
GI:
GU:
Endocrine:

FAMILY HISTORY:

LABORATORY EVALUATION (GIVE DATES, RESULTS):

Relevant blood, urine tests:
Neurodiagnostic studies (e.g., EMG, nerve conduction studies, autonomic function studies):
Imaging studies (e.g., radiographs, bone scans, CT, MRI):

GI, gastrointestinal; GU, genitourinary; TENS, transcutaneous electrical nerve stimulation; PT, physical therapy; CNS, central nervous system; OTC, over-the-counter medicine; EMG, electromyogram.

General Appearance

Orient[3] states that the general appearance portion of the physical examination should provide " . . . sufficient succinct material to permit a stranger, should he walk on the wards, to identify the patient you are describing immediately." While the frequently used "WN, WD, WM in NAD" is succinct, it otherwise falls short of Orient's ideal. The general appearance should be a documentation of the patient's motor activity, behavior, body habitus, nutritional status, salient abnormalities (which are described in more detail in the per-

tinent section of the physical examination), and speech. The clinician should also note whether the patient appears well or ill.

The general appearance is also an appropriate section for noting whether the patient's demeanor is appropriate to the presenting complaint, if the general behavior is consistent with behavior during the examination, and the patient's interaction with any companions, if present. Some clinicians recommend inspecting the patient's shoes to see if the wear and tear is consistent with any apparent gait abnormalities noted.

Integumentary System

The clinician should describe cutaneous lesions by the following attributes:

1. Anatomic distribution of lesions.
2. Configuration of groups of lesions.
   a. Annular, aciniform, or polycyclic (circular, arc-like, or a combination)
   b. Serpiginous
   c. Iris (bull's eye)
   d. Irregular
   e. Zosteriform
   f. Linear
   g. Retiform (network-like)
3. Morphology of individual lesions.

Musculoskeletal System

The pertinent joints should be compared to the contralateral joint, and the following observations should be noted:

1. Erythema
2. Swelling
3. Temperature
4. Deformity
5. Crepitus
6. Active and passive range of motion

NEUROLOGIC EXAMINATION

The report of the neurologic examination may be recorded in any systematic way, but the following is the method used in DeGowin[1]:

1. Cranial nerves.
2. Motor function.
   a. Mass/bulk
   b. Tone
   c. Strength
   d. Abnormal movement
3. Reflexes.
4. Spinal automatisms: these are not relevant to most chronic pain problems, but may be important in patients with spinal cord injuries.
5. Associated movements (e.g., normal swinging of the arms while walking, the protective position of the arm in reflex sympathetic dystrophy).
6. Meninges: Kernig's and Brudzinski's signs.
7. Coordination.
8. Gait.
9. Sensation.
10. Autonomic nervous system.
    a. Vasodilatation
    b. Sweat
    c. Temperature
    d. Capillary perfusion
11. Mental status examination.

A template for a pain-directed physical examination is shown in Box 5-2. If there are concerns about the patient's mental status because of clinical behavior or the report of family or friends, the clinician should perform a mental status examination to screen for the need for more sophisticated evaluation. A useful examination is administered and scored as follows[3]:

1. Ask the patient for the year, month, date, and day: one point for each correct answer.
2. Ask the patient for the state, county, town, and clinical facility: one point for each correct answer.
3. Ask the patient to remember three objects. Score one point for each correctly recalled immediately. Then go over the objects until the patient can repeat them. Go on to other parts of the exam. After several minutes ask the patient to repeat the objects. Score one point for each correct answer.
4. Ask the patient to perform serial 7s (count backward by sevens). Score one point for each of the first five numbers that are correct.
5. Spell "earth" backwards. Five points.
6. Ask patient to name two objects. One point for each correct answer.
7. Ask the patient to repeat the sentence, "No ifs, ands, or buts." One point.
8. Ask the patient to perform a three-step task. One point for each successfully completed step.

A normal score is at least 20 out of 30 possible points. Many practitioners are reluctant to perform this examination out of fear of embarrassing or irritating the patient. Orient recommends telling the patient that some questions will be asked, some of which can be answered, some of which may not answerable; the results will provide important information.

COMPLIANCE

While assessing compliance may not be a part of the initial evaluation, the clinician may need to assess it during follow-up visits. The assessment of compliance is a multistep process beginning with the initiation of therapy[9]; other steps include:

1. Patient education and assessment of understanding.
   a. The medication or other therapeutic modality.
   b. The purpose of the intervention.
   c. Dosing.
   d. The duration of therapy.
2. Physician steps to enhance compliance.
   a. Provide few medications or other interventions at one time.

Box 5-2 Template for Pain-Directed Physical Examination

General Appearance:
Gait:
Range of Motion:
Tenderness (e.g., muscle, bone, tendon, scar):
Provocative Test (e.g., Tinel's SLR, Spurling's):
Sensory Exam (i.e., anesthesia or hypoesthesia, allodynia, hyperalgesia):
Motor Exam (e.g., muscle bulk, symmetry, strength, spasm, abnormal movement, reflexes):
Vascular Exam (e.g., skin temperature, color, sweating; edema; pulses; venodilation; ulcers, stasis)
Other Findings:
    Head and Neck:
    Chest:
    Abdomen, Pelvis:
    Back:
    Extremities:

SLR, Straight leg raising.

    b. Use few doses, not more doses.
    c. Use least expensive interventions as possible.
    d. Use interventions likely to be effective.
3. Follow-up evaluation.
    a. Have patient bring **all** medications to appointments evaluate for omissions and redundancies.
    b. Use pill containers to make discussion more concrete.
        1. Ask patient about dosing schedule.
        2. Ask patient about problems.
        3. Perform pill count.
    c. Determine reason for noncompliance and proceed accordingly.
        1. Misunderstanding.
        2. Forgetfulness (perform mental status examination).
        3. Adverse effect.
        4. Cost.
        5. Other.

COUNSELING ABOUT LIFESTYLE CHANGES

Many chronic pain patients must make important changes in lifestyle such as exercise habits and substance use. The clinical assessment is a natural take-off point for this discussion.

Chronic pain patients should improve their aerobic capacity, strength, and flexibility. Among the benefits to regular exercise are an improvement in anxiety and depression. Many chronic pain patients may have suffered prior injury during exercise and are reluctant to undertake this activity. The physician should counsel the patient about the importance of gradual increases in duration and intensity.[10]

The clinician may also use the FRAMES mnemonic to guide a discussion of substance use[11]:
1. F: **F**eedback of clinician concern: aberrant behavior, urine drug test incompatible with therapy
2. R: encourage **R**esponsibility on the part of the patient for addressing the problem
3. A: **A**dvise the patient to make the necessary changes
4. M: provide a **M**enu of options
5. E: be **E**mpathic
6. S: encourage the patient to be **S**elf-efficacious

DIFFICULT SITUATIONS[3,12]

Patients who provide vague answers. The clinician can try to use the bracketing technique or persist in asking the same question. If three attempts at asking the question are unsuccessful, the clinician should specifically address the difficulty the patient has in answering the questions.

Patients (or requesting physicians) who just want a procedure without an evaluation. The clinician can explain that another evaluation will provide a fuller picture of the patient's problem and suggest directions that can be taken if the initial therapy is inadequate.

Patients who are evasive or refuse to answer certain questions. The clinician should note the evasion and ask why the patient is reluctant to answer the question. If the patient has legitimate concerns, the clinician can address these. If the patient still refuses to answer, the clinician should ask the patient to outline the goals for care. The clinician should then explain the reason the information is needed to accomplish the goals. If the patient is still evasive, the clinician should evaluate if a therapeutic relationship is possible.

Hostile patient. The clinician should note the hostility and ask about the reasons for it. Depending on the answer, the practitioner should deal with the situation as appropriate.

Demanding patients. The practitioner should explain the reasons for procedures and explore why the patient is so demanding.

Patients who press for a diagnosis when none is forthcoming. The physician should explain to the patient that some diseases elude diagnosis, but the monitoring and evaluation of the patient for serious disease will be ongoing to prevent harm. The physician should then discuss the patient's feeling about the importance of a diagnosis.

COMPLETING THE PATIENT VISIT[9]

1. Before proceeding with the wrap-up the physician should ask the patient, "Is there anything that you want to tell me?"
2. The physician should discuss any special studies, the reason for getting them, and a plan to provide the patient with the results.
3. The physician should discuss any prescriptions or other recommendations.
4. The patient should be apprised of what to do if any problems arise prior to the follow-up appointment.
5. The physician should provide written documentation of the physician's name and contact information.
6. The physician should offer to answer any questions the patient has.

CONCLUSION

Patients who suffer from chronic pain can provide the clinician with many challenges during the entire clinical encounter. The preceding suggestions will help smooth the course of clinical assessment of the patient with chronic pain

REFERENCES

1. DeGowin RL: DeGowin and DeGowin's Bedside Diagnostic Examination, 5th ed. New York, Macmillan Publishing Co., 1987.

2. Loeser JD: Medical evaluation of the patient with pain. In Loeser JD, Butler SH, Chapman CR, Turk DC (eds): Bonica's Management of Pain, 3rd ed. Philadelphia, Lippincott Williams & Wilkins, 2001, pp 267-278.

3. Orient JM: Sapira's Art and Science of Bedside Diagnosis, 2nd ed. Philadelphia, Lippincott Williams & Wilkins, 2001.

4. American Medical Association. Current procedural terminology, 2004. Chicago, AMA Press, 2004.

5. McKibbon A, Hunt D, Richardson WS: Finding the evidence. In Guyatt G, Rennie D (eds): User's Guide to the Medical Literature: Essentials of Evidence-Based Clinical Practice. Chicago, AMA Press, 2002, pp 21-71.

6. Crum RM: The epidemiology of addictive disorders. In Graham AW, Schultz TK, Mayo-Smith MF, Ries RK, Wilford BB (eds): Principles of Addiction Medicine, 3rd ed. Chevy Chase, American Society of Addiction Medicine, Inc., 2003, pp 17-31.

7. Goldberg D, Bridges K, Duncan-Jones P, et al: Detecting anxiety and depression in general medical settings. BMJ 297:897-899, 1988.

8. Personality Disorders. The Merck Manual [monograph on the Internet]. Whitehouse Station, NJ, Merck and Company. Available from: http://www.merck.com/mrkshared/mmanual/section15/chapter191/191a.jsp. Accessed July 11, 2004.

9. Fletcher SW: Clinical decision-making: approach to the patient. In Goldman L, Bennett JC (eds): Cecil Textbook of Medicine, 21st ed. Philadelphia, W.B. Saunders Co., 2000. pp 77-79.

10. Pratt M: Physical activity. In Goldman L, Bennett JC (eds): Cecil Textbook of Medicine, 21st ed. Philadelphia, W.B. Saunders Co., 2000, pp 31-33.

11. Samet J: Drug abuse and dependence. In Goldman L, Bennett JC (eds): Cecil Textbook of Medicine, 21st ed. Philadelphia, W.B. Saunders Co., 2000, pp 54-59.

12. Block P: Flawless Consulting: A Guide to Getting Your Expertise Used, 2nd ed. San Francisco, Jossey-Bass/Pfeiffer, 2000.

CHAPTER 6

Drugs in Chronic Pain Management

HARIHARAN SHANKAR

INTRODUCTION

Research in pain has been extensive, and with our increasing knowledge, new therapeutic strategies are continually being developed. Pharmacological management of pain continues to be an evolving field with the introduction of newer drugs. However, attempts to treat chronic pain by targeting the symptom and anatomical site of origin have not always been successful. This chapter will discuss the common drugs used in chronic pain management.

ACETAMINOPHEN

Basic Science

Being an aniline derivative, acetaminophen, or N-acetyl-p-aminophenol (APAP), has the potential to cause methemoglobinemia but is the least toxic among the anilines. APAP is highly lipid soluble and poorly protein bound (10% to 25%). It crosses the blood-brain barrier. Based on animal studies, the following central and peripheral mechanisms of actions have been proposed:

1. A central action through the noradrenergic/serotoninergic systems.
2. Direct and indirect effects on the opioidergic systems by modulating dynorphin release and κ-receptor function.
3. Via a direct action Cyclooxygenase (COX)-2 may inhibit spinal PGE_2 release.
4. Through free radical uptake scavenging, thereby decreasing COX-1 activity.
5. Spinally, it may inhibit nitric oxide (NO) generation impairing N-methyl-D-aspartate (NMDA) release or NK-1 activation.

Clinical Science

APAP is an antipyretic and analgesic with weak anti-inflammatory action. APAP reaches peak plasma concentration in 30 to 60 minutes with a plasma half-life of approximately 2 hours. Rectal bioavailability is roughly half the oral dose. Its primary metabolic pathway is via conjugation with glucuronic acid and oxidation via cytochrome P-450 CYP2E1 isoenzyme. It crosses the placenta but is safe for use in pregnancy. Two percent of the maternal dose is excreted in breast milk. The recommended oral dose is 325 to 650 mg every 4 hours, with a maximum of 4 gm in 24 hours.

APAP has been proven effective in arthritis pain, headache, postsurgical pain, dysmenorrhea, muscle aches, cancer pain, and sore-throat pain. It is first-line therapy in osteo-arthritis pain.

Adverse effects include anemia, hemolysis, methemoglobinemia, syndrome of inappropriate secretion of antidiuretic hormone (SIADH), gastric bleeding, impaired liver function, liver failure, asthma, and rash. IgE mediated anaphylactic type reactions to APAP has also been reported. Habitual appropriate use of APAP alone does not cause renal toxicity. Major APAP toxicity is on the liver, producing acute centrilobular necrosis. This is a complex and multi-factorial reaction. Oxidative stress seems to play a key role. Severity of liver damage is reduced by pretreatment with calcium antagonists. Protection against hepatic injury is also offered by clofibrate, chlorpromazine, 4-amino benzamide, stiripentol, gadolinium chloride, and dextran sulfate. Features of toxicity include nausea and vomiting in a few hours, abdominal pain, tenderness (16 to 72 hours), oliguria, renal failure, back pain (24 to 48 hours), and fulminant hepatic failure (3 to 6 days).

NONSTEROIDAL ANTI-INFLAMMATORY DRUGS

Basic Science

The chemical classes of different nonsteroidal anti-inflammatory drugs (NSAIDs) are listed in Box 6-1. The primary mechanism of nociception for all NSAIDS is inhibition of production of the prostaglandin E series. They also inhibit formation of prostacyclin and thromboxane, which accounts for some of their adverse effects.

COX inhibition by NSAIDs reduces the conversion of arachidonic acid to prostaglandin G_2. Acetylsalicylic acid (ASA) acetylates the COX enzyme, whereas the other NSAIDs are reversible inhibitors. Salicylates are classified into acetylated and nonacetylated groups, with nonacetylated salicylates being less potent and causing less gastrointestinal (GI) mucosal injury.

The COX-1 isoenzyme is present in many cell types and is expressed constitutively. Products of the COX-1 isoenzyme play an important role in maintaining the integrity of the gastric mucosa. While prostaglandins and prostacyclins are important for maintaining intrarenal blood flow, COX-2 specific inhibitors as well as NSAIDs can cause renal damage. COX-2 is inducible at times of stress. Analgesic and anti-inflammatory effects of NSAIDs are believed to be due to mainly to COX-2 inhibition. By

Box 6-1 Common Nonsteroidal Analgesics

Class	Generic	Brand Name
Salicylates	Acetylsalicylic acid	Aspirin
	Salsalate	Disalcid
	Choline magnesium trisalicylate	Trilisate
Propionic acid	Naproxen	Naprosyn, Anaprox
	Ibuprofen	Motrin, Advil
	Ketoprofen	Orudis, Oruvail
	Flurbiprofen	Ansaid
	Oxaprozin	Daypro
Indoleacetic acid	Indomethacin	Indocin
	Etodolac	Lodine
	Sulindac	Clinoril
Phenylacetic acid	Diclofenac	Voltaren, Cataflam
Pyrrole acetic acid	Tolmetin	Tolectin
	Ketorolac	Toradol
Anthranilic acid	Mefenamic acid	Ponstel
Pyrazolone	Phenylbutazone	Butazolidin
Naphthylalkanone	Nabumetone	Relafen
Oxicam	Piroxicam	Feldene

inhibiting prostaglandin synthesis, NSAIDs normalize cell-cycle responses including apoptosis (programmed cell death). Various animal models have shown the involvement of central nervous system COX-2 and prostanoids in inflammatory pain hypersensitivity in arthritis models.

NSAIDs are lipophilic and interrupt signal transduction. They reduce recruitment of phagocytic cells and production of free oxygen radicals, inhibit phospholipase C activity in macrophages, inhibit rheumatoid factor production, and block NO synthase.

Clinical Science

Relevant pharmacological properties of commonly used NSAIDs are shown in Box 6-2. Most NSAIDs are completely absorbed after oral administration. Greater than 95% of the absorbed dose is protein bound. Metabolism is predominantly by the CYP2C9 isoform of the cytochrome P450 system and excreted in the urine, thus requiring dose adjustments in patients with renal or hepatic disease. Some NSAIDs (e.g., indomethacin, sulindac, and piroxicam) with prominent enterohepatic circulation should be used with caution in the geriatric population. Indomethacin crosses the blood-brain barrier at a high rate, making it ideal for chronic paroxysmal hemicrania but also predisposing to central nervous system (CNS) side effects. The serum half-life ranges from 1.1 ± 0.2 hours for Diclofenac to 57 ± 22 hours for piroxicam. Sulindac and Nabumetone are unique in that they are prodrugs releasing active metabolites after first pass metabolism in the liver.

Although at equipotent doses, the clinical efficacy and tolerability of the approximately 20 different NSAIDs available in the United States are similar, individual responses vary. NSAIDs have differing potency of analgesic, anti-inflammatory, and anti pyretic properties. NSAIDs are indicated in myalgias, headache, joint pain, mild to moderate pain of any etiology including osteoarthritis, rheumatoid arthritis, ankylosing spondylitis, cancer pain, and metastatic bone pain. COX-2 specific inhibitors are indicated in dysmenorrhea, osteoarthritis, rheumatoid arthritis, and other inflammatory pain conditions. Ketorolac, the only injectable NSAID currently available, has been found effective in reducing peri-operative opioid consumption. Its use should be limited to 5 days due to its potential for renal toxicity at recommended perioperative doses.

The following adverse effects of NSAIDs and COX-2s have been reported:

1. Increased risk of myocardial events and stroke with rofecoxib prompted its withdrawal from the market. It has yet to be seen whether it is likely to be a side effect of COX-2 selectivity. For the present, it is prudent to encourage low-dose aspirin therapy with selective COX-2 inhibitors.

2. Elevation of hepatic transaminase levels. Significance is attached to levels 2 to 3 times the upper limit, decreased serum albumin, or elevated prothrombin times. When initiating NSAID treatment and at 8-12 weeks, all patients should have biochemical evaluation.

3. Patients with history of allergic rhinitis, nasal polyposis, or asthma are at risk for anaphylaxis.

4. Decreased platelet aggregation. Nonaspirin NSAIDs inhibit COX-1 reversibly, whereas aspirin acetylates COX-1 permanently.

5. Abdominal pain, dyspepsia, nausea and vomiting, esophagitis, stricture, gastritis, erosions, hemorrhage,

Box 6-2 Relevant Pharmacology of NSAIDs

Drug	Peak Concentration	Elimination Half-Life	Dosing Schedule
Etodolac	1–2hrs	6–7hrs	200–400mg/q6-8hrs
Oxaprozin	3–5hrs	50–60hrs	600–1200mg/day
Ketoprofen	0.5–2hrs	1.4–3.3hrs	25–75mg/q6-8hrs
Naproxen	4–6hrs	12–15hrs	275–500mg/q8-12hrs
Tolmetin	20–65min	2.1–6.8hrs	200–600mg/q8hrs
Diclofenac	14–50min	1.1–2hrs	25–75mg/q8-12hrs
Indomethacin	0.5–4hrs	2.2–11.2hrs	25–50mg/q8-12hrs
Ketorolac	40–50min	2.4–9hrs	10mg/q6-8hrs
Nabumetone	3–6hrs	24hrs	1000–2000mg/qDay
Sulindac	2hrs	16–18hrs	150–200mg/q12hrs
Ibuprofen	1.4–1.9hrs	2–2.5hrs	400–800mg/q6-8hrs
Meloxicam	4–5hrs	15–20hrs	7.5–15mg/qDay
Valdecoxib	3hrs	8–11hrs	10–20mg/q12-24hrs
Rofecoxib	2–3hrs	17hrs	12.5–50mg/qDay
Celecoxib	3hrs	11hrs	100–400mg/q12hrs

and peptic ulceration have all been reported. Overall risk of NSAID-induced gastric ulcer development is 2% to 4% per year. Nonacetylated salicylates are safer.

6. Renal effects include retention of sodium, tubular dysfunction, interstitial nephritis, and reversible renal failure.

7. Nonspecific skin rash, photosensitivity, reversible toxic amblyopia, tinnitus, aseptic meningitis, and psychosis are other adverse events.

8. Chronic rofecoxib administration is associated with an increased incidence of adverse cardiac events. It is not known whether this is a drug class effect or whether it is specific to that drug.

Future Possibilities:

1. Nitro aspirins are an amalgam of NO and aspirin, with the advantage of less gastrointestinal and hemorrhagic side effects. NO has cytoprotective properties due to its ability to increase local blood flow and as a free radical scavenger. S-nitroso-diclofenac is a prodrug, which also releases NO and has gastric-protective effects.

2. Parecoxib is a water-soluble prodrug of valdecoxib formulated for parenteral administration. It may be useful in the perioperative setting. Etoricoxib is a long-lasting COX-2 selective inhibitor with a selectivity ration of 106 (COX-1: COX-2). Lumiracoxib is a highly selective COX-2 inhibitor, being 300-fold less potent against COX-1. Its elimination half-life is 3 to 6 hours and achieves peak concentration in 2 hours.

OPIOIDS

Opioids are among the oldest known pharmaceutical agents and have been extensively researched. Opioid receptors belong to three major families: μ, δ, and κ as well as the nociception and orphanin FQ (N/OFQ) receptor. Opioid receptors are dynamic, responding to agonist/antagonist interaction by internalization promoted by β-arrestin. Receptors and ligands are found in laminae I & II, in the spinal cord, spinal trigeminal nucleus, and periaqueductal gray. Other opioid receptor rich areas include amygdala, thalamus, cortex, and locus caeruleus (modulation of affective behavior) globus pallidus, caudate, putamen, (motor control), medulla, and median eminence.

N/OFQ is poorly understood and is selectively activated by endogenous nociceptin. It has been implicated in suppression of pain, but it also may increase substance-P release and mediate hyperalgesia. N/OFQ receptors are found in high concentration in hippocampus and cortex with suggested involvement in drug reward, reinforcement, learning, and memory.

Opiate receptors for the most part are G-protein receptor coupled. Receptor activation produces activation of receptor-operated K^+ currents, suppression of voltage-gated Ca^{++} currents and inhibition of adenyl cyclase. K^+ channel activation leads to hyperpolarization and decreased excitability, while Ca^{++} current suppression is thought to be the mechanism for suppression of excitatory neurotransmitters.

Paradoxically, exogenous opioids are capable of producing hyperalgesia through a CNS sensitizing effect. Persistent activation of the receptor produces activation of protein kinase C (PKC). This is evident in animal experiments within seven days. PKC uncouples the G-protein from the potassium channel, reducing the analgesic effect (tolerance), phosphorylates the NMDA receptor, enhances Ca^{++} influx in response to glutamate release, and produces sensitization of second-order neurons. It is not clear how often this occurs clinically, but there is ample evidence that opioids can produce hyperalgesia in humans, particularly in patients on very high opioid doses. For instance, marked reduction in pain thresholds are seen among patients in methadone maintenance programs.

Another mechanism of opioid-induced hyperalgesia involves glial cell activation. Activation of microglia and astrocytes occurs in response to opioid administration in rats, even in the absence of inflammation or nerve injury. The response is exaggerated in nerve-injured animals. Glial activation leads to the increased production and release of proinflammatory cytokines, NO, and reactive oxygen species followed by sensitization of neurons in the spinal cord and dorsal root ganglia.

Intrinsic Activity of Opioids

Drug efficacy is related to the number of receptors that need to be occupied in order to produce a given effect. Opioids with high intrinsic activity produce substantial analgesia with low receptor occupancy. A highly efficacious drug may produce a given analgesic effect with a 20% receptor occupancy while a weak opioid might require 70% occupancy to produce the same effect. As the intensity of the noxious stimulus increases, the drug with high intrinsic activity can provide analgesia with a small increase in dose, while the weaker agent may require a several-fold increase to control the more intense pain. The same holds true for the individual who has become tolerant. With fewer receptors available the drug with high intrinsic activity can provide satisfactory analgesia by occupation of the available receptors, while the drug with low intrinsic activity may not provide significant analgesia at any dose. In general, the more potent drugs, such as fentanyl and sufentanil, tend to be more efficacious than less potent drugs, such as codeine and meperidine. However, this relationship is not uniform. For instance, buprenorphine is more potent than morphine, but has a low intrinsic activity and is, in fact, a partial agonist.

Commonly Used Opioids

Codeine

Codeine is a weak opioid that is mainly used orally, often combined with acetaminophen. It has a relatively low affinity to the μ-opioid receptor. It undergoes O-demethylation to morphine. This reaction is catalyzed by CYP2D6, which is polymorphically expressed. The usual oral dose is 30 to 60 mg.

Hydrocodone

Hydrocodone is a codeine derivative that is somewhat more efficacious than codeine. It is also usually combined with acetaminophen. It has several active metabolites, including dihydromorphine, hydromorphone, and dihydrocodeine, which can accumulate and produce unexpected side effects in patients with renal impairment. The usual oral dose is 5 to 10 mg.

Oxycodone

Oxycodone is slightly more effective than hydrocodone, but has about the same potency (usual dose 5 to 10 mg). It is metabolized to the active metabolite oxymorphone, catalyzed by CYP2D6. Significant variation in the levels of the active enzyme account for large inter-individual variations in effect. The usual oral dose when combined with acetaminophen is 5 to 10 mg. However, as the dose of the uncombined drug is increased, the analgesic effect increases proportionately. Oxycodone is available as a 12-hour sustained release preparation in doses of 10 to 80 mg. The higher doses are not recommended for opioid naïve patients.

Meperidine

Meperidine is a relatively low efficacy opioid with local anesthetic and anticholinergic properties that is available as oral and parenteral preparations. The usual IM dose for acute postoperative pain is 50 to 150 mg. It is about 1/3 as potent orally. It should not be used in high doses for tolerant patients or for prolonged periods at any dose, as it is metabolized to normeperidine, which has a long half-life and produces CNS toxicity, including myoclonus and seizures.

Morphine

Morphine is effective orally and parenterally, with the oral dose requirement about 3 times the IM or IV dose. The usual postoperative IM dose is 5 to 15 mg. It is available in either 12- or 24-hour oral sustained release preparations. It is intermediate in efficacy. A low proportion is metabolized to morphine-6-glucuronide, which has a high affinity for the μ-opioid receptor and is thought to be somewhat more potent than morphine. A higher proportion is metabolized to morphine-3-glucuronide, which has minimal if any analgesic effect but produces CNS irritability and hyperalgesia. Oral administration produces higher proportions of both metabolites because of first-pass hepatic metabolism. When given intrathecally or epidurally, it produces prolonged analgesia (18 to 24 hours following 0.3 to 0.5 mg IT or 3 to 5 mg epidural) because of its high water solubility. There is also considerable risk of delayed respiratory depression after neuraxial administration because of slow migration to the intracranial portions of the cerebrospinal fluid (CSF).

Methadone

Methadone is intermediate in its efficacy. It is available in both oral and parenteral preparations. The IM or

IV dose is roughly equivalent to that of morphine. The oral dose is generally lower than that of oral morphine, as the drug has an extremely long, unpredictable terminal half-life (up to 36 hours) and accumulates with repeated dosing. The usual oral dose in opioid naïve patients is 5 to 10 mg bid. Dosing is reassessed after several days, and dosage increases are made very slowly. The risk of life-threatening respiratory depression is high, especially in elderly or debilitated patients.

In addition to its μ-opioid effect, methadone is a weak, noncompetitive NMDA antagonist. In animal models, NMDA receptor antagonism reduces the rate of opioid tolerance development. It is not clear how important this effect is clinically. The fact that tolerance and hyperalgesia develops almost uniformly in patients on methadone maintenance suggests that it is not an important property.

Hydromorphone

Hydromorphone is about 4 to 5 times more potent than morphine and is somewhat more efficacious. The usual oral dose is 2 to 8 mg and the parenteral dose for postoperative pain is about 1 to 2 mg (5:1 oral-parenteral ratio). It is a highly polar molecule and has a long duration of action (about 12 hours) when given spinally or epidurally. Like morphine, it is partially metabolized to a 3-glucuronide, which can accumulate with chronic administration, producing CNS irritability.

Fentanyl and Sufentanil

Fentanyl is about 80 times as potent as morphine. It has been used for many years as a parenteral perioperative analgesic. It is highly lipid soluble and very short acting. It is extensively metabolized in the liver, utilizing the enzyme CYP3A4. It is available as a transdermal formulation in units that deliver from 25 to 100 μg/hr. Opioid naïve patients should be cautiously started at the lowest dose. Fentanyl is rapidly absorbed from mucous membranes, and a transmucosal preparation is available in doses ranging from 200 to 1600 μg. Fentanyl's high intrinsic activity and versatile dosage forms make it a logical choice for patients who are opioid tolerant or who have poorly controlled pain and intolerable side effects from other agents. Its high lipid solubility limits its efficacy as a neuraxial analgesic. Epidural fentanyl infusions do not appear to provide better analgesia than IV infusions. Intrathecal administration provides only 2 to 4 hours of analgesia compared to many hours with morphine or hydromorphone.

Sufentanil is only available as an injectable drug. It is 5 times as potent as fentanyl. It may have a slightly better intrinsic activity, but its very short duration of action and exclusively injectable form make it a less versatile drug. Occasionally, it is helpful as an IV infusion for cancer patients who have become very opioid tolerant.

Adverse Effects of Opioids

Constipation

This is the most prevalent and often the most troublesome side effect. Unlike other adverse effects of opioids, tolerance to constipating effects of opioids does not develop. Mild cases may respond to stool softeners and adequate hydration. Severe cases require the addition of a stimulant laxative and an osmotic agent such as lactulose.

Nausea and Vomiting

Nausea is often transient, resolving within a few days after initiation of treatment. Severe or persistent cases may respond to rotation to a different agent. Most antiemetics are helpful, including serotonin antagonists (e.g., ondansetron), butyrophenones (e.g., droperidol), and anticholinergics (e.g., scopolamine), and antihistamines (e.g., hydroxyzine). Metoclopramide has also been used successfully.

Sedation

Sedation may occur at minimally effective doses in some patients. If it occurs late in treatment, it may be related to increasing doses or accumulating metabolites. Rotation to a more efficacious drug is sometimes helpful. Dextroamphetamine, methylphenidate, and modafinil may be used in cases in which satisfactory analgesia can not be achieved without some CNS depression. These drugs are most often used in cancer patients who require high opioid doses and are generally not used for chronic pain patients who are on very long-term analgesic therapy.

Respiratory Depression

This is the most concerning adverse effect of opioids and can be fatal, especially in elderly or debilitated patients. It is uncommon in patients who have been on chronic opioid therapy unless the dose is rapidly escalated. Methadone is particularly worrisome, since it may take several days at a given dose to reach steady state tissue and blood levels. Intrathecal or epidural administration of water-soluble drugs such as morphine can produce delayed respiratory depression associated with cephalad drug migration in the CSF.

A2 AGONISTS

Basic Science

The α_2 adrenergic receptor is a single polypeptide chain glycoprotein with the cytoplasmic side coupled to G-protein. There are three subtypes, α_2A, α_2B, and α_2C, located both presynaptically and postsynaptically. Most α_2 receptors in human dorsal horn cell bodies are

α_2A and α_2B subtypes, whereas α_2B and α_2C are predominantly seen in the dorsal root ganglion. Animal studies indicate that the α_2A subtype is involved in anti-hyperalgesia, and the presence of intact sympathetic fibers along with α_2A subtype is required in thermal hyperalgesia. Three major classes of agonists act on these receptors:

1. Phenylethylamines (e.g., a methylnorepinephrine)
2. Imidazolines (e.g., clonidine, tizanidine, dexmedetomidine)
3. Oxaloazepines (e.g., azepexole)

Imidazolines also bind to imidazoline receptors; for example, I_1, and I_2, which contribute indirectly via interactions with cannabinoid receptors or α_2 or both. Activation of α_2 receptors results in inhibition of cyclic AMP formation and opening of K^+ channels.

The possible mechanisms of analgesia by α_2 agonists include:

1. Reduced sympathetic outflow by direct effect on pre-ganglionic outflow at spinal level and by decreasing norepinephrine levels via adrenals.
2. Inhibition of transmitter release from primary afferent neurons probably via effects on pertussis toxin sensitive G-protein.
3. Gi/o subunit activation decreasing transmitter release and C-AMP formation.
4. Stimulation of Gi/o coupled inwardly rectifying potassium channels (GIRK) causing hyperpolarization thereby inhibiting dorsal horn neurons.
5. α_2 adrenoceptor agonists increase acetylcholine concentration in dorsal horn and CSF leading to increased NO synthesis. NO increases norepinephrine release and regulates COX-2 activity.

Clonidine

Clinical Science

Clonidine is a partial agonist with α_2/α_1 affinity ratio of 200-1. It is available as oral, transdermal, epidural, and intrathecal preparations. Clonidine achieves peak plasma concentration in 3 to 5 hours with a half-life of 12 to 16 hours. Peak concentration is achieved in 2 days with the transdermal patch and in 19 minutes with neuraxial administration. The liver contributes to 50% of the drug's metabolism and 40% to 60% of the drug is excreted unchanged in the urine in 24 hours. Hepatic or renal insufficiency does not require any dose adjustments.

It is currently the most widely used among this group. It is used in postop pain, cancer pain, complex regional pain syndrome (CRPS), postherpetic neuralgia, peripheral neuropathy, and chronic headache. It has been used with local anesthetics and opioids in nerve blocks and neuraxial infusions. To avoid a withdrawal syndrome, a gradual decrease is recommended.

The common adverse effects include dry mouth, nausea, sedation, orthostasis, hypotension, bradycardia, dizziness, confusion, and fever. Features of withdrawal syndrome include hypertension, nervousness, tremor, agitation, and headache. Caution should be used in patients with coronary artery disease, recent myocardial infarction, cerebrovascular disease, chronic renal failure, and the elderly because of orthostatic hypotension. Patients on calcium channel blockers, digitalis, or β-blockers may experience AV block or bradycardia, with the use of clonidine responsive to atropine.

Tizanidine

Tizanidine reaches peak plasma concentration in 1 to 5 hours and has an elimination half-life of 4 to 8 hours. It is primarily hepatically metabolized to inactive metabolites and renally excreted. Clearance of tizanidine is decreased by oral contraceptives.

Tizanidine is used in painful conditions with spasticity, myofascial pain, headache syndromes, acute low back pain, and trigeminal neuralgia paroxysm. When combined with NSAIDs, it may have a gastro-protective effect.

The most commonly reported adverse effect is dry mouth. Other adverse effects include somnolence, asthenia, dizziness, hypotension, and bradycardia. Sedation and hypotension are dose related. Hepatic injury is a worrisome effect with about 5% having elevated liver enzymes. Manufacturer recommends aminotransferase level monitoring at baseline and 1, 3, and 6 months.

Dexmedetomidine

This drug reaches peak levels in 6 minutes with an elimination half-life of 2 to 5 hours. Dexmedetomidine is almost completely metabolized by glucuronidation and cytochrome P450 pathway. Dose reduction is necessary with hepatic insufficiency or renal impairment.

Although currently approved only for short-term (<24 hours) sedation in the ICU, it may also be useful in postop pain and as an adjunct to general anesthesia. It provides the most potent antinociception among the current α_2 agonists. It can attenuate responses to laryngoscopy and intubation. It decreases the requirements of thiopental, isoflurane, and fentanyl. Dexmedetomidine has a α_2/α_1 affinity ratio of 1600:1. α_2 selectivity is lost with rapid infusions or high doses.

Common adverse effects include dry mouth, nausea, and hypotension. Adverse effects include significant bradycardia and sinus arrest responsive to anticholinergics. Hence, caution is advised with heart block, severe ventricular dysfunction, hypovolemia, diabetes mellitus, and hypertension. Other adverse effects include hypertension, vomiting, fever, bronchospasm, hypoxia, tachycardia, and anemia. Although sedation is seen with higher doses, respiratory depression is not encountered. Dexmedetomidine also has the potential for abrupt withdrawal syndrome.

GLUTAMATE RECEPTOR ANTAGONISTS

Glutamate is a major excitatory neurotransmitter of the CNS associated with chronic pain and opioid tolerance, dependence, and addiction. It activates NMDA, α-amino-3-hydroxy-5-methyl-4-isoxazole propionate (AMPA), and kainate receptors, causing opening of ion channels or by coupling to intracellular signal transduction systems via G-protein. It plays an important role in central sensitization and "wind-up" leading to allodynia and hyperalgesia. NMDA antagonists reduce spontaneous pain and hyperalgesia, acute postop pain, and chronic neuropathic pain. Physical dependence and tolerance to opioids are reduced in experimental animals by combination with NMDA antagonists.

KETAMINE

Basic Science

NMDA antagonists with affinity at the phencyclidine site include ketamine, which is a noncompetitive receptor antagonist at the open calcium channel pore. It increases peripheral monoaminergic transmission and possibly modulates descending inhibitory pathways, interacts with opioid receptors, inhibits central and peripheral cholinergic transmission, blocks sodium channels at high doses, and possibly has effects on calcium channels. The S-Ketamine is 2 to 3 times more potent. The major limitation is the narrow therapeutic window as they cause memory impairment, sedation, psychotomimetic effects, ataxia, and motor incoordination.

Clinical Science

Ketamine achieves peak serum levels in 5 to 30 minutes after intramuscular and in 30 minutes after oral administration. It has an elimination half-life of 2 to 3 hours. It is primarily metabolized in the liver and hydroxylated and conjugated metabolites are excreted in the urine.

In humans, it has been shown to relieve glossopharyngeal neuralgia and cancer pain in subanesthetic doses. It has also been found useful in postherpetic neuralgia, acute postop hyperalgesia, phantom pain, orofacial pain, central pain, chronic ischemic pain, and mixed neuropathic pain syndromes. Most pain relief occurs at doses producing unpleasant psychotomimetic effects. Oral ketamine may have a better side-effect profile. Prior to initiating oral ketamine, an intravenous trail of ketamine in a dose up to 0.25 mg/kg infused over 20 minutes with pain assessment before and after is undertaken. Poor responders to the trial are unlikely to benefit from oral ketamine.

Adverse effects of subcutaneous and intravenous ketamine are dose-dependent nausea, tachycardia, hypertension, hypersecretion, elevation of intracranial pressure, nystagmus, skin rash, confusion, hallucinations, visual disturbances, unpleasant dreams, delirium, and other psychotomimetic effects. Cortical and limbic system activities are suggested as responsible for these effects. Oral ketamine has been associated with hepatic damage, gastric ulcer, and memory impairment. It results in higher levels of nor-ketamine, the main metabolite, which is equipotent as the parent drug.

Miscellaneous

Low affinity channel blocking NMDA receptor antagonists like dextromethorphan, amantadine, memantine, and magnesium have a better side-effect profile, but are often less effective analgesic agents. Dextromethorphan and its main metabolite, dextrorphan, also antagonize voltage dependent calcium channels. Conflicting results of dextromethorphan's efficacy may be due to genetic polymorphism of cytochrome P450 enzymes. Its elimination half-life ranges from 2 to 19 hours depending on metabolism. Reported adverse effects include dizziness, fatigue, confusion, depression, GI disturbances, and nystagmus.

By blocking ion channels, magnesium prevents extracellular calcium from entering NMDA-regulated calcium channels. Although animal studies showed that magnesium reduces mechanical allodynia and heat hyperalgesia, human studies have been conflicting. Adverse effects include flushed feeling, heat sensation, sedation, and pain at injection site.

Opioids with NMDA activity include methadone, dextropropoxyphene, and meperidine. They have low affinity for the PCP site. The D-isomer of methadone seems to have analgesic activity mediated through the NMDA receptor. Methadone has a long half-life, excellent absorption following oral and rectal administration, and has no known active metabolites. Its activity in both opioids and NMDA receptors may be useful in decreasing opioid induced tolerance.

Topiramate, an anticonvulsant, acts by decreasing activity of glutamate at AMPA/kainate receptors. One of the proposed mechanisms of action of lamotrigine is to reduce glutamate release from the primary afferent nerve terminal.

ANTIDEPRESSANTS

Basic Science

Analgesia produced by antidepressants has been shown not to be a result of their antidepressant properties, although most chronic pain patients have a component of depression. The doses used for antinociception are somewhat lower than the antidepressant doses and the onset of analgesia tends to be more rapid. The classes of antidepressants include tricyclic antidepressants, monoamine oxidase inhibitors, selective serotonin reuptake inhibitors, and the newer atypicals like serotonin, norepinephrine reuptake inhibitors. Tricyclic antidepressants (TCAs) have been in use for the longest period. The disadvantages of monoamine oxidase inhibitors (MAOIs) include: (a) adverse effect profile, including weight gain, orthostatic, hypotension, and sexual dysfunction; (b) dietary restrictions to prevent hypertensive crisis; (c) potentially fatal drug interactions; and (d) toxicity with overdose.

Amitriptyline, doxepin, desipramine, imipramine, and clomipramine produce concentration-dependent suppression of neuronal sodium channels of longer duration than bupivacaine. TCAs inhibit naltrexone binding and imipramine induced analgesia was partially reversed by naloxone suggesting a role for opioid receptors in TCAs antinociception. Desmethylimipramine and imipramine decreased the binding of MK801 (NMDA antagonist) and decreased calcium influx into neurons. Intrathecal amitriptyline's antihyperalgesic action was shown to be partly related to NMDA receptor blockade. It has also been shown that α_2 receptor antagonists blocked the antinociceptive action of antidepressants. TCAs potentiate adenosine-induced antinociception. They also inhibit the release of inflammatory mediators like IL-6, IL-1β, TNF-α, NO, and PGE$_2$ and stimulates IL-10. Venlafaxine at higher doses shows more norepinephrine action. Although capable of producing nerve block, antidepressants induce apoptosis in lymphocytes and are toxic to neurons. To summarize mechanisms of antinociception is thought to be due for the most part to serotonin and norepinephrine reuptake inhibition. α_2 adrenergic stimulation, NMDA receptor blockade, sodium channel blockade, adenosine, potentiation, and effects on inflammatory mediator release are the other mechanisms.

Clinical Science

As a group, TCAs are much more likely to produce analgesic or antihyperalgesic effects than the selective serotonin reuptake inhibitors (SSRIs). They tend to be more effective for neuropathic than for visceral or somatic pain. Clinical effects usually begin 1 to 3 weeks after initiation. TCAs achieve peak plasma concentration in roughly 1 to 6 hours and their elimination half-life ranges from 10 to 35 hours. Tertiary amines are more effective than secondary amines and have more side effects. Clinical uses include a variety of pain syndromes like painful diabetic neuropathy (number needed to treat [NNT] of 3.4), postherpetic neuralgia (NNT of 2.1), can-

cer pain, fibromyalgia, central pain, tension-type headache, and migraine.

Adverse effects of all antidepressants depend on their receptor affinities and can be decreased by slow titration. Overall, adverse effects of TCAs include constipation, dry mouth, hypotension, tachycardia, sedation, aplastic anemia, heart block, SIADH, seizures, weight gain, and sexual dysfunction. Adverse effects of venlafaxine include anxiety, headache (16%), insomnia (20%), somnolence (9%), asthenia, dry mouth, nausea, vomiting, diarrhea, weight loss, constipation, mydriasis, hypertension, and activation of mania. MAOIs are contraindicated in CHF, phaeochromocytoma, and hepatic disease. Overdose of antidepressants may be lethal and hence should be avoided in acutely suicidal patients. TCAs are better avoided in patients with heart block, prolonged QT$_C$, narrow angle glaucoma, and prostatic hypertrophy.

Serotonin Syndrome

Acute onset of 3 of the following 10 symptomatology coincident with the addition or increase of a serotoninergic agent defines Serotonin Syndrome: mental status changes, hyperreflexia, diaphoresis, agitation, tremor, diarrhea, myoclonus, fever, dyscoordination, and shivering. When severe, it can include hyperthermia, coma, convulsions, and death. It is seen in combinations of MAOIs, TCAs, SSRIs, SNRIs, and rarely with meperidine, tramadol, and sumatriptan.

ANTICONVULSANTS

Antiepileptic drugs (AEDs) have been in use for analgesia for a few decades. Neuropathic pain states possibly have redistribution of certain sodium channels to the peripheral axon at the site of injury. This results in spontaneous ectopic discharges and lowering of threshold for mechanical stimuli. Sodium channel blockers like phenytoin and carbamazepine may block these ectopic discharges. Calcium channel subunit α_2-δ is upregulated in dorsal root ganglion after peripheral nerve ligation and potentials through NMDA receptors have been found to cause the "wind-up" phenomenon. AEDs with calcium channel blocking properties like gabapentin, lamotrigine, and oxcarbazepine could help decrease this effect. AEDs have differing modes of action but similar therapeutic effects. The mechanism of action of AEDs is listed in Box 6-3. The choice of a particular AED is made based on prior experience, comorbid conditions, and side-effect profile (see Box 6-4). Once a therapeutic limit is achieved with no pain relief an alternate AED from another class is chosen. AEDs are indicated in neuralgias, cancer pain, central pain, postsympathectomy pain, painful diabetic neuropathy, paroxysmal pain in multiple sclerosis, migraine, phan-

Box 6-3   Mechanism of Action of Antiepileptic Drugs

Mechanism of Action	Drug
GABA enhancement	Gabapentin, topiramate, valproic acid, zonisamide, tiagabine
NA^+ current blockade	Carbamazepine, oxcarbazepine, phenytoin, lamotrigine, sodium valproate
Ca^{2+} current blockade	Gabapentin, oxcarbazepine, pregabilin
Decrease excitatory amino acid	Phenytoin, topiramate, lamotrigine
Anti-inflammatory effect	Gabapentin, lamotrigine

Box 6-4   Recommended Treatment Strategies of Antiepileptic Drugs

Pain Disorder	First Line	Second Line	Third Line
Painful diabetic neuropathy	Gabapentin, Pregabalin	Topiramate, Oxcarbazepine, Zonisamide	Phenytoin
Trigeminal neuralgia	Oxcarbazepine	Gabapentin, Carbamazepine	Topiramate, Lamotrigine
Postherpetic neuralgia	Gabapentin	Carbamazepine, Oxcarbazepine, Topiramate	Valproate, Lamotrigine
Migraine	Valproate	Gabapentin, Levetiracetam	Tiagabine, Topiramate
Cranial neuralgias	Gabapentin	Oxcarbazepine	Lamotrigine
Central pain	Gabapentin	Oxcarbazepine, Zonisamide, Topiramate	Lamotrigine, Valproate, Clonazepam
Neuropathy/Radiculopathy	Gabapentin	Oxcarbazepine, Topiramate, Zonisamide	Valproate, Tiagabine

tom pain, stump pain, and peripheral neuropathy. It is more useful for paroxysmal lancinating pain than continuous pain. A 6-week trial for most agents is the minimum required to assess analgesic efficacy.

Carbamazepine

Basic Science

Carbamazepine is an iminostilbene derivative, causing blockade of voltage dependent sodium channel channels. Carbamazepine (CBZ) is chemically related to TCAs. It suppresses spontaneously firing A-δ and C fibers. It acts through both central and peripheral mechanisms. The central effect is through γ-aminobutyric acid (GABA)-ergic systems in periaqueductal grey. CBZ decreased nociceptive behavior in animal models through an A1 adenosine receptor agonist action. It possibly has some anti-inflammatory effects as well. It can elevate brain serotonin levels and decrease pain threshold in rats.

Clinical Science

After oral administration, CBZ achieves peak plasma concentration in 4 to 8 hours. Its half-life ranges from 10 to 20 hours. About 40% of the drug is biotransformed by epoxidation. It induces its own metabolism. Metabolism of CBZ is via cytochrome-p 450 3A4 isoenzyme and its metabolite has equipotent anticonvulsant activity with a shorter half-life.

Most frequent use of CBZ is in trigeminal neuralgia and painful diabetic neuropathy. Less frequent uses include postherpetic neuralgia, tabetic pain, and central pain.

Starting doses are 200 mg/day, increased by 100 mg/wk to a maximum of 1200 mg/day in divided doses. During therapy with CBZ, blood counts are monitored at baseline and periodically thereafter.

Common adverse effects are somnolence, dizziness, and gait disturbances. Other side effects include agranulocytosis, aplastic anemia, hyponatremia, erythema multiforme, Steven Johnson's syndrome, jaundice, oliguria, hypertension, and acute left ventricular failure.

Oxcarbazepine

This drug is a keto derivative of CBZ. Oxcarbazepine (OBZ) is prodrug for 10-hydroxy oxcarbazepine.

OBZ produces both sodium and calcium channel blockade. OBZ has a half-life of 8 to 10 hours and is excreted unchanged in the urine or as a glucuronide. It is dosed at 150 mg/day and increased weekly by 150 to 1800 mg/day in 2 divided doses.

OBZ is a first-line therapy for trigeminal neuralgia. It is also useful in patients unresponsive to CBZ and in other neuropathic conditions. Common adverse effects include dizziness, vertigo, weight gain, and edema. GI symptoms, fatigue, agranulocytosis, and allergy type reactions have also been reported. There is a 25% cross reactivity with CBZ allergy.

Gabapentin

Basic Science
Gabapentin (GBP) is a structural GABA analogue with possible effects on $\alpha_2\text{-}\delta$ calcium channel and inhibits voltage dependent sodium channels. It has both peripheral and central actions. Increased spinal neuronal activity was blocked by GBP. By selectively modulating the facilitation of spinal nociceptive processing, hyperalgesia was reversed by intrathecal GBP. Dose-dependent blockade of allodynia by GBP was shown in rats. It increases the threshold for mechanical allodynia. It has been shown to have peripheral as well as central nervous system effects.

Clinical Science
GBP has a bioavailability of 60%. It achieves peak plasma concentrations in 2 to 3 hours. Its elimination half-life is between 4 and 22 hours. It undergoes no appreciable metabolism and is excreted renally.

It is used in neuropathic pain states including painful diabetic neuropathy and postherpetic neuralgia. It is also useful in CRPS, central pain, phantom pain, and other neuropathic pain conditions.

Starting dose is 100 to 300 mg/day, gradually increased to 1800 mg/day in divided doses. Pain relief not obtained at 1800 mg is unlikely to be seen by dose escalation. Doses over 3600 mg/day rarely provide additional benefit.

Common adverse effects include dizziness, somnolence, GI disturbances, fatigue, poor concentration, anorexia, nausea, nystagmus, and ataxia. Other side effects include rash, peripheral edema, stuttering, anxiety, paraesthesias, arthralgias, tremor, twitching, abnormal vision, and headache.

Lamotrigine

Basic Science
Lamotrigine is a phenyltriazine derivative. It blocks voltage-dependent sodium channels and inhibits glutamate and aspartate release. It may have a neuroprotective effect. Inhibition of neuronal sensitization leading to decrease in hyperalgesia was demonstrated in animal models. Cold allodynia was reversed by both agents in a study comparing GBP and lamotrigine.

Clinical Science
It achieves peak plasma concentration in 1 to 4 hours. It is metabolized in the liver by glucuronidation. Lamotrigine is started in a dose of 25 mg twice a day, gradually increased every 2 weeks. Doses less than 200 mg are unlikely to be of any benefit.

Most common adverse effects include dizziness, ataxia, constipation, nausea, somnolence, and diplopia. Rash develops in 10% and can progress to Stevens-Johnson Syndrome. Long-term use can rarely lead to blindness.

Zonisamide

Basic Science
Zonisamide belongs to the sulfonamide group of drugs. It is a sodium and T-type calcium channel blocker and possibly increases GABA release. Other effects include scavenging of hydroxyl radicals, NO synthase inhibition, and stabilization of neuronal membrane. It facilitates dopaminergic and serotoninergic transmission. In a cat model trigeminal complex modulation of descending excitation was demonstrated with Zonisamide

Clinical Science
Zonisamide has a plasma half-life of 63 hours. Metabolism is by cytochrome p-450 system. It is started at 100 mg and increased weekly by 100 mg to a maximum of 400 mg/day. It is used in some neuropathic pain states unresponsive to other AEDs.

Adverse effects include abnormal thinking, asthenia, dizziness, nausea, headache, somnolence, dyspepsia, constipation, paresthesia, anorexia, ataxia, nystagmus, induction of SLE-like syndrome, renal tubular acidosis, and renal calculi.

Sodium Valproate

Basic Science
Sodium valproate attenuates neuronal excitation induced by glutamate receptors. Valproate blocks degradation and increases synthesis of GABA. c-fos activity is suppressed. It also has direct effects on sodium channels, calcium dependent potassium channels, and possibly T-type calcium channels.

Clinical Science
It is highly protein bound and crosses blood brain barrier easily. It achieves peak plasma concentration in 1 to 4 hours with an elimination half-life of 6 to 16 hours. It is started at a dose of 250 mg/day, gradually increased to 1200 mg/day in 2 divided doses. Maximum dose is 60 mg/kg

It is used for migraine prophylaxis, chronic daily headache, and cancer-related neuropathic pain. Clinical efficacy in neuropathic pain is not well-established. It has multiple drug interactions and a *Physicians' Desk Reference* black box warning for hepatotoxicity, teratogenicity, and pancreatitis. Other side effects include GI upset, weight gain, tremor, rash, ataxia, hair loss, and hematological toxicity. In women of childbearing age, it can cause "fetal valproate syndrome."

Topiramate

Basic Science
Topiramate is a sulfonamide relative. Besides blockade of sodium channels, it can also produce enhancement of GABA inhibition and attenuate kainate induced responses at glutamate receptors.

Clinical Science
Less than 15% of topiramate is protein bound. It has a half-life of 18 to 24 hours. It is primarily cleared by the kidney with a small hepatic component. There has been a reduction in migraine frequency with the use of topiramate. It has also been tried in refractory intercostal neuralgia, trigeminal neuralgia, and painful diabetic neuropathy. It is started at a dose of 25 to 30 mg at night and increased over 8 weeks to 400 mg in 2 doses.

Side effects of topiramate include fatigue, anorexia, weight loss, asthenia, dizziness, tremor, headache, cognitive dysfunction, and urolithiasis. Weight loss is seen 10% and peaks in 15 to 18 months.

Tiagabine

Basic Science
Tiagabine is derived from nipecotic acid. Antinociceptive effect of tiagabine is due to activation of GABA-B receptors secondary to raised endogenous GABA levels. Tiagabine inhibits uptake presynaptically.

Clinical Science
Tiagabine achieves peak plasma concentration in 45 minutes. Its elimination half-life is 7 to 9 hours. It is metabolized by cytochrome-P 450, CYP3A isoenzyme. Limited human data is available on its effect in neuropathic pain.

Dosing schedule is 4 mg once a day increased by 4 to 8 mg/day at weekly intervals to a maximum of 50 mg in 2 to 4 doses.

Its side effects include asthenia, tremor, dizziness, hypertension, tachycardia, abdominal pain, diarrhea, difficulty concentrating, depression, nervousness, seizures, pruritus, increased appetite, and emotional lability.

Clonazepam

Basic Science
Clonazepam is a benzodiazepine, which potentiates inhibitory GABA transmission. Being a GABA-B agonist combination with other GABA-B agonists can increase sedation. Analgesic effect may also be due to decrease in anxiety and spasticity.

Clinical Science
Peak plasma concentration is achieved in 1 to 4 hours. Clonazepam's elimination half-life is 18 to 36 hours. It is hepatically conjugated into inactive metabolites and excreted in the urine.

It has been found useful in cranial neuralgias including glossopharyngeal neuralgia and cluster headache. It may be beneficial in phantom pain especially the shooting pain. It is started at a dose of 0.5 mg/day and increased gradually to 4 mg/day.

Its common side effect is sedation. Drowsiness, mood disturbances, dizziness, and fatigue are not uncommon. Monitoring for liver enzyme elevation and blood dyscrasias is recommended. It can produce a withdrawal syndrome.

Levetiracetam

Basic Science
Levetiracetam is a pyrrolidine derivative with a specific binding site at synaptic plasma membranes in CNS. Its mechanism of action is unknown. Appears to have some GABA mediated effects and selectively inhibits N-type calcium channels.

Clinical Science
It is currently approved for partial seizures and may have an effect in neuropathic pain. It is started at 1000 mg/day in 2 doses and increased over a month to 2000 mg/day. Its side effects include nausea, ataxia, headache, dizziness, asthenia, somnolence, and sedation.

Phenytoin

Basic Science
This was the first AED reported effective in trigeminal neuralgia. It blocks sodium channels, and at high concentration may inhibit presynaptic glutamate release.

Clinical Science
Enteral administration is unreliable and slow. Peak plasma levels are achieved in 3 to 12 hours. Metabolism is by hepatic endoplasmic reticulum to inactive metabolites. Plasma half-life ranges from 6 to 24 hours. Efficacy has been shown in trigeminal neuralgia, painful diabetic neuropathy, and various other neuropathic pain syndromes. Usual dose is 100 mg thrice daily. Side effects include ataxia, nystagmus, slurred speech, gingival hypertrophy, facial hair thickening, allergic skin rash, vestibular dysfunction, hepatotoxicity, and fetal hydantoin syndrome.

Pregabalin

Basic Science
Pregabalin is a 3-alkylated GABA analog released in late 2004. It has been shown to increase rate of GABA synthesis, bind to α_2-δ subunit of calcium channels, and

reduce potassium induced monoamine release. Animal studies have shown decreased mechanical allodynia in chronic constriction injury model. Pregabalin seems less sedating than GBP. Reduction in joint swelling and prevention of heat hyperalgesia were seen in rat model of arthritis. It may also be effective in postop pain.

Clinical Science

It achieves peak plasma levels in 1 hour after administration. Its plasma half-life is 6 hours. It has negligible hepatic metabolism and is mostly renally excreted. It is useful in painful diabetic neuropathy, and probably has the same spectrum of use as GBP.

Side effects include dizziness, somnolence, myoclonus, headache, asthenia, ataxia, confusion, and GI symptoms.

MISCELLANEOUS AGENTS

Tramadol

Basic Science

Tramadol is a centrally acting drug available as a racemic mixture with the L-isomer having activity at opiate receptors and D-isomer acting at other sites. Its major mechanism of action is by inhibiting uptake of serotonin and norepinephrine, which is less than TCAs. It also has a weak interaction at μ-opioid receptor, almost 6000 times less than morphine. There is evidence to show that Tramadol's analgesic effect is due to inhibition of norepinephrine transporter (NET) function by blocking Desipramine binding sites. NET suppression facilitates descending inhibitory system and was absent in NET knockout mice. There may possibly be some antinociception due to its effect on cholinergic receptors.

The major active metabolite of tramadol, mono-O-desmethyl tramadol (M1) has 200-fold more potent binding at μ-opioid receptor. In animals it has been found to be 3 times more potent than tramadol. The clinical effect, although, may not be due to M1. Tramadol has been studied in nerve blocks with local anesthetics, for regional anesthesia, and epidural analgesia. Intrathecal administration has also been shown to be effective in animals. It stimulates natural killer cells.

Clinical Science

Tramadol administered orally is almost completely absorbed and achieves peak concentration in 2 hours. It has an elimination half-life of 6.3 hours. It is metabolized by N- and O-deethylation, through CYP2D6 and 3A4 isoenzymes and conjugation into 11 metabolites. Only M1 has weak antinociceptive properties. It is excreted renally (90%) and in feces.

It is used in painful diabetic neuropathy, fibromyalgia, musculoskeletal pain, and postcraniotomy pain. Its advantages include less respiratory depression and less effect on sphincter of Oddi.

Adverse effects most commonly are nausea, vomiting, constipation, dizziness, headache, light-headedness, and drowsiness. These are dose-related and transient and are avoided by slow titration. It produces seizures in higher than recommended doses and it lowers the seizure threshold in patients on MAOIs, TCAs, SSRIs, Bupropion, and neuroleptics. It can lead to physical dependence and psychological dependence. It has significant drug interactions.

Baclofen

Basic Science

Baclofen is a p chlorophenol derivative of GABA with a GABA-B agonist effect. It is a racemic mixture with L-Baclofen being the active form. It produces GABA mediated decrease in calcium currents. It has both presynaptic and postsynaptic effects. In addition, substance-P release is inhibited. The mechanism of skeletal muscle relaxation is unknown but could be due to its GABA effect. In animal models it has been found effective in neuropathic pain.

Clinical Science

Baclofen achieves peak plasma concentration in 2 hours. Its elimination half-life is 3 to 7 hours. It undergoes minimal hepatic metabolism, and the majority is excreted unchanged in urine. It is started at 5 mg 2 to 3 times a day and its maximum dose is 80 mg/day. Baclofen is effective in trigeminal neuralgia. It has also been used in spasticity, chronic low back pain, muscle spasms, multiple sclerosis, atypical facial pain, cluster headaches, and CRPS-1.

Side effects include sedation, weakness, confusion, hypotension, blurred vision, nausea, vomiting, and headache. Abrupt withdrawal can produce seizures, hallucinations, tachycardia, and anxiety.

Lidocaine

Basic Science

Its mechanism of action is by sodium channel blockade and membrane stabilization. It is used in chronic pain management as a topical agent and as an intravenous agent.

Clinical Science

Topical 5% patch is approved for postherpetic neuralgia. It has also been found to decrease allodynia in other neuropathic pain states including HIV neuropathy, postmastectomy, and thoracotomy pain besides CRPS. Intravenous lidocaine has been found useful in some neuropathic pain states such as painful herpetic neuralgia, phantom limb pain, CRPS, and painful diabetic neuropathy. A trial of IV lidocaine is necessary to assess efficacy with a 50% or greater reduction in pain warranting a trial with oral Mexiletine. Side effects during trail include tinnitus, perioral paraesthesia, metallic taste hypotension, arrhythmias, and seizures.

Mexiletine

Basic Science

It is an analog of lidocaine structurally modified to reduce hepatic first pass metabolism. It is also a sodium channel blocker.

Clinical Science

Elimination half-life is 9 to 15 hours and dosing is 150 mg orally 3 times daily. It has been found useful in painful diabetic neuropathy, central pain, and CRPS. Predominant side effects are GI dysfunction and CNS effects.

CONCLUSION

Potential future targets for drug development include antagonists of inflammatory pain mediators, purinoceptors, vanilloid receptors, and NR_2B subunit of NMDA receptors. Free radicals contribute to hyperalgesia maintenance; hence, antioxidants like α-lipoic acid may likely have a role. Integrating over current knowledge of receptors and ion channels may pave the way for the ideal pain drug. For the present combination therapy targeting pain transmission at multiple levels seems to be the ideal compromise.

SUGGESTED READING

Backonja MM, Beydoun A: Mechanistic stratification of antineuralgic agents. J Pain Symptom Manage 25:S18-S30, 2003.

Hocking G, Cousins MJ: Ketamine in chronic pain management: an evidence-based review. Anesth Analg 97:1730, 2003.

MacPherson RD: The pharmacological basis of contemporary pain management. Pharmacol Ther 88:163-185, 2000.

Martin TJ, Eisenach JC: Pharmacology of opioid and nonopioid analgesics in chronic pain states. JPET 299:811-817, 2001.

Smith HS: Drugs for Pain, 1st ed. Philadelphia, Hanley & Belfus, 2002.

Walia SK, Khan EA, Ko DH, et al: Side effects of antiepileptics: a review. Pain Practice 4(3):194-203, 2004.

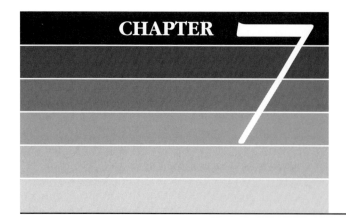

INTRODUCTION

There is probably no therapeutic endeavor more vexing to physicians than providing long-term opioid therapy to patients with chronic non-cancer pain. Most patients genuinely need relief of suffering. Most clinicians genuinely want to provide these patients with optimal and compassionate care, yet they are often not able to do this simply. An organized approach using prospectively established guidelines would facilitate patient care while providing practitioner peace of mind. Unfortunately, like most statements related to this form of therapy, there is no published evidence to support this claim.

This chapter discusses patient evaluation and selection and establishment of a therapeutic plan including monitoring and contingency plans for therapeutic misadventures. The pharmacology of opioids and general principles of therapeutics, although important, will not be discussed in detail; however, since these concepts provide much of the foundation for the principles laid out in this chapter, readers unfamiliar with these concepts should consult any number of monographs that discuss these issues in detail.[1,2,3]

PATIENT EVALUATION

The evaluation of the pain patient is covered in a number of textbooks,[4,5,6] so only relevant points will be reiterated here.

An important objective of the clinical evaluation of the pain patient is to identify processes that may be amenable to medical interventions. Opioids are likely to be ineffective for pain that has no nociceptive component. The role of opioids in the management of neuropathic pain is controversial, but they have no role in the management of chronic anxiety or depression accompanying chronic pain. Another important objective of the clinical evaluation is to establish a baseline for use in monitoring the results of therapy. Finally, clinical evaluation may have important effects in building rapport with the patient and in providing reassurance to the patient that he is being monitored for progression of a disease that must be treated definitively.

A Venn diagram (Fig. 7-1) can represent the situation of patients with chronic pain.[7] The circle labeled "B" represents the biologic component of the pain problem: the nociceptive or neuropathic component. This component can be managed by pharmacologic techniques among other medical modalities. The circle labeled "I" represents the illness component of the pain problem: the psychological distress. This component can be managed by psychological interventions, including psychotropic medications. The circle labeled "S" represents the sickness component of the pain problem: the loss or diminution of function, which is most appropriately managed by physical modalities. As much as possible, the practitioner must address only the biologic component of the patient's pain problem with opioids. This is admittedly a qualitative assessment, but one the practitioner must consciously make for each patient (Box 7-1).

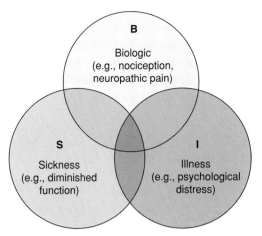

Figure 7-1   Venn diagram.

The epidemiology of substance abuse is composed of conflicting literature for a number of methodological reasons, but a modicum of familiarity with it will allow the practitioner to be aware of patients who should be considered at an increased risk for abuse of opioid therapy. Those patients at increased risk seem to be those who have a degree of anomie in their social background, those with psychopathology (i.e., anxiety, borderline personality disorder, depression, and sociopathy), and those who have multiple family problems. While these are considered risk factors for substance abuse in the general population, the current literature does not indicate if it is reasonable to extrapolate from the general population to the chronic pain population. While some have recommended using various instruments like the CAGE questionnaire, most of these instruments have been most useful in the evaluation of the risk of alcohol abuse and their relevance to opioid abuse in the chronic-pain patient population has not been established.[8] Another risk factor for opioid abuse that the practitioner must be mindful of is the speed of onset of the opioid; fast onset opioids are more likely to be abused.

Box 7-1   Definition of Addiction

Characterized by persistent pattern of dysfunctional opioid use involving:
Adverse consequences associated with opioid use
Loss of control over opioid use
Continued opioid use despite harm
Preoccupation with obtaining opioids despite adequate pain control—craving

---

In summary, the clinical evaluation of the pain patient can provide information to make an assessment of the effectiveness of opioid therapy for the patient's pain problem, a baseline from which to measure progress in treating the problem, and an estimate of the patient's risk of substance abuse.

THE ROLE OF PRACTICE PARAMETERS

A number of medical societies have established various practice parameters to assist practitioners. (In this chapter the author is using the definitions and categories of practice parameters proposed by the American Society of Anesthesiologists.[9]) While a number have been published for opioid therapy in the chronic pain patient, they tend to be rather general, reflecting the current lack of strength of evidence in support of opioid therapy. It is helpful to have a method to evaluate them for methodological rigor when considering whether to adopt them.[10] Those parameters that use a rigorous methodology will provide a systemic summary of the evidence, consider all relevant options and outcomes, and provide an explicit discussion of the utility of the outcomes to the decision makers. As practice parameters decline in methodological rigor, they fail to adhere to the preceding criteria. Many evaluations of opioid therapy in chronic pain seem to have a low level of rigor, failing especially to explicitly consider the utility of outcomes. While the practitioner should regularly seek practice parameters, they may be of little assistance in the near future.

In the absence of rigorous practice parameters, the practitioner should try to determine if there is literature support for the type of opioid therapy contemplated. The practitioner can best accomplish this by a systemic approach to the literature that involves asking an answerable, clinically useful question[11]:

1. **P:** Be as specific as possible about the **P**atient, **P**opulation, or **P**roblem to be treated.
2. **I:** Be as specific as possible about the **I**ntervention contemplated.
3. **C:** Look for studies that used a **C**ontrol group.
4. **O:** Be as specific and complete as possible about the **O**utcome of interest.

For example, the practitioner could search the literature by asking and trying to answer the question: Of patients with fibromyalgia (**P**), what percent of patients treated with long-acting opioids on a chronic basis (**I**) are able to maintain a program of exercise 5 times a week (**O**) compared to patients treated with tricyclic antidepressants (**C**)?

TREATMENT GOALS

The practitioner and the patient should agree on prospectively established treatment goals. The current literature is silent on whether analgesia by itself is a sufficient goal for long-term opioid therapy, or if other goals such as improved function or quality of life is necessary as well.[12] The "Five As" represent a useful way to summarize the important goals of opioid therapy: analgesia, activity, affect, adverse effects, and aberrant behavior. If there is inadequate progress in any of the components, the practitioner must re-evaluate the therapy.[13]

There are a number of instruments that can be used to assess analgesia. Because none of them have been shown to be superior, the practitioner may select the one(s) that best work in the clinical setting. When patients do not improve (or deteriorate) in the analgesia component three possibilities should be considered progression of disease, inadequate dosing or tolerance, and development of hyperalgesia. The practitioner can monitor for progression of disease by regular clinical assessment of the patient. There is no reliable, practical way to differentiate inadequate dosing, tolerance, and hyperalgesia. The practitioner can assess the probability of inadequate dosing, tolerance, or hyperalgesia by titration of the opioid dose to either analgesia or unacceptable side effects. If the patient improves with an increase, or decrease, in dose, the patient is maintained on the minimal effective dose. If the patient develops unacceptable side effects in the face of inadequate analgesia, the opioid is tapered and possibly eliminated.[12]

There are likewise a number of ways of documenting increases in activity; a diary may be useful for this.

The practitioner can assess changes in affect by clinical assessment or by using psychometric instruments.

Clinical assessment will be sufficient for monitoring side (adverse) effects. Many of the adverse effects of opioid therapy can be managed expectantly (by allowing the patient to develop tolerance to the side effect) or directly by administering a medication that will ameliorate the side effect.

The presence of aberrant behavior is the untoward effect that is probably most challenging for the practitioner. Early refills, lost prescriptions or medications, increased consumption of medications, urine drug tests incompatible with therapy are behaviors that rapidly become time-consuming and increase cynicism on the part of the practitioner. A reasonable approach to aberrant behavior is to increase the level of control present in the therapeutic plan. For example, the patient is scheduled for more frequent follow-up, the various goals are broken down into more manageable components, or the patient is called in for unannounced urine drug tests and pill counts. These are always difficult situations, and the practitioner must handle with tact and diplomacy emphasizing that these steps are being taken in the patient's best interest (Box 7-2).

Urine drug testing is an important monitoring technique. The practitioner should develop a close relationship with a colleague in the clinical laboratory who can assist with proper interpretation of the results of such tests. Because the threshold for a positive result may vary, care and judgment must be exercised in interpreting and acting on the results.

OPIOID TAPERING

When it becomes apparent that the dose of the opioid analgesic agent must be reduced or eliminated, the dose of opioid can be reduced by 10% of the initial dose per week over 10 weeks or more gradually by 3% of the initial dose per week over about 30 weeks.[14] Adjuncts to tapering may include alternative methods of analgesia and clonidine. If the practitioner believes the patient has

---

Box 7-2   Behaviors indicative of addiction[15]

Behaviors more prevalent in patients with addictive disease:
Obtaining prescriptions from >1 provider
Patient increased dose, frequency
Calling for early refills
Obtaining opioids from emergency rooms
Losing prescriptions, medications
Forging prescriptions
Use of street drugs
Hoarding unused medications
Use of opioid for other symptoms (insomnia, anxiety, depression)
Supplement with alcohol or psychoactive drugs
History of physician or dentist terminating care because of concerns about analgesic use
Family members concerned about patient addiction
Use of opioids prescribed for family members
Personal (not family) history of addiction
History of undergoing detox
Preference for route of administration
Behaviors *not* more prevalent in subjects with addictive disease:
Coexisting psychopathology
History of physical or sexual abuse (31% overall)
Receiving disability, involved in litigation
Mistrust of past healthcare providers
Family member, spouse with substance abuse history or chronic pain history
Somatoform disorder

a substance abuse problem, detoxification should be managed by an addictionologist.

SELECTION OF OPIOID

The results of basic research have implied a number of advantages for various opioids and for opioid rotation (the practice of changing the opioid prescribed); however, none of these advantages have been established in the clinical literature.[12] The rapidity of onset of effect of a drug has been implicated as a risk factor in substance abuse, so this characteristic is probably the most important trait to be considered in selection of an opioid for long-term therapy. It would be prudent to prescribe long-acting opioids as the mainstay of therapy, reserving fast-onset opioids for activity-related pain.

In switching from one opioid to another, it is essential to know equianalgesic doses. Unfortunately, there can be variations in the absorption and metabolism of certain drugs, so it is prudent to begin with doses that are lower than calculated. This is particularly true for methadone, which is now thought to be more potent than some of the older conversion tables indicate. A conservative dose of a long-acting opioid should be started and a rescue dose of a short-acting drug can be prescribed until the appropriate dose of the long-acting drug is reached. Short-acting "breakthrough" medications can be continued if there are periods of activity-related pain not controlled by the background drug. A conversion chart for several commonly used opioids is shown in Table 7-1.

OPIOID CONTRACT

The utility and purpose of an opioid contract (written agreement specifying the responsibilities of the patient and practitioner during opioid therapy) have not been established by rigorous evidence. If the practitioner wishes to use such a document, there are numerous examples available in the medical literature. Some of the common components of opioid contracts are shown in Box 7-3.

CONCLUSION

Long-term opioid therapy for chronic pain is probably the best example of a schism between basic research and clinical practice. While a great deal is known about the basic pharmacology of opioids, there are major gaps in our knowledge of clinical use of opioids. Much of this is due to the complicated problems of chronic pain and the secondary gain that opioids can provide. However, there are patients who may well benefit from chronic opioids. Pain management practitioners can best serve their patients by regularly reviewing the literature critically and using a combination of pharmacologic principles and common sense.

Table 7-1	Conversion chart for commonly prescribed opioids (Doses shown are roughly equianalgesic. The starting doses in opioid naïve patients are generally lower than those shown.)

Opioid	Oral Dose	Parenteral Dose
Morphine	30mg	10mg
Oxycodone	20mg	NA
Hydrocodone	30mg	NA
Methadone*	10-15mg	10mg
Meperidine	200-300mg	75mg
Levorphanol	4mg	2mg
Hydromorphone	7.5mg	1.5mg
Fentanyl**	NA	50-100µg
Codeine	200mg	130mg

*Methadone has a very long half-life. It accumulates slowly, so dose adjustments should not be made any more often than every three days. Dosing is usually b.i.d.

**Transdermal fentanyl 25µg is equivalent to about 75 to 120 mg oral morphine per 24 hours. Oral transmucosal fentanyl is available in doses of 200 to 1600 µg. It is indicated only for opioid tolerant patients.

Box 7-3 Issues that may be addressed in an opioid contract or agreement

Treatment goals (e.g., pain relief, function, activity)
Evaluation of treatment goals
Appointment intervals
Consequences of not adhering to agreement
Plan for taper and D/C if treatment ineffective, intolerable side effects, agreement broken
Frequency and type of lab studies, including random drug screens
Responsibility to take drugs as directed, safeguard drugs, management of lost or stolen drugs
Conditions for refilling prescriptions—office hours, only during scheduled visits
Situations prompting consultations
Reporting of side effects
Avoiding hazardous activities if impaired
Prescribing source (one group, one physician)
Permission of physician to communicate with other providers, pharmacists, regulators, law enforcement regarding contract
Statement by patient regarding history of substance abuse
Adherence to state and federal regulations
Initiation of bowel regimen
Address suicidal ideation—mechanism for dealing with suicidal thoughts
Use of birth control for female patients

REFERENCES

1. Gutstein HB, Akil H: Opioid analgesics. In Hardman JG, Limbird LE, Gilman AG (eds): Goodman & Gilman's The Pharmacological Basis of Therapeutics, 10th ed. New York, McGraw-Hill, 2001, pp 569-619.

2. Myoshi HR, Leckband SG: Systemic opioid analgesics. In Loeser JD, Butler SH, Chapman CR, Turk DC (eds): Bonica's Management of Pain, 3rd ed. Philadelphia, Lippincott Williams & Wilkins, 2001, pp 1682-1709.

3. Nies AS: Principles of therapeutics. In Hardman JG, Limbird LE, Gilman AG (eds): Goodman & Gilman's The Pharmacological Basis of Therapeutics, 10th ed. New York, McGraw-Hill, 2001, pp 45-66.

4. Loeser JD: Medical evaluation of the patient with pain. In Loeser JD, Butler SH, Chapman CR, Turk DC (eds): Bonica's Management of Pain, 3rd ed. Philadelphia, Lippincott Williams & Wilkins, 2001, pp 267-78.

5. DeGowin RL: DeGowin and DeGowin's Bedside Diagnostic Examination, 5th ed. New York, Macmillan Publishing Co., 1987.

6. Orient JM: Sapira's Art and Science of Bedside Diagnosis, 2nd ed. Philadelphia, Lippincott Williams & Wilkins, 2001.

7. Sharpe M, Mayou R, Bass C: Concepts, theories, and terminology. In Mayou R, Bass C, Sharpe M (eds): Treatment of Functional Somatic Symptoms. Oxford, Oxford University Press, 1995, pp 3-16.

8. Crum RM: The epidemiology of addictive disorders. In Graham AW, Schultz TK, Mayo-Smith MF, Ries RK, Wilford BB (eds): Principles of Addiction Medicine, 3rd ed. Chevy Chase, American Society of Addiction Medicine, Inc., 2003, pp 17-31.

9. American Society of Anesthesiologists. Statement on practice parameters. 1999.

10. Guyatt G, Hayward R, Richardson WS, et al: Moving from evidence to action. In Guyatt G, Rennie D (eds): User's Guides to the Medical Literature: Essentials of Evidence-Based Clinical Practice. Chicago, AMA Press, 2002, pp 271-310.

11. McKibbon A, Hunt D, Richardson WS, et al: Finding the evidence. In Guyatt G, Rennie D (eds): User's Guides to the Medical Literature: Essentials of Evidence-Based Clinical Practice. Chicago, AMA Press, 2002, pp 21-71.

12. Ballantyne JC, Mao J: Opioid therapy for chronic pain. New England Journal of Medicine 349:1943-53, 2003.

13. Savage SR: Opioid medications in the management of pain. In Graham AW, Schultz TK, Mayo-Smith MF, Ries RK, Wilford BB (eds): Principles of Addiction Medicine, 3rd ed. Chevy Chase, American Society of Addiction Medicine, Inc., 2003, pp 1451-63.

14. Kosten TR, O'Connor PG: Management of drug and alcohol withdrawal. New England Journal of Medicine 348:1786-95, 2003.

15. Compton P, Darakjian J, Miotto K: Screening for addiction in patients with chronic pain and "problematic" substance use: evaluation of a pilot assessment tool. J Pain Symptom Manage, 16(6):355-63, 1998.

CHAPTER 8

Chronic Spinal Drug Administration

MARK S. WALLACE

HISTORY OF SPINAL DRUG DELIVERY

The earliest reports of spinal drug delivery involved the single injection of local anesthetics. In 1885, James Leonard Corning demonstrated that cocaine delivered intrathecally in a dog resulted in an intense sensory motor blockade. In 1899, Bier injected local anesthetics into himself, his assistant, and several patients; this resulted in potent anesthesia. By 1901, there had been nearly 1000 reports of local anesthetics delivered both intrathecally and epidurally in the caudal, lumbar, thoracic, and cervical canals. The first spinal cannulation was achieved by Love in 1935 using a 5 French ureteral catheter, and in 1942 Manalan performed a continuous caudal anesthesia using a malleable Lemmon spinal needle. A major breakthrough for continuous intraspinal drug delivery occurred in 1942 with the introduction of smaller catheters, and in 1945 with the description of the use of a needle with a side-opening tip developed by Huber to place an intrathecal catheter. In 1949, the Tuohy needle was used for epidural cannulation.

In the following decades, there was a significant increase in the understanding of the physiology of nociceptive processing at the spinal cord level, and it was determined that drugs delivered spinally were capable of producing powerful antinociception. As these discoveries were made, spinal canal cannulation evolved to the point where long-term spinal drug delivery was possible. In 1982, the first programmable pump delivering morphine was successfully implanted. In 1984, the same programmable pump was implanted for the delivery of baclofen for the treatment of spasticity and in 1988, the SynchroMed programmable pump (Medtronic Neurological, Minneapolis) was released on the market. Technological advancements continue to refine spinal drug delivery (Box 8-1).

RATIONALE

In 1965, Melzack and Wall[1] noted that the spinal cord was the "gatekeeper" of nociceptive processing. In the following decades, the spinal dorsal horn pharmacology and physiology was studied intensely, and the importance of excitatory amino acids, such as glutamate, in nociception was discovered. In addition, the identification of substance P release evoked from C fibers stimulation and the inhibition of this release with the spinal delivery of morphine set the trend for spinal drug delivery in the treatment of acute and chronic pain.

In the late 1980s, changes in spinal function secondary to peripheral nerve injury were beginning to be understood and animal models of neuropathic pain were developed that permitted the assessment of the pharmacology of nociception at the spinal level. These models have allowed for a better understanding of the role of different transmitter-receptor systems (i.e., neuropeptides) and ion channels (i.e., sodium, and N-type calcium) in nociceptive processing. This has led to the development and utilization of a variety of agents delivered spinally for the treatment of acute and chronic pain [i.e., opioids, sodium channel blockers, N-type channel blockers, adenosine agonists, and γ-aminobutyric acid (GABA) agonists].

With improvements in the technology of spinal drug delivery, it is now possible to deliver a variety of therapeutic agents via implanted ports, pumps, and externalized catheters (described below).

Box 8-1   History of Spinal Drug Delivery

1885: Corning delivered intrathecal cocaine in the dog
1899: Bier injected local anesthetic intrathecally
1935: First spinal cannulation by Love using a 5 French ureteral catheter
1942: Manalan performed a continuous caudal anesthesia using a malleable Lemmon needle
1942: Introduction of smaller catheters
1945: Intrathecal catheter placed using a Huber needle
1949: Tuohy needle used for epidural cannulation
1982: First programmable pump delivering morphine implanted
1984: Implanted programmable pump used to deliver baclofen
1988: SynchroMed programmable pump released for market

PHARMACOLOGY

Drug Kinetics: Epidural Versus Intrathecal

Current knowledge of the pharmacokinetics of spinal delivered drugs arises from studies after acute delivery; very few studies exist regarding drug kinetics during chronic delivery. Factors such as the presence of a spinal catheter, fibrosis, granuloma formation, drug concentration and volume affect chronic drug delivery but not acute delivery. The following discussion is our current knowledge on acute spinal drug delivery; however, there are general principles that still apply to chronic drug delivery into the spinal canal.

After epidural administration of drugs, vascular absorption appears to be affected by the lipid solubility of the drug and the dose administered. The higher the lipid solubility, the earlier the peak plasma level. However, the higher the lipid solubility, the more variable the plasma levels, which may be attributed to varying epidural fat between patients. Epidural fat acts as a depo for the more lipid-soluble drugs. The exception to the rule of lipid solubility is meperidine, which has peak plasma levels occurring later than morphine. This may be due to the larger doses of meperidine administered; this phenomenon has also been demonstrated in animals. After epidural meperidine, there is an initial rapid increase in plasma levels in the first 10 minutes followed by a gradual increase that occurs between 10 to 45 minutes. This phenomenon is not seen with epidural morphine.

When compared to an intravenous and intramuscular injection, epidural opioids tend to resemble an intravenous injection. After epidural administration, peak plasma levels tend to occur earlier than with intramuscular injections and are less sustained. Except for the first 2 minutes, epidural opioids follow kinetics very similar to the intravenous route. This demonstrates the rapid and extensive absorption of the epidural opioids into the vasculature. Thus, epidural opioids given in sufficiently high doses will begin to act systemically as well as locally on the spinal cord. Increased blood flow through the epidural venous plexus will increase the vascular absorption. This increase in vascular absorption will reduce the concentration gradient between the epidural space and cerebrospinal fluid (CSF). Also, increased intra-abdominal and intrathoracic pressure can redirect blood flow up the basi-vertebral system to deliver potentially high doses of opioids directly to the brain. This is the most likely explanation of the systemic effects seen with epidural opioids because only a small fraction (perhaps as low as .1%) of morphine found in the plasma is able to penetrate into the central nervous system. This low penetration is unlikely to have much of a systemic effect through systemic redistribution unless large doses are given. It has also been demonstrated in human and animal studies that meperidine administered intravenously partitions from the plasma to the CSF. Although there is a much more favorable partitioning into the central nervous system after intraspinal administration, opioids administered in repeated doses will eventually result in enough systemic accumulation to result in systemic side effects because of the concomitant partitioning from plasma to the central nervous system. The same holds for the concomitant systemic and intraspinal administration of opioids.

The potentially high level of opioid in the basi-vertebral plexus may account for early peak cisternal levels of the lipid-soluble opioids. Since blood in the basi-vertebral system is so close to the site of administration of the opioid, levels will most likely be high while blood samples taken at more peripheral sites (such as the extremities) may be much lower and may not reflect transfer of the opioid from the blood to cisternal CSF. Peak plasma levels after intrathecal administration of opioids tend to occur later than after epidural administration, as demonstrated with morphine and sufentanil. Again, the exception to this rule applies to meperidine (one study showed earlier peak plasma levels).

The same factors that apply to vascular absorption also apply to meningeal penetration. Both animal and human studies demonstrate that the more lipid-soluble drugs have earlier peak CSF levels. Peak pain relief after epidural opioids seems to coincide with peak CSF levels, which demonstrates that the analgesia associated with epidural opioids is due to an action at the spinal cord level. The exception to this is meperidine, which has a peak pain relief that coincides with peak plasma levels. It has been hypothesized that epidural narcotics are delivered to the dorsal horn of the spinal cord via the radicular arteries. But if this were the case, then peak analgesia would coincide with peak plasma levels, which is not true. The effect of injectate volume and adrenaline on vascular uptake and dural transfer are probably minimal; however, further studies on the more lipid-soluble drugs are needed.

Due to the difficulty in sampling cisternal CSF, there are unanswered questions on the extent of rostral spread of intraspinal narcotics. It is generally accepted that the more water-soluble narcotics have a more rostral spread due to a decrease rate of vascular absorption. After epidural morphine, human studies demonstrate that peak cisternal CSF levels occur much later than peak plasma levels. Of interest is that after epidural fentanyl in humans, peak cisternal levels occur much earlier than after morphine. This same phenomenon is demonstrated in animals after epidural sufentanil. These studies appear to point toward vascular redistribution of the more lipid-soluble opioids to the cisternal CSF; however, both animal and human studies refute the possibility of this vascular redistribution as peak cisternal CSF levels are much higher than peak plasma levels. As mentioned ear-

lier, this redistribution may be through the basi-vertebral venous plexus in the epidural space. Levels of opioid in this system would be much higher than blood levels from sites more peripheral from the site of opioid administration. Therefore, blood levels measured in these studies would not reflect the transfer of the opioid from the vasculature to the cisternal CSF.

Many factors influence the CSF distribution of opioids after subarachnoid administration. Advanced age may influence rostral spread because of decreased vascular absorption of the opioid from the CSF. The height of the patient, anatomic configuration of the spinal column, positioning of the patient, and baricity of the opioid solution influences rostral spread of intrathecal local anesthetics; therefore, it is likely that these influence rostral spread of intrathecal opioids. The effect of changes in intra-abdominal/thoracic pressure on rostral spread of intrathecal opioids is due to changes in the CSF volume. As previously discussed, the effects of intra-abdominal/thoracic pressure on the vascular redistribution of epidural opioids are by another mechanism. Due to the turbulence created by direct intrathecal injections, the rate and volume of injection influence rostral spread. With the slow delivery of implanted pumps, turbulence is not a factor in the distribution. Direct intrathecal administration results in very high concentrations of opioid at the site of administration; therefore, higher doses will create higher concentration gradients, thus greater rostral spread. Finally, the lipid solubility is an important factor in rostral spread since the more lipid-soluble drugs are absorbed more rapidly into the spinal cord and vasculature, thus limiting rostral spread. Due to the low vascular absorption of intrathecal opioids, it would appear unlikely that vascular redistribution accounts for rostral spread. However, one study demonstrated that after intrathecal meperidine peak ventricular levels occurred later than peak plasma levels, but vascular redistribution accounted for the movement of meperidine into the ventricular CSF. It may be that cisternal levels are due to rostral spread in the CSF, while ventricular levels are due to vascular redistribution. Animal studies demonstrate that after intrathecal administration of morphine, the rostral spread is highly variable and unpredictable.

Clinical Utilization of Spinally Administered Drugs (Box 8-2)

Opioids and Sodium Channel Antagonists
Through the μ, κ, and δ receptors spinally administered opioids induce a postsynaptic hyperpolarization of the cell membrane by increasing potassium conductance. In addition, activation of these receptors results in a presynaptic inhibition of voltage sensitive calcium channels resulting in decreased neurotransmitter release

---

Box 8-2 Drugs Used for Chronic Spinal Delivery

Current Drugs:
Opioids—Morphine, Hydromorphone, Fentanyl, Sufentanil, Meperidine, Methadone
Local Anesthetics—Bupivacaine, Tetracaine, Ropivacaine
α-2 Adrenergic antagonists—Clonidine
GABA agonists—Baclofen, Midazolam
Future Drugs:
N-type voltage sensitive Calcium Channel Blockers—Ziconotide
Somatostatin
NMDA receptor antagonists
Adenosine
Cholinergic antagonists—neostigmine

---

from C fibers. The effects on the presynaptic and post-synaptic membranes result in a potent analgesia. The potent effects of μ and δ agonists upon small sensory afferent terminal excitability provide a functional explanation for the potent effects of these agents upon pain resulting from small afferent input (e.g., acute nociception) as well as the facilitated states that arise from persistent small afferent activation (e.g., as in the "wind-up" of dorsal horn neurons). The effects of spinal opiates on the thermal hyperalgesia induced by nerve injury but not the allodynia may result from the absence of opiate receptors on the spinal terminals of low-threshold mechanoreceptors that are believed to mediate the evoked allodynic state.

Opioids are the most commonly used drugs for long-term spinal drug therapy for pain control. Morphine is the only opioid with Food and Drug Administration (FDA) approval for long-term intrathecal delivery and is the "gold standard." Morphine has been demonstrated to be safe and effective for chronic delivery. When intrathecal morphine is no longer effective for pain relief, the physician may choose other opioids. Although these alternative opioids are commonly used chronically, there are very few reports on efficacy and safety. The rationale supporting the chronic use of these alternative agents is derived from the acute delivery for postoperative and labor pain.

Wide variations in the total daily dose of morphine are reported in the literature. For continuous delivery, the limitation to the total daily dose partly depends upon the drug solution concentration. The higher the concentration, the longer the pump can deliver between refills. Higher daily doses will require more frequent refills. The upper dose for morphine sulfate is limited by the apparent solubility (approximately 60 mg/ml). No systematic studies exist on the safety of such concentrations; however, there is evidence in animal studies that high concentrations of morphine predispose to granuloma formation. Compounding drugs near the limit of their solubility raises further concern of the potential risk of precipitation within the pump and the possibility of unexpected precipitation in drug mixtures.

Other opioids that are used intrathecally include hydromorphone, fentanyl, sufentanil, and meperidine. Hydromorphone is an attractive, alternative choice because the kinetics are similar to morphine. It is available in concentrations up to 10 mg/ml but can be compounded to higher concentrations. Sufentanil and meperidine are thought to have local anesthetic properties that may contribute to the analgesic effect. The δ opioid agonist DADL (d-ala-2-d-leu 5 enkephalin) has been shown to be effective in long delivery in a single case study with cancer pain and in single-dose trials with cancer patients. Butorphanol, a modestly selective κ-agonist, has been reported to have activity in postoperative pain.

Determining the efficacy of long-term intraspinal drug therapy remains one of the greatest challenges in chronic pain management. To date, there is only one published and one unpublished controlled study evaluating efficacy of long-term intrathecal morphine. All other studies rely on retrospective reviews of large numbers of patients with limited follow-up. Therefore, the true efficacy of long-term intrathecal therapy with morphine has yet to be determined.

One of the reasons for the lack of controlled trials is that the high cost and invasiveness of such treatment ethically precludes a double-blind, placebo controlled study design. Therefore, we can only rely on the retrospective reviews of patients receiving this therapy and attempt to make conclusions on the efficacy of this treatment. Future studies may focus on open label prospective trials with carefully designed algorithms for drug dosing or randomized controlled trials comparing intrathecal drug therapy with conventional medical management. This may allow for better conclusions on the true efficacy of long-term intraspinal drug therapy.

Many studies have attempted to determine efficacy of long-term intraspinal morphine therapy based on classification of the pain. However, a review of these articles reveals large discrepancies in pain classification between studies. Because pain is often multifactorial (i.e., failed back syndrome), and it is difficult to determine what pain syndromes are the most responsive to this therapy.

Even with high-dose intraspinal opioids, some pain syndromes do not respond, and a logical next step is the addition of local anesthetics. Several reports in the literature use this method, with most of them reviewing cancer pain. However, like the studies on intraspinal morphine alone, studies on opioid/local anesthetic mixtures are very limited and no strong conclusions can be made. Reports of morphine/bupivacaine combination therapy demonstrate that patients with pain refractory to intraspinal opioids alone may respond to the addition of a local anesthestic. These studies report a wide range of daily bupivacaine doses with few side effects.

There are many drug-related side effects with intraspinal delivery. Rarely are these side effects serious or life-threatening, and they are usually reversible on decreasing the dose or discontinuing the drug. Most side effects spontaneously resolve with the exception of sweating and peripheral edema, which persist. Other less common side effects reported in the literature include paranoia, hyperalgesia/myoclonus Meniere-like symptoms, nystagmus, and polyarthralgia.

Whereas most side effects of intrathecal morphine are not dose-related, bupivacaine-induced side effects are dose-related. These side effects are related to the anesthetic effects of the bupivacaine at the spinal level and include paresthesias, motor and sensory blockade, arterial hypotension, and urinary retention. Diarrhea has also been reported with the use of intrathecal bupivacaine. All of these side effects begin occurring at daily doses of > 45 mg/day. However, these dosing recommendations were acquired from cancer patients with limited follow-up. End-stage cancer patients are often bedridden, making it difficult to make conclusions on efficacy and side effects.

α-2 Adrenergic Agonists

Like the opioids, α-2 agonists depress the release of C fiber transmitters such as substance P and calcitonin gene related peptide and hyperpolarize the post-synaptic membrane through a Gi coupled potassium channel. As with opiates, they are active in models of thermal hyperalgesia, but unlike opiates, they display considerable potency in models of nerve injury evoked tactile allodynia. The known mechanism of action for the α-2 agonists does not explain why these agents are effective against tactile allodynia in contrast to the spinal opiates.

Clonidine (Duraclon) is FDA-approved for epidural use in cancer pain only. However, there are reports of the use of intrathecal clonidine for both cancer and non-malignant pain. Daily intrathecal doses as high as 400 µg have been reported with no untoward effects. Tramadol produces analgesia through both opiate and adrenergic mechanisms. Epidural administration of doses sufficiently high to provide a significant systemic analgesic effect (50 to 100 mg) were shown to produce postoperative analgesia in humans, but it is not clear from these clinical studies whether the epidural route is associated with a significant spinal mechanism of action.

The most convincing studies on the efficacy of intraspinal clonidine are from Rauck in 1993 and Eisenach in 1995. Rauck et al[2] reported on a series of 19 patients with reflex sympathetic dystrophy who received a continuous epidural infusion of clonidine. All patients were screened with a single epidural injection of clonidine in a placebo-controlled blinded fashion, and those who responded were given the option of a continuous infusion. The mean follow-up was 43 days with an average daily clonidine dose of 768 µg. The mean pain scores decreased from 7.1 out of 10 pre-infusion to 5.1 out of 10 postinfusion. Side effects were mild and transient and did not result in any patient discontinuing therapy.

The largest study to date was published by Eisenach et al[3] who used a double-blind placebo controlled trial of epidural clonidine for the management of cancer pain. They used epidural morphine as a rescue. The mean follow-up was 8 weeks and the total daily dose used was 720 µg. They reported that pain relief was better in the clonidine group, but there was no difference in morphine requirements between the groups. They also noted that clonidine was quite effective in the management of neuropathic pain.

There are few side effects associated with clonidine even at higher doses. The most common side effects are hypotension, bradycardia, and sedation. These side effects are often well-tolerated and do not necessitate discontinuation of the drug. The hypotensive effect of intrathecal clonidine likely occurs secondary to the effects of the drug on the preganglionic fibers in the thoracic spinal cord. The sedative effect most likely occurs secondary to actions primarily in the locus ceruleus in the brainstem.

γ-Aminobutyric Acid Agonists

The GABA receptor is a G-protein-coupled receptor. Activation of a GABA receptor evokes a hyperpolarization of the membrane mediated by Gi protein coupled with an increase in potassium conductance, or a decrease in the opening of voltage sensitive Ca^{2+} channels that serve to attenuate terminal transmitter release. Receptor autoradiography indicates that GABA sites are found throughout the spinal cord with the highest concentrations in the substantia gelatinosa. Unilateral rhizotomy and capsaicin treatment both reduced GABA binding, suggesting a location both presynaptic and post-synaptic to the primary afferent; however, baclofen has no effect upon the spinal release of substance P.

Baclofen is FDA-approved for the treatment of spasticity, although it has been shown to have analgesic properties. There are a few reports on the use of intrathecal baclofen both as a single agent and in combination with other drugs for chronic pain management.

Future Drugs

N-Type Voltage Sensitive Calcium Channel Blockers: Localization studies with SNX-111 binding or subunit antibodies indicate that N-type channels are in high levels in the substantia gelatinosa and are frequently found on membranes of profiles that contain substance P. Extensive characterization of the role of N-type calcium channels in dorsal root ganglion cells emphasizes their role in transmitter release. Blockade of N-type channels will reduce dorsal horn glutamate release. This effect upon glutamatergic transmission and the role of spinal glutamate in facilitatory states is thus consistent with the observed profile of intrathecal N type voltage sensitive calcium channel blockers. Studies have shown that an intrathecal N-type Ca channel antagonist (Ziconotide) will attenuate neuropathic pain conditions in patients suffering from neuropathic and cancer pain. Daily doses range from 2.5 to 25 µg. It is being evaluated in a multicenter study as an intrathecal agent for the treatment of chronic malignant and nonmalignant pain. Common side effects with Ziconotide include dizziness, nausea, nystagmus, gait imbalance, confusion, constipation, and urinary retention.

Somatostatin: The effects of intrathecal somatostatin (SST) are likely mediated by one or more of the five somatostatin receptors referred to as SSTR1-SSTR5. Several of these receptors are found in the primary afferents and in the spinal gray matter, while others show significant concentration in the ventral horn. Electrophysiologically, somatostatin can hyperpolarize a cell though a G protein coupled inwardly rectifying K current and block the opening of coupled calcium channels that serve to reduce transmitter release. Conversely, it should be emphasized that somatostatin can produce significant depolarization in part by augmenting the synaptic actions. The literature on the spinal analgesic actions of SST or an analogue (SST) in humans is largely anecdotal and controversial. Somatostatin was reported to have analgesic actions in postoperative and cancer pain states, though such efficacy was considered controversial when examined in blinded studies.[4] Intrathecal Octreotide was reported effective in two nonmalignant pain patients. In 6 of 8 patients suffering in the terminal stages of malignancy, somatostatin was able to produce some degree of pain relief. All patients showed a very rapid escalation of drug dose over the brief period of infusion, perhaps reflecting either the rapidly escalating pain state or a very rapid tolerance development.

There is little doubt that SST can influence spinal nociceptive processing. It is reasonable, however, to hypothesize that its controversial effects and potential toxicity may be associated with one or more of the five subtypes of receptors, given the multiple receptor populations that exit in the spinal cord. The development of appropriate analogues for these classes of receptors may provide insight and appropriate prospects for development.

N-Methyl-D-Aspartate (NMDA) Receptor Antagonists: The NMDA receptor, a calcium ionophore, is activated by glutamate. The release of glutamate and occupancy of the NMDA receptor serves to depolarize the membrane and increase intracellular calcium. The opening of the channel is regulated by several additional components:

1. A magnesium block that is removed by membrane depolarization.
2. Allosterically coupled sites occupied by glycine and polyamines required for channel activation.
3. Phosphorylation sites that serve to enhance glutamate-evoked NMDA receptor opening. The opening of the channel may be prevented by: competitively antagonizing the occupancy by glutamate of the receptor; blocking the channel; or by blocking the allosterically coupled glycine site.

Tissue injury evokes a significant increase in spinal glutamate release and results in well-defined allodynia and hyperalgesia, mediated by the activation of the NMDA receptor (wind-up). Ketamine, a noncompetitive NMDA antagonist, has been given epidurally for postoperative pain with modest results. There is little information regarding the use of intrathecal NMDA antagonists in chronic pain states. Spinal administration of CPP, a competitive NMDA antagonist, suppresses allodynia but not spontaneous pain in a patient with a peripheral nerve injury. Most of the reports on the efficacy of long-term intraspinal ketamine are anecdotal. There are several reports on the use of ketamine/morphine combinations for terminal cancer pain with good results. There are also questions about the toxicity of chronic intraspinal ketamine. Karpinski et al[5] reported on a case of a terminal cancer patient who received a 3-week intrathecal infusion of ketamine prior to death. An autopsy demonstrated subpial vascular myelopathy. The long-term safety of intrathecal ketamine is unclear.

Adenosine: A1 receptors are located in high concentrations in the substantia gelatinosa, but they appear to be largely on nonprimary afferent terminals, a finding consistent with the inability of A1 agonists to block substance P release from primary afferents. Evidence suggests that adenosine, through the A1 receptor, may diminish glutamate release from spinal systems. Consistent with this effect upon spinal glutamate release, a single unit recording from dorsal horn wide dynamic range neurons emphasizes that A1 agonists can diminish wind-up without altering Aa evoked activity. Consistent with the preclinical observations, acute delivery of the adenosine A1 selective agonist in humans has been shown to diminish the allodynia elicited by vibration and touch in neuropathic pain patients. Rane and colleagues[6] have recently reported that the bolus intrathecal delivery of adenosine in human volunteers will reduce the areas of secondary allodynia after local skin inflammation and forearm ischemic pain ratings. Eisenach[7] demonstrated that the intrathecal but not the intravenous delivery of an adenosine agonist suppressed allodynia of neuropathic pain. At present there are no reports of chronic spinal delivery of adenosinergic agents in humans.

Cholinergic Agonists: M3 binding sites have been localized in laminae I to III of the dorsal horn. M2 binding sites are present throughout the dorsal and ventral horns and background levels of M1 binding are noted. M4 binding has also been observed. Studies have shown that Muscarinic receptors in dorsal horn can enhance GABA release. Others have shown that muscarinic agonists' activity can also enhance nitric oxide release. Electrophysiologically, muscarinic receptors appear to mediate a presynaptic inhibition that can regulate monosynaptic reflex activity. Tolerance to the analgesic effect of cholinomimetics occurs rapidly in animal models of antinociception. Intrathecal neostigmine (an acetylcholinesterase inhibitor) produces analgesia in humans; however, at doses that are analgesic in human volunteers, IT neostigmine is associated with nausea and vomiting and lower extremity weakness as well as increases in blood pressure and heart rate.

Combination Spinal Drug Therapies

There are several persuasive reasons to anticipate that codelivery of agents with distinct mechanisms of action may be therapeutically advantageous. First, as indicated above and discussed in detail elsewhere, many clinical pain states are a composite of several mechanisms (e.g., acute afferent drive from the injury site, the persistent ongoing input that leads to a facilitated state, and the central changes after nerve injury that lead to anomalous pain processing not dependent upon small afferent input). In such states, it is reasonable to presume that an agent with a defined mechanism of action may include a component but not all components of the systems that underlie the specific pain state. Secondly, there is strong evidence that the agents may not display cross tolerance (e.g., μ and ∂

and μ and α_2) and attenuate the concurrent development of tolerance otherwise associated with an equipotent dose of a single drug given alone. Finally, even for pain states that are mediated by the same mechanism, agents that act on different elements of the systems may display nonlinear interactions that enhance the therapeutic ratio. Numerous studies have emphasized that spinally delivered agents may show positively synergistic interactions regarding modulation of nociceptive processing. For example, in the interaction between spinal μ-opioid and α_2 agonists, an enhanced nociception can result without an attendant increasing respiratory depression or hypotension.

INTRASPINAL DRUG DELIVERY TECHNIQUES

There are basically three types of intraspinal delivery techniques: (1) an externalized system; (2) a partially externalized system; and (3) a totally implanted system. Each technique has different risks and costs that are taken into account when deciding which approach to use. Parameters of drug delivery (e.g., infusion rates and bolus injection volumes) depend on a variety of factors (Box 8-3).

Externalized Systems

Externalized epidural catheters are the most widely used techniques for delivering drugs to the perispinal space. Such systems are designed for short-term (hours to days) use, but have been successfully used for longer-term delivery (weeks to months). The use of an externalized catheter leads to a possible concern that the catheter will develop a local infection at the exit site and that the catheter may serve as a favorable access track for either an epidural or intrathecal infection. Because of the potential risk of infection, extended placement of externalized systems are usually reserved

---

Box 8-3 Intraspinal Drug Delivery Techniques

Current Systems
Externalized systems
Partially externalized systems
Totally implanted systems:
    SynchroMed Infusion System (programmable, battery operated)
    Arrow Continuous Flow Infusion System (constant flow rate)
    IsoMed Infusion System (constant flow rate)

for the epidural route only. In the terminally ill patient, the risk: benefit ratio may justify the intrathecal route with an externalized system. The incidence of infection is reviewed below. Some practitioners tunnel these catheters under the skin for some distance to provide stability and reduce the likelihood of inadvertent withdrawal. It is postulated that this maneuver will decrease the chance of infection. There is currently only one FDA-approved externalized intrathecal delivery system, which is the Algoline Intraspinal catheter. It is approved for use up to 30 days. Extensive work with percutaneous catheters for parenteral drug delivery for cancer patients led to the development of the Hickman catheter, which possesses a Dacron cuff for antimicrobial protection. Epidural catheters for chronic placement, such as the DuPen, Algoline (Medtronics, Inc.), SKY (PMT, Inc.), and E-Cath catheter have such fittings. Dacron cuffs at the exit site are believed to minimize catheter site and catheter-related infection risks. The Dacron cuff also results in catheter anchorage to the subcutaneous tissue at the exit site.

Partially Externalized Systems

Partially externalized systems are those in which the catheter is placed by a needle inserted into the target site through a small incision of the skin. The external end of the catheter is then connected to an access port, which is placed under the skin. The port is secured by suture loops. The incision is then sutured closed. Injections are made by placing a needle though the skin and into the access port. The Port-a-Cath epidural port system (Pharmacia-Deltec, Inc., St. Paul, MN) is the only FDA-approved implanted port system.

While it is clear that the subcutaneous systems permits freedom of movement, reduces the risk of catheter removal, and eases the impediment to patient movement, it may be asked whether the use of the subcutaneous port confers any safety benefit compared to a well-maintained percutaneous system. A study by deJong and Kansen[8] considered the infection rate of three epidural catheter techniques: a subcutaneous port, a non-tunneled externalized catheter, and a tunneled externalized catheter. They concluded that when the infection rate was indexed to catheter days, the number of infections per 1000 catheter days in the injection port group was half that of the percutaneous group (2.86 infections vs 5.97 for percutaneous catheters). No injection port became infected in the subcutaneous group during the first 70 days of treatment, whereas infections occurred in the percutaneous group as early as the first week. Another study showed no infections in 252 patients using the subcutaneous port system. From these studies, it appears that subcutaneous port systems are superior to externalized systems if long-term use is

anticipated. There are no currently approved externalized or partially externalized systems for intrathecal use. However, the Port-a-Cath system has been successfully used for intrathecal drug delivery.

Totally Implanted Systems

Totally implanted systems are those with the catheter and delivery system completely implanted. They have the advantage of a lower risk of infection and allowing the patient more independence. The totally implanted systems are more expensive and require a greater surgical intervention than the externalized or partially externalized systems. Accordingly, patients should be carefully selected. These systems are generally reserved for patients with a life expectancy of greater than one year, although some physicians have routinely decreased this to 6 months (see Economics section).

There are currently three approved commercially available devices; these include the SynchroMed Infusion System (Medtronic Neurological, Minneapolis, MN), Arrow Constant Flow Implantable System (Arrow Int., Reading, PA), and the IsoMed Constant Flow System (Medtronic Neurological, Minneapolis, MN). These systems are accessed percutaneously for pump refills. Pump refills are required at intervals depending on the infusion rates and the size of the pump reservoir. All three pumps have direct access ports to the cerebrospinal fluid for bolusing or aspiration. The infusion systems are implanted in the lower abdominal wall and connected to a catheter that is tunneled subcutaneously around the abdominal wall into the cerebrospinal fluid (CSF).

The SynchroMed Infusion System (SIS) is the only implantable pump that is programmable. The pump is programmed externally through a radio-telemetry link. The programmability allows for a variety of infusion modes, which includes continuous infusion, continuous-complex infusion (increases and decreases throughout the day), single bolus, and intermittent bolus. It comes in two models, one with a 10ml and one with an 18ml reservoir. These reservoir volumes are smaller than the other two pumps but because of the extremely low flow rates that can be achieved, pump refills may only be required up to 60 days. The pump reservoir is accessed through a centrally located access port. The side port that has direct access to the CSF is some distance from the refill port. Pump refills of the reservoir use a 22-gauge needle, and the CSF side port requires a 25-gauge needle for entry, thus providing an additional safety mechanism. The battery life is from 3 to 5 years after which the pump must be removed and replaced. The SIS is approved for intrathecal morphine and baclofen.

The Arrow Continuous Flow Infusion System (ACFIS) is only approved for intrathecal morphine. This pump is not programmable and has a factory preset flow rate (low, medium, or high). The flow rate is controlled by a flow restrictor that controls the flow rate based on the drug viscosity. Therefore, flow rates may vary for different drugs based on differences in viscosity. A significant increase in drug viscosity may occur with very high concentrations, thus impairing the flow rate (e.g., the flow rate for water in a medium flow pump is 1.1 ml/day and for morphine sulfate it is 1.0 ml/day). In addition, changes in body temperature and atmospheric pressure will change the flow rate by affecting the gas pressure within the system. Because it is not programmable, to increase the amount of drug delivered, the pump must be refilled with a higher or lower drug concentration. This usually results in more frequent pump accessing initially. The infusion is driven by Freon; therefore, it does not require replacement, as does the SIS. The pump is available in two reservoir volumes of 16 ml and 30 ml. Whereas the SIS and the Infusaid System have a direct access side port to the CSF separate from the pump refill access port, the ACFIS direct CSF and pump refill port are accessed through the same septum. There is a built-in safety mechanism that prevents direct injection into the CSF when filling the pump.

The IsoMed Infusion System (IMIS) (Medtronic Inc., Minneapolis, MN) is similar to the ACFIS in all aspects except that it has a CSF access port separate from the central reservoir fill port. As with the SIS, the CSF side port requires a 25-gauge needle for access. The pump is available in three factory preset flow rates of 0.5, 1.0, or 1.5 ml/day. It is also available in three reservoir sizes, 20 ml, 35 ml, and 60 ml.

Future Directions

One disadvantage of the totally implanted spinal drug delivery systems is the lack of control of drug delivery by the patient. For the SIS system, there is one device in clinical trials that is a hand-held programmer that allows the patient to self-administer drug boluses. Restrictions and lockouts are programmed into the system to enhance patient safety and prevent drug overdose.

Although the currently available systems are only FDA-approved for the use of morphine (SIS, ACFIS, IMIS) and baclofen (SIS), it is common practice to use drug combinations off label. The disadvantage of this is that when infusion rates are increased, both drugs are increased. A pump that has a duel reservoir with the ability to independently increase or decrease the infusion of each drug is in development.

PATIENT SELECTION

Before considering implantable therapy, the patient should have progressed through the pain treatment con-

tinuum of the World Health Organization ladder. This assures that the patient has been given a fair trial of more conservative therapies before embarking on invasive pain treatment therapies. One area of controversy is when a spinal cord stimulator should be utilized versus spinal drug delivery. Spinal cord stimulation is considered a more conservative therapy since there are no drugs involved and there is less utilization of the healthcare system for management. As discussed below, with newer spinal agents for neuropathic pain, the decision to use spinal cord stimulation versus spinal drug delivery should be based more on pain distribution. With advancements in the technology of spinal cord stimulation, this view may become obscure. The current recommendation is spinal cord stimulation for axial pain with extremity pain and spinal drug delivery for axial or truncal pain.

Nociceptive pain is mediated by an intact and functioning nervous system. Neuropathic pain is elicited by a damaged peripheral or central nervous system. Historically, it was thought that nociceptive pain is more responsive to intrathecal drug therapy, whereas neuropathic pain is more responsive to spinal cord stimulation. However, with the development of nonopioid drugs, this consensus may not necessarily be true. Preclinical studies have demonstrated that the spinal delivery of agents such as clonidine, sodium, and calcium channel blockers is more effective than the opioids in treating neuropathic pain. With these better drugs and better technology for spinal cord stimulation, definite lines between spinal cord stimulation and spinal drug delivery are obscured.

Another area of controversy is the absence or presence of a known pain generator. Should patients without an identified pain generator be managed with implantables? An example is the low back pain patient with normal imaging studies, no physical findings, and negative diagnostic injections. These patients present a dilemma since undiagnosed psychological disorders may be overshadowing the problem. Objective evidence of pathology is more important for nonmalignant pain than for malignant pain because of psychological issues that surround pain of unknown etiology. It is not to say that patients without objective evidence of pathology should be excluded, rather they should be evaluated closely for psychological issues (discussed below). If they are declared psychologically stable for implantation, then the clinician should proceed even in the absence of objective pathology.

Inclusion/Exclusion Criteria (Box 8-4)
Inclusion Criteria
1. Pain type and generator appropriate (see discussion above).
2. Demonstration of opioid responsiveness. This is another area of controversy. Historically, it has been a requirement to demonstrate some response to

systemically administered opioids. The decision to proceed with spinal drug delivery was usually made if the patient experienced a partial, unacceptable response or unacceptable side effects in spite of adequate pain relief. In the absence of any appreciable pain relief at reasonable doses of an opioid in a nociceptive pain patient probably precludes the use of intraspinal opioids. However, this criterion is controversial for neuropathic pain. It has been demonstrated in the Chung model of neuropathic pain that intrathecal opioids are ineffective in relieving pain, whereas systemic opioids are effective.[9] This is an example of where a partial response of a systemically administered opioid in no way predicts the effect of the intrathecal opioid. This explains why some patients still require systemic opioids in addition to the spinal nonopioid agents. However, most patients that demonstrate some response to systemic opioids will respond to spinal opioids. A general rule of thumb is that the closer the injury is to the central nervous system, the less likely pharmacological therapy will be effective, whether you are using opioids or nonopioids. Demonstration of opioid responsiveness is a strict criterion, but if used, there will be fewer failures. It is unlikely that neuropathic pain will be able to be managed with a nonopioid alone. The nonopioid is usually added to the opioid to enhance analgesia.

3. Psychological clearance (see discussion below).
4. Successful completion of a screening trial (see discussion below).

Exclusion Criteria

1. Absolute: Aplastic anemia; systemic infection; allergy to implant materials; allergy to intended medications

(this is rarely a problem since there are a number of drugs to choose from); or certain psychological-behavioral features (see discussion below).

2. Relative: Emaciated patient (the size of the pump precludes implantation into an emaciated patient due to the risk of wound breakdown and extrusion; there must be an appropriate amount of fat tissue to create a pocket); ongoing anticoagulation therapy; child before fusion of the epiphyses; occult infection possible; recovering drug addict; lack of social or family support; socioeconomic problems; or lack of access to medical care.

Psychological Screening

Most experts will agree that psychological screening is mandatory prior to embarking on chronic intraspinal drug therapy. In spite of this consensus, there are few reports on the efficacy of psychological screening in predicting outcome. This probably reflects the research challenges in this area and the difficulties in predicting long-term success based on psychological screening. However, there are some reports in the literature supporting psychological screening.[10] In general, these studies find that patients with a psychological profile deemed appropriate for implantable therapy have better outcomes than those deemed inappropriate. However, there are some early reports that question the utility of a psychological evaluation in predicting outcome. Several studies state that depression, hysteria, and hypochondriasis are very common in pain patients and do not constitute a contraindication to implants. Burton[11] went as far as to question the need for psychological evaluation per se, but did admit that psychological testing can identify significant problems that may interfere with long-term success. There have been others that have agreed with this belief; however, specialists with the most experience with implantables for pain relief hold strong to the belief that psychological screening is crucial to the long-term success of implantables for chronic pain management. Most of this literature involves spinal cord stimulation; however, this information can be applied to chronic intraspinal drug delivery.

Most of the studies in this area use the Minnesota Multiphasic Personality Inventory (MMPI) as a predictor of outcome with spinal implantables. North et al[12] reported on the predictive value of psychological testing on the outcome of spinal cord stimulation. He concluded that low scores on two psychological traits, anxiety and problems with authority (as measured by the Derogatis Affects Balance Scale and the Wiggins scales of the MMPI, respectively) predicted pain relief following a spinal cord stimulation trial but not 3 months after permanent electrode implantation. They pointed out that their sample could have been biased, but they still supported psychological screening. Burchiel et al[13] studied

---

Box 8-4 Inclusion/Exclusion Criteria for Chronic Spinal Drug Delivery

Inclusion criteria
    Pain type and generator appropriate
    Demonstration of responsiveness
    Psychological clearance
Exclusion criteria
    Absolute:
        Aplastic anemia
        Systemic infection
        Allergy to implant materials or intended drug
    Relative:
        Emaciated patient
        Ongoing anticoagulation therapy
        Child before fusion of the epiphyses
        Socioeconomic problems
        Lack of access to medical care

40 patients with chronic low back and leg pain who underwent spinal cord stimulation. They used the MMPI, the visual analogue pain rating scale (VAS), the McGill Pain Questionnaire (MPQ), the Oswestry Disability Questionnaire, the Beck Depression Inventory, and the Sickness Impact Profile to predict treatment outcome. Regression analysis revealed that increased patient age and MMPI D subscale scores correlated with poor outcomes. Higher scores on the evaluative subscale of the MPQ correlated with an improved outcome. From this study, they developed the following equation, which correctly predicted success or failure at 3 months in 88% of their patients: % delta VAS = 112.57 − 1.98 (D) − 1.68 (Age) + 35.54 (MPQe). Brandwin and Kewman[14] found that treatment-resistant patients had relatively lower hysteria and hypochondriasis scores than the successful patients. They also concluded that higher elevations of the depression scale were associated with treatment failure. Daniel et al[15] used a 6-point rating scale based on the results of a psychological interview, a pain questionnaire, a health index, the Cornell Medical Index, the MPQ, the Beck Depression Inventory, and the MMPI. They reported 76.5% accuracy in the psychologists predicting outcome based on this scale.

In a focus article, Nelson et al[16] summarized certain psychological-behavioral features that would exclude a patient from further consideration for implantable therapy (Box 8-5). These include:

Active psychosis: A psychotic patient can have very real pain but their perception of the pain is often distorted. If the psychotic patient is stabilized on neuroleptics, they may be reconsidered for implantation but carefully monitored.
Active suicidality: Stabilization of the suicidal thoughts and associated mood disturbances is necessary before further consideration.
Active homicidality: It is quite difficult to stabilize these individuals, and they are often too unstable to engage in any treatment of this sort.

Box 8-5 Psychological-Behavioral Features Precluding Implantable Therapy

Active psychosis
Active suicidality
Active homicidality
Major uncontrolled depression or other mood disorders
Somatization disorder or other somatoform disorders
Alcohol or drug dependency
Compensation of litigation resolution
Lack of appropriate social support
Neurobehavioral cognitive deficits

Major uncontrolled depression or other mood disorders: Patients with severe depression may experience increases in pain. If the depression is treated, their pain may decrease significantly to eliminate the need for invasive therapy.
Somatization disorder or other somatoform disorders: These patients are at risk of developing other symptoms in response to the implant. These exclusionary criteria should be used with caution as many chronic pain patients have vague pain complaints with no identifiable etiology.
Alcohol or drug dependency: Patients with major alcohol or drug problems who demonstrate a minimum of 3 months of appropriate control of substance use may be reconsidered.
Compensation or litigation resolution: Although treatment obstacles may occur if the patient has a monetary incentive to remain disabled by pain, most pain experts agree that these patients should be evaluated on a case-by-case basis for implantable therapy.
Lack of appropriate social support: This is not an absolute exclusionary criterion but should be considered, as the pain treatment team cannot assume all responsibility for the patient's needs.
Neurobehavioral cognitive deficits: Severe cognitive impairments may interfere with the patient's reasoning and judgment, making it difficult for them to assume the shared responsibility required for implantable therapy.

In summary, psychological testing serves as a screening tool to identify the appropriateness of invasive therapy for the management of chronic pain. Using the exclusionary criteria of Nelson et al,[16] the psychological evaluation should focus on identifying these problems that may interfere with a successful outcome. As our medical judgment on the treatment of chronic pain is not infallible, neither is psychological screening. However, when the two are used together, only positive results will follow.

Screening Techniques
Although most clinicians recommend a screening trial prior to pump placement, a screening protocol that accurately predicts a successful outcome has not been established. In general, screening trials can be divided into the following: single injection, multiple injections, or continuous infusion. There are no studies supporting one over the other, and the clinician should decide which technique is best. It is recommended that the initial screening be done as an inpatient in a monitored setting. After 24 hours of observation, the patient may have the drug continuously infused in the comfort of his or her home. In a retrospective review of 429 physicians,[17] 33.7% used a single intrathecal injection technique, 18.3% used

a multiple injection with a blinded placebo technique, and 35.3% used a continuous epidural infusion technique. The most common technique appears to be a continuous intrathecal infusion technique.

Single Injection

The single injection technique involves a single administration of drug intrathecally or epidurally. The morphine dose is usually 0.5 to 1.0 mg intrathecally or 5 to 10 mg epidurally. An intrathecal or epidural equivalent of the patient's daily systemic dose may also be used. It has the advantages of low cost, low risk, and ease of use. In addition, it probably overestimates side effects. Therefore, in the absence of side effects, it is likely that the drug will be tolerated long-term and at higher doses. Disadvantages are lack of correlation with a continuous infusion and a placebo response is more likely.

Multiple Injections

With the multiple-injection technique, the patient is administered a series of injections, either intrathecally or epidurally. Morphine doses are similar for the single-injection technique. Advantages of this technique are that the patients may receive a placebo injection for comparison with actual drug administration. A disadvantage is lack of correlation with a continuous infusion.

Continuous Infusion

A continuous infusion may be administered intrathecally or epidurally through a temporary catheter connected to an external pump. The response to therapy can be determined over days to weeks. The initial morphine dose is 20 µg/hour intrathecally or 200 µg/hour epidurally or the equivalent to the patient's daily systemic dose. The dose may be increased every 12 to 48 hours until pain relief or unacceptable side effects are reached. The advantage of this method is that it more closely mimics the implantable system. In addition, the response to therapy can be more accurately assessed in the patient's own environment while performing normal daily activities. Single injection and multiple injections are performed in the clinic or hospital setting, making it more difficult to accurately assess the patient's response.

Drug Selection and Dose

There is much uncertainty in the decision-making process surrounding intraspinal drug therapy. According to an Internet survey[18] consisting of 413 physicians who represented management of 13,342 patients, responding physicians chose morphine most often, but many other drugs were selected without clear indications. There was evidence of wide variations in clinical practice among physicians who use this modality. This led to an interdisciplinary panel with extensive clinical experience in intraspinal infusion therapy that evaluated the results of the Internet survey, the systematic reviews of the literature, and their own clinical experience. This panel proposed a scheme for the selection of drugs and doses for

intraspinal therapy. They developed a hierarchy of therapeutic strategies that can be used during the screening process. It is controversial whether one should proceed past the second line approach during the screening process. This decision should be carefully determined on a case-by-case basis (Box 8-6).

Daily Dose Limit and Concentration

There are many complicating factors that should be weighed in determining the upper daily dose limit and concentration. These factors include:

1. Availability of compounding. If one is limited to commercially available drugs, then there are limitations on drug concentrations. If a patient requires higher doses, then there will be frequent refills. Commercially available concentrations include: Morphine 50 mg/ml; Hydromorphone 10 mg/ml; Fentanyl and Sufentanil 50 µg/ml; Meperidine 100 mg/ml; Bupivacaine 7.5 mg/ml; Clonidine 500 µg/ml; and Baclofen 2000 µg/ml.
2. Refill intervals. As discussed above, higher drug dose requirements will result in frequent refills. The upper limit of doses will depend on the availability of drug compounding. The goal is to try and keep the refill intervals between 1 to 3 months.
3. Side effects.
4. Risk of inflammatory mass formation. A concern with chronic intraspinal drug delivery is the development of catheter tip inflammatory masses. It has been suggested that the risk of granuloma formation is dependent upon the concentration of the drug delivered. The exact drug concentration that will predispose to granuloma formation is unknown; however, it is recommended that the lowest concentration possible be used. In addition, preclinical studies suggest that the coadministration of clonidine may protect against granuloma formation (Yaksh, personal communication).

When performing the screening infusion trial, the clinician should mimic the long-term delivery as closely as possible. Chronic daily infusion rates may range from as low as 0.1 ml/day (with the SynchroMed pump) to 1.5 ml/day (with constant flow rate pumps). The lower limit of commonly used infusion pumps is 0.1 ml/hour, which equals 2.4 ml/day. It is unclear if there is much difference in the analgesic outcome with the same dose delivered as 0.1 ml/day versus 2.4 ml/day. However, preclinical pharmacokinetic studies have demonstrated that the drug spread through the CSF is volume dependent. Therefore, a larger volume may result in a higher dermatomal spread of the drug, which may affect analgesia. This explains why some patients report excellent analgesia during the screening trial when higher volumes are infused but find this pain relief disappears when the infusion pump is implanted and the

Box 8-6   Drug Selection for Chronic Spinal Drug Delivery

First-line approach
  a. Defined as clearly established via data and extensive clinical experience
  b. Morphine
Second-line approach
  c. Defined as limited trial data but extensive clinical experience
  d. If pain has a neuropathic component
       i. Morphine/bupivacaine
       ii. Morphine/clonidine
  e. Adequate analgesia but morphine-related toxicities
       i. Hydromorphone
Third-line approach
  f. Defined as agents that show promise but lack sufficient base of scientific data and clinical experience
       i. Morphine/bupivacaine/clonidine
       ii. Fentanyl or sufentanil
       iii. Hydromorphone, or fentanyl, or sufentanil/bupivacaine or clonidine
Fourth-line approach
  g. Defined as agents used based on physician judgment in patients with intractable pain because evidence too meager to recommend regular use
  h. For select patients only
  i. Category 1: Data supporting safety but little information on efficacy
       i. Meperidine
       ii. Methadone
       iii. Ropivacaine
       iv. Neostigmine
  j. Category 2: Anecdotal evidence of pain relief with related spasticity
       i. Baclofen
  k. Category 3: Unresolved safety issues
       i. Tetracaine
       ii. Midazolam
       iii. NMDA receptor antagonists

same dose is infused at a lower volume. The best method to mimic chronic infusion therapy is with a microinfusion pump with a lower volume of 20 mcl/hour. However, these infusion pumps are expensive, thus limiting their use.

Pump Selection

Pump selection depends on several factors. What was the final dose of drug that achieved analgesia? Is the patient limited to commercially available drugs? What daily volume of drug will be required and what will be the refill interval? Will the patient need complex continuous infusions? The answer to these questions will need to be evaluated to determine which pump is best for the patient. For example, if the patient is limited to commercially available drugs and fails morphine but responds to hydromorphone at a daily dose of 3 mg/day, a constant flow rate pump of 35 ml at 1 ml/day infusion rate would be reasonable because this would allow doses of up to 10 mg/day. A patient who is limited to commercially available drugs, fails morphine and hydromorphone, but responds to fentanyl at 50 µg/day would do well with a

constant flow rate pump of 35 ml at 1.5 ml/day that would allow a dose of up to 150 µg/day.

COMPLICATIONS

In general, the morbidity from intraspinal drug delivery is uncommon, although the risk of infection is more common with the external systems as opposed to the totally implanted systems. The morbidity can be divided into those associated with the drug delivered, those associated with the catheter system, those with the pump or port pocket, and pump system complications (Box 8-7). The risk of inflammatory mass from high concentrations of drugs was discussed above and will not be discussed further. Although there are few formal spinal toxicity studies on most spinal drugs, clinical experience demonstrates minimal if any spinal toxicity even with high concentrations of local anesthetics that have previously been shown to be toxic with acute delivery. However, high concentrations of drugs (commonly seen with drug compounding) should be used with caution. High doses of spinal opiates have been reported to induce hyperalgesia and myoclonus. These reports are consistent with the preclinical literature.

Catheter Associated Morbidity

The most serious morbidity of intraspinal catheterization is related to the catheter system. These complications include neurological complications secondary to the catheter or epidural fibrosis, catheter infection, catheter fibrosis/inflammation leading to pain on injection, obstruction, altered diffusion kinetics of the drugs delivered, and catheter malfunction.

Neurological Complications

Neurological complications from placement of an epidural or intrathecal catheter are a rare occurrence. Most severe neurological complications from epidural catheterization occur from an epidural abscess or epidural fibrosis. Even these are rare occurrences. Transient neurological abnormalities following lumbar epidural blockade are much more common than permanent abnormalities (0.1% vs 0.02%, respectively). There have been reports of paralysis associated with epidural anesthesia in the presence of spinal stenosis. The mechanism of nerve injury in spinal stenosis may be secondary to the injection of fluid into a space of limited volume, or the development of edema resulting in acute compression of the cauda equina at the level of the stenosis.

Infection

Catheter infection represents a potentially serious but infrequent complication of intraspinal catheterization. It is most common with externalized long-term catheters and patients who are immunosuppressed. With long-term catheters, the incidence of catheter insertion site infection is higher than actual nervous system infection (4.3 vs <1%). Infections may involve mild catheter colonization, deep paraspinous muscle infections, clinical meningitis, or epidural abscess. The catheter hub is regarded as the main point of entry of bacteria leading to catheter colonization; however, hematogenous spread and tracking of bacteria from the insertion site may also occur. The most common microorganisms that have been isolated from intraspinal catheters include coagulase-negative staphylococci, Staphylococcus aureus, and Gram-negative bacilli. Gram-negative bacilli and S. aureus tend to cause more serious infections. Although rare, case reports of epidural abscesses have been made with long-term epidural catheters. S. aureus is the most common bacteria isolated from epidural abscesses, followed by gram-negative rods. Patient selection and strict aseptic techniques are the most important factors in preventing catheter infection. Caution should be exercised when using intraspinal catheters in the immunocompromised or diabetic patient. Other methods that may be used to prevent catheter infection include antimicrobial dressings and the use of bacterial filters.

Catheter Fibrosis/Inflammation

Over time, both intrathecal and epidural catheters can become difficult to inject and cause pain on injection. Foreign bodies placed within the epidural and intrathecal space can induce some degree of local reactivity. The nature and magnitude of the reaction may depend upon the catheter material; however, as discussed above, the inflammatory reaction is likely due to the drug rather than the catheter. Considerable work remains to be accomplished regarding this inflammatory process. The local reaction can have two consequences. First, fibrosis/inflammation can potentially become a space-occupying intrusion into the respective space. Secondly, the fibrosis/inflammatory mass may result in altered diffusion kinetics of the drugs delivered in the epidural and intrathecal space. Fibrosis and inflammatory masses can occur with either epidural or intrathecal catheters. Most patients can achieve long-term catheterization without significant fibrosis and altered drug delivery.

Catheter Malfunction

Previous studies of intrathecal delivery systems have found catheter malfunction occurring at rates varying from 10% to 40%. Catheter malfunction can be divided into the following categories: (1) disconnection from the pump or port; (2) large to small catheter disconnect (if present); (3) kinks or holes in the catheter; (4) catheter breaks; and (5) catheter dislodgements. The implantable infusion pumps have two locations where the catheter may become disconnected, from the pump or port, or from the large to small catheter disconnect. Over time, the catheters may develop a kink or hole and may also break anywhere along the catheter. Penn et al[19] performed a prospective study of thin and thick walled intrathecal catheter reliability in 102 patients. Sixty percent of the patients had no catheter complications; the remaining patients had one to five complications. Most of the complications occurred in the thin-walled Silastic catheter. The authors concluded that the thin-walled Silastic catheter does not perform well and the larger, thick-walled catheters should be used. Presently, most of the catheters in use are thick walled.

Pump or Port Pocket Problems

Complications that can occur in the pocket include hematoma, seroma, and infection. Hematomas usually occur immediately postoperatively. Meticulous care should be taken to control all bleeding prior to surgical incision closure as the development of a hematoma provides a nidus for infection and the pocket may require surgical exploration to evacuate the hematoma. Hematomas can be prevented by appropriately screening the patients for coagulopathies prior to pump implantation.

Seromas may also develop around the pump or port. As with hematomas, seromas may also increase the chances of infection in the presence of a foreign body. If the patient develops a seroma, it can be drained percutaneously, taking care to use strict aseptic technique. Seromas can be prevented by requiring the patient to wear an abdominal binder for 1 month after the implantation.

Infections may occur in the pump pocket or back incision. Not all wound infections require pump or catheter removal and, if superficial, can be treated with antibiotics. If an infection of the pocket is suspected, careful aspiration is useful to provide a culture and sensitivity. If the infection is deep and severe (associated with fever and leukocytosis), the system should be removed. It may be necessary to leave the wound open in this case and allow it to close secondarily. Consultation with an infectious disease specialist may be helpful.

Pump System Problems

Programmable pump complications include filling errors, pump failure, programming errors, and torsion or flipping of a freely moveable pump. Complications that can occur when filling the pump include inadvertent side port access, overfilling the pump, and inadvertent placement of the drug in the pump pocket. Many of the intrathecal pumps contain a side port with direct access to the intrathecal space. If this side port is inadvertently accessed when refilling the pump, a large dose of med-ication will be delivered directly into the CSF leading to a drug overdose. The SynchroMed 8615 and 8615-S pumps and the Infusaid Model 400 pump contain side ports. The SynchroMed 8615-S pump has a screened side port that will only allow entry of a 25-gauge needle. This will prevent access from the usual 22-gauge Huber type needle used for pump refill. Also, the side ports are located on the periphery of the pump, whereas the refill port is located in the center. The refill kits contain a template that can be used to locate the two different ports. The Arrow Model 3000 pump has a special bolus needle for bolus injections directly into the CSF. The needle is designed with a sealed tip and a slot opening midway up the needle cannula. When the needle is inserted through the double stacked pump septums within the pump, the closed tip is in contact with the needle stop and the slot opening is automatically at the level of the bolus pathway allowing bolus injection or infusion. If the pump is overfilled, the reservoir will be over-pressurized, which may lead to pump damage, failure, or overdose. Most pump refill kits come with a manometer system to alert the physician or nurse of an overpressurized system. If the pump or port pocket is inadvertently accessed and the drug deposited directly into the pocket, a drug overdose can result. Most of the drugs used for intrathecal drug delivery are highly concentrated and can lead to very high plasma levels and drug overdose.

Pump failure most often occurs with battery failure. The SynchroMed Infusion System is the only system that is battery operated. The normal battery life depends on the flow rate but is usually 3 to 5 years. The pump has a battery alarm that will alert the patient and physician when the battery is getting low. When the battery fails, the entire pump must be replaced. By the time the battery requires replacement, most patients are on a stable flow rate and do not require many rate changes. At this point it is may be more cost-effective to use one of the constant flow rate systems (Arrow or IsoMed) that are not battery operated. These systems are also less expensive than the SynchroMed Pump. However, these systems also have disadvantages unique from the SynchroMed Pump (as discussed above) that should be weighed.

Another cause of pump failure is failure of the electronic telemetric receiving module, which prevents the pump from receiving programming instructions. This converts the pump to a constant flow system (like the Arrow and Infusaid Systems). If the patient is at a stage where programmability is not important, the pump may be left in and adjustments in drug dosing made by changing drug concentration.

Programming errors can lead to inadequate pain relief, abstinence syndrome, or drug overdose. Programming a drug concentration that is higher than the actual drug concentration may lead to under dosing and increased pain or drug abstinence syndrome. Programming a drug concentration that is lower than the actual drug concentration may lead to drug overdose and death. The newer software that is available with Medtronic programmable pumps asks the programmer if the right choices have been made, which the programmer should carefully check. Also, the software has certain constraints that do not allow extreme changes in drug concentration or rates.

Pumps or ports that are not secured with sutures inside the pocket can flip or torque. Pumps that torque within the pocket may kink the catheter or pull the catheter out of the intrathecal space. If the pump flips on itself, the pump will be unable to be refilled or programmed. This problem is usually discovered at the time of refill when the pump cannot be accessed or programmed. If this happens, the pump will require surgical revision. The pumps and ports have anchors that can be sutured in the pocket, thus preventing this complication.

ECONOMICS

De Lissovoy et al[20] looked at the cost-effectiveness of long-term intrathecal morphine for failed back syndrome and presented the most comprehensive assessment of this issue. They used a cost-effectiveness analysis to compare the direct costs of intrathecal pain therapy via an implanted pump to medical management alone for failed back surgery patients over a 5-year period. Base-case, worst-case, and best-case scenarios were developed by a panel of experts. Charges for repeat back surgery were not included in the analysis. They concluded that the costs for medical management exceeded the base-case costs for intrathecal drug therapy at 22 months.

Other studies have compared the costs of different routes of delivery. Bedder et al[21] compared the cost of the epidural morphine delivered via an external pump or intrathecal delivery. They concluded that although the initial costs for an intrathecal pump implant are higher (1.67 times higher), the break-even point appeared at 3 months; at 1 year the total charges for the epidural group were about twice as high as the intrathecal group. Another similar study compared different routes of delivery for opioids in the management of cancer pain. The authors believe this model could be applied to nonmalignant pain. Five different routes of administration were studied: oral, transdermal, subcutaneous/intrathecal via an external infusion pump, epidural via an external infusion pump, and intrathecal delivery via an implanted infusion pump. They used an empirical dose rate of 10 mg/hour of intravenous morphine equivalent for the cost comparison. If the dose remains constant, they concluded that at 25 months oral and transdermal delivery were the least expensive, followed by the intrathecal delivery with an implanted infusion pump, followed by the

epidural and subcutaneous delivery via an external infusion pump. If one assumed a 5% per month increase, they concluded that at 25 months intrathecal delivery was the least expensive, followed by the oral and transdermal delivery, and then followed by the epidural and subcutaneous delivery via an external infusion pump.

These studies demonstrate cost savings with intrathecal drug delivery using an implanted infusion system over a few years. It is yet to be determined if there are cost savings over the life of the patient but these studies suggest savings. However, only a portion of the picture is captured with these studies and there may be far-reaching significance to the patient, payer, provider, and society as a whole.

REFERENCES

1. Melzack R, Wall PD: Pain mechanisms: a new theory. Science 150(699): 971–979, 1965.
2. Rauck RL, Eisenach JC, Jackson K, et al: Epidural clonidine treatment for refractory reflex sympathetic dystrophy. Anesthesiology 79(6):1163–1169, 1993.
3. Eisenach JC, DuPen S, Dubois M, et al: Epidural clonidine analgesia for intractable cancer pain. Pain 61(3):391–399, 1995.
4. Desborough JP, Edlin SA, Burrin JM, et al: Hormonal and metabolic responses to cholecystectomy: comparison of extradural somatostatin and diamorphine. Br J Anaesth 63(5):508–515, 1989.
5. Karpinski N, Dunn J, Hansen L, Masliah E: Subpial vacuolar myelopathy after intrathecal ketamine: report of a case. Pain 73(1):103–105, 1997.
6. Rane K, Segerdahl M, Goiny M, Sollevi A: Intrathecal adenosine administration. Anesthesiology 89(5):1108–1115, 1998.
7. Eisenach JC, Rauck RL, Curry R: Intrathecal but not intravenous adenosine reduces allodynia in patients with neuropathic pain. Pain 105(1–2):65–70, 2003.
8. de Jong PC, Kansen PJ: A comparison of epidural catheters with or without subcutaneous injection ports for treatment of cancer pain. Anesth Analg 78(1):94–100, 1994.
9. Lee YW, Chaplan SR, Yaksh TL: Systemic and supraspinal, but not spinal, opiates suppress allodynia in a rat neuropathic pain model. Neurosci Lett 199(2):111–114, 1995.
10. Kupers RC, Van den Oever R, Van Houdenhove B, et al: Spinal cord stimulation in Belgium: a nationwide survey on the incidence, indications and therapeutic efficacy by the health insurer. Pain 56(2):211–216, 1994.
11. Burton C: Dorsal column stimulation: optimization of application. Surg Neurol 4(1):171–176, 1975.
12. North RB, Kidd DH, et al: Prognostic value of psychological testing in patients undergoing spinal cord stimulation: a prospective study. Neurosurg 39:301–311, 1996.

13. Burchiel KJ, Anderson VC, Wilson BJ, et al: Prognostic factors of spinal cord stimulation for chronic back and leg pain. Neurosurg 36(6):1101-1111, 1995.

14. Brandwin MA, Kewman DG: MMPI indicators of treatment response to spinal epidural stimulation in patients with chronic pain and patients with movement disorders. Psychol Rep 51:1059-1064, 1982.

15. Daniel MS, Long C, Hutcherson WL, Hunter S: Psychological factors and outcome of electrode implantation for chronic pain. Neurosurg 17(5):773-777, 1985.

16. Nelson DV, Kennington M, Novy DM, et al: Psychological selection criteria for implantable spinal cord stimulators. Pain Forum 5:93-103, 1996.

17. Paice JA, Penn RD, Shott S: Intraspinal morphine for chronic pain: a retrospective, multicenter study. J Pain Symptom Manage 11(2):71-80, 1996.

18. Hassenbusch SJ, Portenoy RK: Current practices in intraspinal therapy—a survey of clinical trends and decision making. J Pain Symptom Manage 20(2):S4-S11, 2000.

19. Penn RD, York MM, Paice JA: Catheter systems for intrathecal drug delivery. J Neurosurg 83:215-217, 1995.

20. De Lissovoy G, Brown RE, Halpern M, et al: Cost-effectiveness of long-term intrathecal morphine for pain associated with failed back surgery syndrome. Clin Ther 19(1):96-112, 1997.

21. Bedder MD, Burchiel K, Larson SA: Cost analysis of two implantable narcotic delivery systems. J Pain Sympt Manage 6:368-373, 1991.

SUGGESTED READING

Bennett G, Burchiel K, Buchser E, et al: Clinical Guidelines for Intraspinal Infusion: Report of an Expert Panel. J Pain Sympt Manage 20:S37-S43, 2000.

Coffey RJ, Burchiel K: Inflammatory mass lesions associated with intrathecal drug infusion catheters: report and observations on 41 patients. Neurosurgery 50:78-86, 2002.

Du Pen SL, Peterson DG, Williams A, et al: Infection during chronic epidural catheterization: diagnosis and treatment. Anesthesiology 73:905-909, 1990.

Du Pen SL, Williams AR: Spinal and peripheral drug-delivery systems. Pain Digest 5:307-317, 1995.

Follet KA, Hitchon PW, Piper J, et al: Response of intractable pain to continuous intrathecal morphine: a retrospective study. Pain 49:21-25, 1992.

Hassenbusch SJ, Paice JA, Patt RB, et al: Clinical realities and economic considerations: Economics of intrathecal therapy. J Pain Sympt Manage 3:S36-S48, 1997.

Hassenbusch SJ, Portenoy RK: Current practices in intraspinal therapy—a survey of clinical trends and decision making. J Pain Sympt Manage 20:S4-S11, 2000.

Hassenbusch S, Burcheil K, Coffey RJ, et al: Management of intrathecal catheter-tip inflammatory masses: A consensus statement. Pain Med 3:313-323, 2002.

Krames ES: Intraspinal opioid therapy for chronic nonmalignant pain: Current practice and clinical guidelines. J Pain Sympt Manage 11:333-352, 1996.

Krames ES: Intrathecal infusional therapies for intractable pain: patient management guidelines. J Pain Sympt Manage 8:36-46, 1993.

Nitescu P, Sjoberg M, Appelgren L, et al: Complications of intrathecal opioids and bupivacaine in the treatment of "refractory" cancer pain. Clin J Pain 11:45-62, 1995.

Oakley J, Staats P: The use of implanted drug delivery systems. In PP Raj (ed): The Practical Management of Pain. Mosby, St. Louis, 2000, pp 768-778.

Staats P, Mitchell V: Future directions for intrathecal analgesia. Prog Anesthesiol 19:367-382, 1997.

Wallace M: Human Spinal Drug Delivery: Methods and Technology. In Yaksh TL (ed): Spinal Drug Delivery, Elsevier, New York, 1999, pp 345-370.

Wallace MS, Yaksh TL: Long-term intraspinal drug therapy: a review. Reg Anesth Pain Manage 25:117-157, 2000.

Yaksh TL (ed): Spinal Drug Delivery. Elsevier, New York, 1999.

CHAPTER 9

Local Anesthetics

CARIDAD BRAVO-FERNANDEZ

INTRODUCTION

Local anesthetics can be introduced into a variety of sites—subcutaneous, intramuscularly, intravenous, epidural, and spinal—in order to block the action potentials needed for nerve conduction in a reversible manner. The specific action at the nerve site depends on which local anesthetic is used and how it is used.

HISTORY[1]

For hundreds of years the inhabitants of the Andes Mountains have been chewing leaves from the coca plant to enable them to work at high altitude with a minimum of fatigue. The "conquistadors" brought the plant to Europe. In 1860 Niemann isolated bitter crystals that numbed his tongue. A Peruvian physician described the pluses and minuses of cocaine in 1868.

In 1884 it was Carl Koller who first described cocaine's use as a local anesthetic for eye surgery. Also in 1884, Sigmund Freud proposed cocaine as a treatment for morphine addiction. Along with cocaine's benefits as a local anesthetic, its toxic and addictive properties became known. Halsted used cocaine as an anesthetic in hundreds of cases at Johns Hopkins Hospital with excellent results.

The impetus to find a "safer" local anesthetic resulted in Einhorn's synthesis of procaine in the 1904. Alterations to procaine yielded tetracaine and chloroprocaine. In the 1940s Lofgren synthesized lidocaine. From there, bupivacaine, and later ropivacaine were developed.

On the commercial side, in 1886 John Styth Pemberton patented a new beverage. In 1892 A.G. Chandler bought the rights to this patented beverage and founded the Coca-Cola Company. In 1906 caffeine replaced cocaine in the "enjoyable drink."

MECHANISM OF ACTION OF LOCAL ANESTHETICS

Nerves carry impulses generated by stimuli—electrical, mechanical, thermal, chemical. These messages are relayed along nerves to different parts of the body, peripherally and centrally. The nerve membrane consists of a framework of phospholipids. The membrane has a charged outer surface that is hydrophilic and a charged inner surface that is hydrophobic. Nerve impulses depend on the concentration gradient of ions along the nerve membrane and the permeability of the membrane to specific ions.

The prevalent ion inside the cell is potassium. There is a 10 to 1 difference in its concentration inside and outside the cell membrane. The ion prevalent outside the cell membrane is sodium. This concentration gradient is actively maintained by Na+-K-ATP pump. The hydrolysis of ATP to ADP provides energy for the pump to function in order to maintain the balance of ions. Sodium is actively transported out of the cell while potassium is transported inward. This state of rest depends on many factors. This resting potential is a –70mV inside the cell.

A stimulus will lead to depolarization. Depolarization occurs with the opening of the sodium channels. The membrane potential becomes progressively less negative with the influx of sodium ions across the membrane and efflux of potassium.

Repolarization starts as this sodium movement into the cell begins to slow down while the gate is still open. The inactivation of the sodium channel begins quickly. Potassium permeability also increases to restore the resting membrane state. The sodium-potassium pump is also at work to expel sodium ions from inside the cell. During this refractory period the nerve has a much diminished capacity to respond to new stimuli or to conduct impulses in a retrograde fashion.

Calcium plays a role in maintaining membrane readiness to respond to stimuli. It helps maintain the potential across the membrane. If extracellular calcium is low, spontaneous firing can occur. If external calcium is too high, cell firing is sluggish. This is of great importance in muscle, especially cardiac muscle.

Local anesthetics have a role in nerve transmission. Local anesthetics bind to transmembrane proteins. This binding closes the sodium channel and inactivates transmission in a reversible fashion.

Local anesthetics block the generation and propagation of nerve action potentials. Local anesthetics interfere with the permeability of cell membranes to Na+. The Na+ receptor channel is bound on the inner surface of the membrane by local anesthetics.

The potency of local anesthetics is directly related to its lipid solubility. Protein binding of local anesthetics affects the duration of action and the toxicity. The binding to the receptor increases duration, but the binding to plasma proteins makes it unavailable to the receptor site. On the other hand, free local anesthetic drug in plasma increases toxic potential.

The local anesthetic molecule can exist in two forms—ionized base and cationic form. The base form is more lipid-soluble, and the cation is more water-soluble. This is determined by the pKa of the individual local anesthetic and the pH of the solution that it is in. (The pKa is the pH at which the basic and cationic forms are in 50:50 proportions.) The ionized form can diffuse across membranes, but the ionized form bind the Na+ receptor channel.

Fiber Size, Function, and Local Anesthetic Sensitivity

Historically, it was widely believed that sensitivity to local anesthetic blockade was related to fiber size, with larger fibers being most resistant and small fibers being most sensitive. With the advent of single fiber recording studies, it was determined that C-fibers are actually the most resistant to local anesthetic blockade. This is mainly related to the Schwann cell sheath that encloses bundles of C-fibers, as unsheathed fibers in vitro are much more sensitive. While there is great variability among A-fibers, there is no real pattern linking size to local anesthetic sensitivity. B-fibers, which are mainly preganglionic sympathetic fibers, are slightly more sensitive than A-fibers, but the differences are small and are dependent on the local anesthetic used, with the differences being greater for bupivacaine than for lidocaine.

On the other hand, the onset of block is dependent upon fiber size. The onset of blockade is faster for small fibers than for large fibers. This phenomenon is related to the fact that for small fibers, blockade of a short segment will produce failure of conduction, while blockade of a longer segment is required for larger fibers. Blockade of at least three nodes of Ranvier is required to produce consistent blockade. As the anesthetic diffuses into the nerve, the length of axons blocked gradually increases, causing the smaller fibers to be interrupted initially. Onset for individual local anesthetics is dependent to some extent on the pKa of the agent (i.e., the pH at which half of the drug is ionized and half is unionized). Drugs with a high pKa have a low proportion of drug unionized and tend to have a slow onset of action, as it is the unionized portion that can diffuse across biologic membranes. An exception is chloroprocaine, which has a very high pKa but a fairly rapid onset.

These concepts are important for interpreting differential spinal block. It has been proposed that by injecting low concentrations of local anesthetic it is possible to interrupt sympathetic fibers while preserving the function of somatic afferent fibers, including nociceptors. Thus, the injection of 0.25% procaine could block B-fibers, selectively interrupting sympathetic preganglionics. We know, however, from single fiber recording studies, that it is nearly impossible to effectively block B-fibers while preserving A-fiber function. Clinically, it is usually observed that there is some degree of somatic blockade achieved when adequate anesthetic is provided to produce a rise in skin temperature. It is also well-established that sub-blocking concentrations of local anesthetic can severely limit maximum firing rates of an axon. Thus, even if there is no detectable change in sensation to cold, touch, or pinprick, there may be pain reduction from partial blockade of nociceptors, which are dependent on high firing rates for activation of spinothalamic pain projection systems.

Another factor affecting the onset and intensity of local anesthetic block is use-dependency. Since local anesthetics gain access to sodium channels most readily when the channel is open, an axon that is firing repeatedly is more likely to become blocked than one that is quiescent. Thus, axons that are tonically active may be blocked more rapidly.

Duration of local anesthetic block is related to lipid solubility. Highly lipid-soluble drugs tend to be long-acting. For procaine and chloroprocaine, their short duration of action is to some extent related to rapid hydrolysis by plasma cholinesterases. While tetracaine is also hydrolyzed by these enzymes, its rate of hydrolysis is much slower (Tables 9-1 and 9-2).

ESTERS

Cocaine is an ester benzoic acid. It is a unique local anesthetic that is also a vasoconstrictor inhibiting norepinephrine reuptake. Its abuse potential and toxicity, particularly its arrhythmogenicity, have limited its use. It is occasionally used as a topical anesthetic, but many practitioners now prefer a combination of 4% lidocaine with 0.25% phenylephrine.

Benzocaine does not have a water-soluble form. It is only used topically. Its rapid hydrolysis to p-aminobenzoic acid can lead to allergic reactions.

Procaine (Novocain) is an amino ester. Its use has decreased because it has low potency, slow onset, and short duration. It is approved for spinal anesthesia. Ten percent procaine diluted with equal volumes of cerebrospinal fluid (CSF) is hyperbaric and produces anesthesia for about 45 minutes. It has been used for differential spinal anesthesia (see discussion above). Its hydrolysis produces para-aminobenzoic acid, which is allergenic in some patients.

2-Chloroprocaine (Nesacaine) has a more rapid onset than procaine. It has a very low potential for systemic toxicity because of its rapid hydrolysis by plasma cholinesterase. Like procaine, it has a short duration. It can be used for local infiltration, peripheral nerve blocks, and epidural anesthesia. It is not approved for spinal anesthesia.

Tetracaine (Pontocaine) is more potent and toxic than procaine. The long duration is enhanced by vasoconstrictors. It does have a slow onset that limits its use in peripheral blocks. It is most often used for spinal anesthesia, but has largely been replaced by bupivacaine, which has better sensory-blocking properties and less profound motor blockade. It is also found in topical preparations. It is slowly hydrolyzed by plasma cholinesterases and

Table 9-1   Local Anesthetic Onset, Duration, pKa, and Lipid Solubility

Local Anesthetic	Onset	Duration	pKa	Partition Coefficient (Lipid solubility)
Procaine	Slow	Short	8.9	100
Mepivacaine	Fast	Intermediate	7.6	130
Prilocaine	Fast	Intermediate	7.9	129
Chloroprocaine	Fast	Short	8.7	810
Lidocaine	Fast	Intermediate	7.8	366
Tetracaine	Slow	Long	8.5	5822
Bupivacaine	Slow	Long	8.1	3420
Etidocaine	Fast	Long	7.7	7317
Ropivacaine	Slow	Long	8.1	775

Table 9-2   Fiber Type, Function, Size, and Conduction Velocity

Type of fiber	Action	Diameter (μm)	Conduction (m/s)
Myelinated			
Aα	Motor, proprioception	12–20	70–120
Aβ	Pressure, light touch	5–12	30–70
Aγ	Muscle spindle afferents	3–6	15–30
Aδ	Pain, cold, touch	2–5	12–30
B	Preganglionic autonomic	<3	3–15
Unmyelinated			
C	Pain, temperature, Postganglionic autonomic	0.3–1.3	0.1–15

has a fairly high potential for systemic toxicity. However, it does not have the high potential for cardiac toxicity seen with bupivacaine and etidocaine (see the following section).

AMIDES

Lidocaine (Xylocaine) has been widely used since the 1950s. It is an extremely versatile agent, which is used clinically for spinal and epidural anesthesia, plexus and peripheral nerve blocks. It is effective topically on mucous membranes. It is rapidly absorbed from gastrointestinal and respiratory tracts as well as transdermally via iontophoresis. It produces local vasodilation, which can be blocked by the addition of epinephrine. It has antiarrhythmic properties and is anticonvulsant at low blood levels. Like other anesthetics, it is neurotoxic in high concentrations. It has been implicated in the causation of cauda equina injury when given intrathecally as a 5% solution via small gauge catheters. The pathophysiology of this injury is related to very slow injection that precludes adequate mixing with CSF, resulting in pooling of anesthetic in the sacral segments of the dural sac. Intrathecal lidocaine has also been reported to produce a condition known as transient radicular irritation, characterized by burning lower extremity and perineal pain lasting 24 to 48 hours. It is unrelated to the concentration used. To date, there have been no reports of permanent neurologic sequelae to this condition.

Mepivacaine (Carbocaine) is slightly longer acting than lidocaine with similar properties. It produces less local vasodilation than lidocaine, and may even have mild vasoconstricting properties. Although it is an effective local anesthetic for nerve blocks, epidurals, and spinals, it is not effective as a topical anesthetic. It is often used without epinephrine for peripheral nerve blocks. It has been studied as a spinal anesthetic and produces a slightly longer block than lidocaine. It does not appear to be neurotoxic spinally, but it can produce transient radicular irritation. It is not currently approved in the United States as a spinal anesthetic.

Prilocaine (Citanest) is intermediate acting and similar to lidocaine. It does not produce much vasodilatation unlike other local anesthetics. It has a lower potential for systemic toxicity because it is rapidly metabolized in the liver. This does not, of course, protect against toxicity associated with accidental intravascular injection. However, its biotransformation to an amino phenol oxidizes hemoglobin to methemoglobin. Its use in children is generally avoided because of its potential for methemoglobinemia. In adults the total maximum dose is limited 600 mg.

Bupivacaine (Marcaine, Sensorcaine) was introduced in 1963. It was the first amide with a truly long-acting effect. It also differed from most existing agents because of its profound sensory blocking effects and relatively lower motor blocking properties. It is approved for local infiltration, peripheral blocks, and epidural and spinal anesthesia. At low epidural concentrations it can produce substantial analgesia with minimal motor blockade. It produces spinal anesthesia lasting up to 3 hours, epidural blockade lasting 3 to 4 hours, and brachial plexus block lasting up to 18 hours. It is highly bound to plasma proteins, potentially reducing its systemic toxicity. However, it does have significant cardiac toxicity because it avidly binds cardiac Na+ channels. In animal studies, there is a 4-fold difference between the central nervous system (CNS) toxic blood levels and cardiotoxic levels for lidocaine. However, for bupivacaine, cardiac arrhythmias often begin at about the same blood levels that can produce seizures. Accidental intravascular injection in human patients can produce fatal ventricular arrhythmias, most commonly of the torsades de pointes variety, which can be very resistant to antiarrhythmic therapy. It has been shown that the levo-isomer is less cardiotoxic than racemic bupivacaine but has essentially the same local anesthetic properties. A preparation of levo-bupivacaine has now been introduced into clinical practice.

Ropivacaine (Naropin) is structurally similar to mepivacaine and bupivacaine (Ropivacaine has a propyl group and bupivacaine has a butyl group substituted for mepivacaine's methyl group). It is a pure levo-isomer with less cardiotoxicity than bupivacaine. Its potency and duration of action are slightly lower than those of bupivacaine, and it appears to be even more motor sparing than bupivacaine. It is not approved for spinal anesthesia. It is effective for local infiltration, peripheral, and epidural blocks.

Etidocaine is a long-acting local anesthetic that is structurally similar to lidocaine. Like bupivacaine, it has the capability of producing life-threatening ventricular arrhythmias when accidentally injected intravascularly. It has not gained widespread popularity, principally because of its potent motor-blocking properties. There have been a number of case reports of motor blockade outlasting the sensory block. When this occurs following epidural blockade, it leads to the suspicion of anterior spinal artery syndrome or epidural hematoma.

Vasoconstrictors

Vasoconstrictors can reduce toxic levels and prolong the duration of local anesthetics by decreasing absorption.

Epinephrine is the most commonly used vasoconstrictor. When used for peripheral nerve block, it is usually added in a concentration of 1:200,000 (the addition of 0.1 ml of 1:1000 epinephrine to 20 ml local anesthetic solution will yield this concentration. When used in conjunction with spinal anesthesia, 0.1 to 0.2 ml 1:1000 epinephrine is usually added to the total volume of local anesthetic injected. When given spinally, epinephrine produces an analgesic effect through activation of α_2 adrenergic receptors, producing a response similar to that of clonidine.

The injection of 3 ml of local anesthetic containing 1:200,000 epinephrine provides a reasonable test dose for detecting intravascular injection. It will fairly reliably produce tachycardia and an increase in blood pressure (N.B.: the rise in BP may not be detected by automated blood pressure devices, as the initial measurement may not inflate above the new systolic pressure. A manual BP device is preferable).

Epinephrine is not recommended for digital or penile blocks. There is concern that a combination of pressure from a ring block plus intense constriction of the arterial supply can produce ischemia. However, there are few if any reports of gangrene following such procedures with epinephrine containing solutions.

Phenylephrine has been used to prolong spinal anesthesia, but has been replaced for the most part by epinephrine (Fig. 9-1).

TOXICITY

Local anesthetics are widely used and have a low side-effect profile. However, reactions have been associated with local anesthetics that are attributed to accidental injections of excessive doses. These reactions involve the CNS and/or the cardiovascular system. The CNS is more susceptible to the actions of local anesthetics than the cardiovascular system. Localized muscle or nerve damage can occur. Rare allergic reactions can also occur.

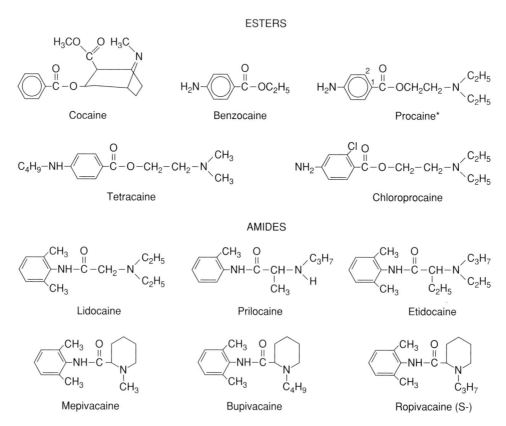

Figure 9-1   Molecular structure of local anesthetics.

Systemic Central Nervous System Toxicity

In the CNS, local anesthetics block inhibitory pathways in the cortex. It is the unopposed excitatory manifestations that are observed.

Symptoms of CNS toxicity begin with tinnitus, light-headedness, visual disturbances, perioral numbness, and confusion. This can progress to muscular twitching and tonic-clonic seizures. Finally, the patient becomes unconscious. Factors that increase the likelihood of systemic toxicity include rapid administration, decreased volume of distribution, and a decreased arterial pH and/or an increased arterial PCO_2.

For lidocaine, CNS symptoms begin at a plasma concentration above 5 µg/ml and seizures generally occur at or above 10 µg/ml. The seizure threshold plasma concentration is similar mepivacaine and prilocaine. Seizures have been reported at venous blood levels of 2 to 4 µg/ml of bupivacaine and etidocaine.

Prevention of Systemic Toxicity

The great majority of systemic toxic reactions are due to intravascular injection. Careful, frequent aspiration during injection is essential. Whenever possible, give a test dose of anesthetic containing epinephrine, and monitor blood pressure and heart rate in the immediate postinjection period. Do not rely on automated blood pressure cuffs to monitor postinjection blood pressure. Use a manual cuff or arterial monitoring.

Calculate the appropriate dose of anesthetic for each patient and procedure. When mixing local anesthetics, toxicity is additive. When supplementing a block with an additional injection, make sure the maximum dose has not been exceeded. Use the lowest effective dose and limit the total dose when injecting highly vascular areas such as intercostal blocks. Inform patients of signs and symptoms of rising anesthetic blood levels and instruct them to inform you if they occur. Do not leave the patient unattended after the block. Peak blood levels occur 20 to 30 minutes after injection in the absence of intravascular injection (Box 9-1).

Treatment of Central Nervous System Toxicity

Antiepileptic drugs were initially used, but were ineffective. Barbiturates (e.g., Pentothal) have been effective in treating seizures, but less so for preventing them. Near-anesthetic doses of intravenous short-acting barbiturates can arrest seizures. Comparable CNS depressants (e.g., propofol) are also effective. Benzodiazepines proved effective in seizure suppression with minimal undesirable side effects. Premedication with diazepam raises the convulsant dose of local anesthetic to trigger a seizure. However, premedication does not reliably prevent seizures from local anesthetic overdose or accidental intravascular injection.

Initial treatment consists of immediate positive pressure ventilation with oxygen. If the patient has a full stomach, immediate intubation facilitated by succinyl choline is indicated. Paralysis with succinyl choline is a reasonable choice if initial ventilation is difficult, which is often the case during a grand mal seizure. The seizure should be terminated promptly with a benzodiazepine, barbiturate, or propofol. Prompt attention must be given to the cardiovascular condition. Cardiovascular depression can occur with all local anesthetics, and ventricular arrhythmias are common with bupivacaine, etidocaine, and ropivacaine (Box 9-2).

Box 9-1 Recommended Local Anesthetic Doses

Theses are general guidelines. Maximum doses vary greatly with site of injections. Intercostal block produces rapid onset of high blood levels; subcutaneous infiltration produces much slower onset and lower peak levels. Plexus blocks and epidural anesthesia result in peak levels between these extremes.

Agent:	Maximum dose (mg)	
	Plain	With Epinephrine
Amides		
Lidocaine	300	500
Prilocaine	600	
Mepivacaine	400	400
Bupivacaine	175	225
Ropivacaine	225	
Etidocaine	300	400
Esters		
Procaine	1000	
Chloroprocaine	800	1000

Peripheral Vascular Effects

Local anesthetics exert effects on peripheral vascular smooth muscle. The effect of lower doses is one of vasoconstriction. As the doses increase, the vasoconstriction changes to vasodilatation. This may be due to competition between local anesthetics and calcium ions in smooth muscle. Cocaine is the only local anesthetic that causes only vasoconstriction through its blockade of norepinephrine reuptake.

Systemic Cardiovascular Toxicity

Local anesthetics affect cardiac function and peripheral vascular smooth muscle. Although lidocaine, a local anesthetic, is used extensively in treating cardiac arrhythmias, other local anesthetics (bupivacaine) appear to precipitate arrhythmias.

Local anesthetics are known to increase pulse rate interval and QRS duration. At higher concentrations local anesthetics can depress pacemaker activity. The primary action is believed to be the inhibition at the sodium channel. Some conflicting evidence also implicates the slow calcium channels. Local anesthetics have additional effects on cardiac muscle itself by depressing contractility, but a clear mechanism is not known.

Bupivacaine, etidocaine, and ropivacaine are of particular interest, since they can produce life-threatening ventricular arrhythmias at concentrations well below those that produce direct myocardial depression. They are capable of generating a unidirectional block and a reentrant dysrhythmia. Ventricular arrhythmias produced by these agents are often resistant to treatment. Other local anesthetics produce dose-related cardiac depression, generally at much higher plasma concentrations than are required to produce seizures.

At extremely high blood levels of nonarrhythmogenic local anesthetics, there is progressive reduction in cardiac output along with peripheral vasodilation. Hypotension and bradycardia can progress to cardiovascular collapse.

Treatment of Cardiovascular Toxicity

Cardiovascular depression from less potent anesthetics such as lidocaine is rarely life-threatening and can usually be managed with ephedrine and atropine. If blood levels are extremely high, epinephrine may be required. Maintaining adequate ventilation and oxygenation is essential.

Overdose with the more potent agents (e.g., bupivacaine) may result in ventricular arrhythmias requiring cardiopulmonary resuscitation. Cardioversion is often ineffective initially, and prolonged circulatory support may be required. Repeated doses of epinephrine may be needed to maintain blood pressure during resuscitation. Bretylium and mg^{++} have been reported to help in some cases (Box 9-3).

OTHER SIDE EFFECTS

Allergic reactions can occur with local anesthetics that have the amino-ester moieties. It appears to be a cross sensitivity with p-aminobenzoic acid, a metabolite of these anesthetics. Some multi-dose preparations of amide local anesthetics contain methylparaben, which can produce allergic reactions in patients sensitive to para-aminobenzoic acid. True allergy to amide local anesthetics is rare, but possible.

Persistent local anesthetic blockade can mask certain pathological conditions. In the early postoperative period, compartment syndromes, which ordinarily produce severe pain, may be masked by the ongoing analgesic effect. Circulatory checks must be carried out frequently whenever the risk of this complication is high. Nerve injury from malpositioning of an anesthetized limb can occur while the local anesthetic persists.

Box 9-2 Symptoms of Local Anesthetic Toxicity

Mild CNS symptoms:	Tinnitus, visual disturbances, numbness of lips and tongue, lightheadedness, confusion
Excitation of the CNS:	Muscular twitching tonic-clonic seizures
Early CV symptoms:	Hypertension and tachycardia (with seizures)
Late CV symptoms:	Hypotension, bradycardia, decreased cardiac output, myocardial depression
Extreme CV symptoms:	Cardiovascular collapse
With etidocaine, bupivacaine, ropivacaine:	Ventricular arrhythmias may occur coincident with onset of seizures: PVCs, ventricular tachycardia, fibrillation, Torsade de Pointes

CNS, central nervous system; CV, cardiovascular; PVCs, premature ventricular contractions.

Box 9-3   Treatment of Systemic Toxicity

Seizure:

Stop anesthetic injection

Hyperventilate with bag, mask, oxygen

Full stomach: Succinyl choline → Intubation

Stop the seizure with anticonvulsant agent:

    Benzodiazepine

    Propofol

    Thiopental

Check cardiovascular status:

    Hypotension → Cardiovascular support

    Ventricular arrhythmia → CPR if required

        Epinephrine, cardioversion

        Consider bretylium, mg++ for intractable

        arrhythmia

        (Do not treat with lidocaine)

REFERENCE

1. De Jong RH: Local Anesthetics. St. Louis, Mosby, 1994.

SUGGESTED READING

Berkun Y, et al: Evaluation of adverse reactions to local anesthetics: experience with 236 patients. Ann Allergy Asthma Immunol Oct:91(4):342-345, 2003.

Catterall W, Macke K: Local Anesthetics. The Pharma-cological Basis of Therapeutics, 10th ed. New York, McGraw-Hill, 2001.

Tucker GT: Local anesthetic kinetics. In Principles and Practice of Regional Anesthesia, 3rd ed. Churchill-Livingstone, 2003.

Wildsmith JAW, Strichartz GR: Peripheral nerve and local anesthetic drugs. Principles and Practice of Regional Anesthesia, 3rd ed. Churchill-Livingstone, 2003.

Wildsmith JAW: Clinical Use of local anesthetic drugs. Principles and Practice of Regional Anesthesia, 3rd ed. Churchill-Livingstone, 2003.

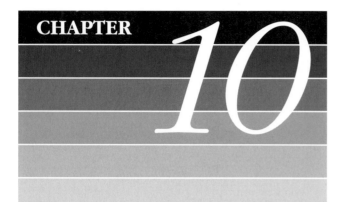

CHAPTER 10

A Practical Approach to Postoperative Pain Management

CONSTANTINE SARANTOPOULOS

INTRODUCTION

"Pain" defines a conscious unpleasant sensory and emotional experience associated with actual or potential tissue damage, described in terms of such damage. The definition applies to acute pain, cancer pain, and chronic pain of nonmalignant states. The sensation of pain is the final result of a complex and interactive mechanisms, integrated at all levels of the nervous system, from the periphery, through the spinal cord, to the higher cerebral structures. Different states or types of pain reflect a wide range of sensory experiences. These can be viewed as the expression of different neurophysiologic mechanisms, not necessarily of absolute teleologic significance. Under normal conditions, a physiologic state exists characterized by a close correlation between the intensity of the noxious stimulus and the conscious perception of a painful response. This is the case in the acute, brief pain. However, changes induced by nociceptive input or by the coexisting conditions can result in variations in the quality, duration, and intensity of the perception of the pain produced by noxious stimulation. These changes tend to be temporary, as homeostatic mechanisms tend to restore the system to the normal interrelationships between stimulation and pain intensity. However, persisting, intense stimuli may produce changes in the central nervous system, overriding these inhibitory mechanisms, and leading to chronic pain.

Acute pain is short-lived and signifies the presence of a noxious stimulus that produces actual tissue damage or possesses the potential to do so. Nonetheless, very intense or prolonged nociceptive input, or disruption or loss of the normal sensory input, distort the nociceptive system to such an extent that the normal correlation between stimulation and pain is lost. Underlying mechanisms, known as *plasticity* and *peripheral* or *central sensitization*, dynamically change the properties of the neural tissue in such a way that prolonged nociception or neuropathy may produce exaggerated responses. These signify the transition to chronic pain states. Pain is considered chronic when it persists 3 to 6 months beyond the resolution of the acute process.

MECHANISMS OF ACUTE PAIN

Acute pain is generated when specialized nociceptors (e.g., Aδ and/or C fibers) are activated mechanically, thermally, or chemically. After loss of tissue integrity, algogenic substances are released at the site of tissue injury or inflammation. These substances include a diverse variety of chemicals and mediators, such as protons (e.g., H$^+$), potassium ions, prostaglandins, bradykinin, serotonin, purines (e.g., adenosine triphosphate), histamine, norepinephrine, etc. They are capable of either sensitizing or stimulating directly the nerve terminals of small fibers (e.g., Aβ and C nociceptors), which subsequently generate action potentials and transmit electrical signals, through synapses, on to neurons at the dorsal horns of the spinal cord. Excitatory neurotransmitters, such as the glutamate and the substance phosphorus (P), synaptically transmit the signal to spinothalamic neurons with ascending axons projecting into the thalamus.

Transmitters (excitatory or inhibitory) are also released from intrinsic neurons or descending fibers. These can modify the neurotransmitter release from the primary afferent terminals, or the postsynaptic responses of the dorsal horn cells, or both.

From the dorsal horns, signals are relayed to certain thalamic nuclei and as well as into specific areas of the brain, mediating the various neural, autonomic, neuroendocrine, and conscious responses to nociceptive input. At the clinical level, nociceptive responses pertinent to acute pain include not only the conscious expression of pain but other manifestations that accompany the former, such as sympathetic stimulation (e.g., tachycardia, hypertension, inhibition of gastrointestinal motility), respiratory changes, insulin resistance, and metabolic changes, immunosuppression, and others. All these responses contribute to adverse sequelae accompanying untreated post-traumatic or postoperative pain (Box 10-1).

Peripheral Sensitization

The peripheral nerve terminals of the nociceptive fibers can be sensitized from inflammatory mediators (e.g., substance P, serotonin, bradykinin, and prostaglandins), while antidromic neural circuits releasing substance P may further enhance and spread sensitization to areas not directly involved in the tissue damage. Such mechanisms provide

---

Box 10-1 Basic Mechanisms Involved in Acute Pain

Substances that can sensitize or directly stimulate the nerve terminals of nociceptors include:
- protons (H$^+$)
- potassium ions
- prostaglandins
- bradykinin, serotonin
- purines (ATP)
- histamine
- norepinephrine

Substances that can sensitize or directly stimulate the pre-synaptic transmitters at dorsal horns include:
- excitatory amino acids, mainly (glutamate)
- substance phosphorus

Substances that can sensitize or directly stimulate postsynaptic receptors include:
- AMPA

Consequences of spinal and ascending transmission and processing:
- spinal reflexes (withdrawal and muscle spasm reflexes)
- central sensitization, possible progression to chronic pain if persistent
- conscious responses of pain
- autonomic responses (tachycardia, hypertension, inhibition of gastrointestinal motility)
- respiratory changes
- insulin resistance and metabolic changes
- immunosuppression

H, hydrogen; ATP, adenosine triphosphate; AMPA, α-amino-3-hydroxy-5-methyl-4-isoxazolepropionate.

the basis of the peripheral sensitization at the neuronal and the primary hyperalgesia (i.e., increased pain after painful stimulation in the injured area). On the contrary, endogenous systems (e.g., upregulated opioid receptors at peripheral nerves) or exogenous interventions (e.g., local anesthetics, antiprostaglandin agents) may attenuate the responses.

Damage or transection of the primary afferent (i.e., peripheral sensory) nerve fibers results in a series of anatomic, physiologic, and biochemical changes leading to hyperexcitability and generation of aberrant spontaneous activity at the nerve axons, their cell somata (at the dorsal root ganglia), and eventually at the dorsal horns.

In addition to peripheral mechanisms, the excitability of the second order neurons in the dorsal horns is subjected to plasticity, which modifies the degree of their responsiveness to incoming stimuli.

Central Sensitization

Prolonged generation and input of intense painful stimuli, through complex synaptic and neuronal interactions, establishes an enhanced responsiveness and hyperexcitability of the dorsal horn neurons. Changes in these neurons are mediated via the activation of the N-methyl-D-aspartate (NMDA) receptor, as a result of excessive excitatory neurotransmitter (i.e., glutamate) release. Subsequently, neurons develop a series of intracellular changes resulting in inappropriately high degrees of excitation, hyperresponsiveness, and generation of spontaneous activity. Painful responses can now occur from larger areas in the peripheral tissues (not necessarily involved in the injury), the response threshold decreases, or pain can occur spontaneously in the absence of any peripheral stimulation. Corresponding clinical phenomena are those of secondary hyperalgesia (i.e., increased pain in response to painful stimuli in areas away from the injured tissues) and allodynia (i.e., pain sensation in response to stimuli—touch, pressure, not associated with pain normally). Similar changes may likewise occur in neurons at higher levels. Interventions aiming to prevent the establishment of central sensitization, by application of analgesics prior to painful stimulation, constitute the basis of *preemptive*

analgesia. However, it seems that a prolonged, intense blockade of the action of all sensitizing and nociceptive mechanisms, continuing throughout the perioperative period, would be necessary in order to be effective.

Advances in basic sciences provide an improved understanding of the mechanisms underlying pain. Significant progress has been made with regards to the management of the acute pain: better education and understanding of relevant phenomena reflect successful management and improvement in perioperative outcome.

CLINICAL MANAGEMENT OF ACUTE PAIN

Acute pain is pain of recent onset and probable limited duration. It usually has an identifiable temporal and causal relationship to surgery, injury, or disease. This is in contrast to chronic pain that lasts for long periods of time, not necessarily associated directly temporally or etiologically with precipitating factors. Chronic pain commonly persists beyond the time of healing of an injury and frequently no identifiable causes can be found.

Transition from acute to chronic pain is not always clear, nevertheless, many differences exist regarding their pathophysiology and management.

Acute pain is a symptom that originates from actual, ongoing, or impending tissue injury. This can be a result of trauma or intentional surgery. Surgical patients suffer from postoperative pain as a result of the surgical procedure, a pre-existing disease, or a combination of disease-related and procedure-related causes. Unrelieved postoperative pain today has been recognized as the cause of many postoperative complications (Table 10-1); however, it is not properly treated in many clinical situations. The traditional common practice of administering intramuscular analgesics (mostly opioids) as needed has been shown to lead into undertreated pain in the majority of the postoperative patients. Other factors related to patients as well as to health professionals have been recognized as causes of poor treatment (Table 10-2). But all of those factors are correctable through appropriate policies and interventions.

Table 10-1   Adverse Sequelae of Acute, Traumatic, or Postoperative Pain

1. Stress-hormone response, insulin resistance, and enhanced catabolism.
2. Sympathetic activation (i.e., hypertension, tachycardia, increased cardiac work).
3. Adverse cardiac effects (e.g., myocardial ischemia, heart failure).
4. Respiratory effects (i.e., impairment in ability to take deep breaths and cough, reduction in respiratory parameters, atelectasis, hypoventilation, hypoxemia).
5. Hypercoagulability and thrombosis.
6. Immunosuppression.
7. Physical deconditioning, mental, and emotional changes.
8. Progression to central sensitization and chronic pain.

Table 10-2   Reasons for Undertreated Postoperative Pain

1. Pain viewed as a symptom, not harmful by itself
2. Fear of addiction to opioids
3. Concerns about side effects
4. Lack of knowledge
5. Inappropriate doses, dosing intervals, or routes of analgesics
6. Misinterpretation of medical orders
7. Patients' difficulties in communicating their needs

Furthermore, effective postoperative pain management is not only an absolute moral obligation toward a most basic human right, but it has been also shown, by numerous studies, to minimize adverse physiologic and psychological sequelae.

PRACTICAL PRINCIPLES OF POSTOPERATIVE PAIN MANAGEMENT

The main focus of management after surgery or trauma is the achievement of fast rehabilitation, recovery of all normal functions, and prevention of complications. In this context, achievement of a pain-free state should be viewed as a fundamental prerequisite of an aggressive regime of postoperative mobilization and early oral feeding. Sufficient evidence supports the fact that effective analgesia may modify many of the adverse sequelae that accompany acute pain and assist recovery. Good pain control, then, may reflect the outcome after surgery (Box 10-2).

A few general principles should guide effective management:

1. Pain should be treated as early as possible. Established, severe pain not only is more difficult to treat, but theoretically can result in progressive central sensitization and vicious circle of self-perpetuation.
2. Flexibility and "tailoring" to individual patient needs produces better outcomes than a rigid application of guidelines.
3. Frequent assessment, reassessment, and charting of pain and analgesia are essential.
4. Although it may be unrealistic to completely abolish pain, it is usually possible to reduce it to comfortable levels.
5. Effective postoperative analgesia (e.g., using systemic analgesics and/or regional techniques, physical therapy) is better planned preoperatively, considering the type of operation, the medical condition of the patient, and needs for early postoperatively mobilization.
6. Multidisciplinary approaches and Acute Pain Services result in more effective relief and better outcomes.

ASSESSMENT OF POSTOPERATIVE PAIN

Effective acute pain relief starts from the careful assessment of the patient. This should take place initially and then regularly throughout the treatment process. Pain is an individual subjective experience and varies markedly among individuals. For this reason patient involvement is essential, and the most reliable indicators of severity are the patients' self-reports, based on appropriate scales.

Verbal pain-scoring methods, such as the verbal rating scale (VRS), use graded descriptors to rate the patient's pain as no pain, mild pain, moderate pain, severe pain, worst possible pain. The verbal numerical rating scale (VNRS) uses numbers. Patients are asked to rate their pain from 0 (no pain) to 10 (worst pain possible). The visual analogue scale (VAS) uses a 10-cm line rated from "no pain" at the left end to "worst pain possible" on the right. Patients are asked to show their pain by marking a representing point on the continuum of the line. Special scales or techniques have also been devised for patients who cannot communicate their pain, such as children, patients with hearing or cognitive impairment, etc. Binary scales are also simple to use and clinically relevant: The patient is asked to answer "yes" or "no" to simple questions about pain changes, such as "Is your pain relieved by at least 50%?" Once a certain scale has been

---

Box 10-2   Basics of Postoperative Pain Management

- Treat postoperative pain as early as possible.
- Consider the type of operation, the medical condition of the patient, and need for early recovery in planning regimen.
- "Tailor" and adjust regimen to individual patient's needs.
- Monitor pain and efficacy analgesia frequently.
- Aim at least at reducing pain to comfortable levels.
- Reduce pain at rest.
- Reduce pain with activity to levels allowing mobilization and function.
- Acute Pain Services produce better outcomes.

selected it should be continued for assessing an individual patient (Box 10-3).

Pain needs to be assessed at rest as well as during activity (e.g., moving, coughing). This is very important since the main purpose of an effective analgesic regimen is to allow function and facilitate early recovery. Analgesia, likewise, should also be adequate to cover pain not only at rest, but also be evaluated according to its efficacy to allow function or to enhance activity.

Pain should be regularly assessed at frequent intervals (e.g., every 2 hours for 48 hours following major surgery), and recorded on visible forms, such as postanesthetic care unit (PACU) records and bedside charts. Increasing pain may result from inadequate analgesia, but may also signify a postoperative complication (e.g., peritonitis, compartment syndrome). In the latter, the vital signs and the qualitative characteristics of the pain may change as well. In any case, a careful history and examination are indicated if any unexpected pain worsening occurs.

METHODS USED TO TREAT ACUTE PAIN

Pharmacologic or other interventions can modulate pain acting at many levels, from the site of injury in the periphery to the brain; anti-inflammatory agents can modify the action of mediators at the site of injury. Local anesthetics can block the transmission of signals in peripheral and neuraxial neural pathways. Other drugs (e.g., opioids, α_2-agonists) can modify the pain control systems via receptors at peripheral, spinal, or supraspinal sites. At the spinal levels, these agents may reduce the release of excitatory neurotransmitters from the afferent terminals or suppress the postsynaptic excitability. Gate control mechanisms can be manipulated using physical modalities [e.g., transcutaneous electrical nerve stimulation (TENS), physical therapy], and the cortical influences may be exploited using cognitive and behavioral manipulations.

Pharmacologic Methods

Opioids for Acute Pain
Opioid analgesics, acting at peripheral, spinal, and supraspinal sites after peripheral, systemic, or neuraxial

administration, are the basis of management of moderate to severe postoperative pain. Traditional methods of administration are via the oral, rectal, intravenous, subcutaneous, or intramuscular route. Novel methods include the peripheral administration, the neuraxial (i.e., spinal or epidural) route, and the use of patient-controlled analgesia (PCA). Other methods such as the intranasal or transmucosal administration of opioid agents have been introduced. The identification of opioid receptors in peripheral nociceptive fibers, and their upregulation after inflammation and tissue injury, has also lead to local application for postoperative pain control, such as the intra-articular injection of morphine after orthopedic joint procedures.

Selection of Agent and Doses of Perioperative Systemic Opioids
Individual opioid requirements vary greatly. For each patient an appropriate agent, dose and dosing interval, and route of administration need to be estimated (Box 10-4). Intermittent opioid injection can provide effective analgesia, but the quality of pain relief after intermittent intravenous (IV) boluses is far superior to that after intermittent intramuscular (IM) injections. Intravenous administration requires appropriate monitoring of the patient and advanced nursing attention. Nevertheless, titration of opioids by giving small IV increments, such as in the PACU, is the best method for estimating optimal starting doses. The dose has to be titrated to the effect, which is effective pain relief. If the patient is still complaining of pain and dose has all been delivered and acted, then it is safe to administer another dose, and if this too is not sufficient, then the process can be repeated.

Provided equianalgesic doses are given, all opioids produce the same analgesia, and there is no evidence that one is better than another (Table 10-3). Doses and dosing schedules depend on the patient's age, concomitant disease, type, site, extent of surgery, use of other drugs, etc.

The type and extent of trauma or surgery should be considered in the context that certain procedures (e.g., upper abdominal, thoracic) may be more painful than others, thus requiring more analgesics.

Box 10-3 Assessment of Postoperative Pain

- Apply consistency in using a suitable measurement scale.
- Assess pain at rest.
- Assess pain during activity.
- Assess analgesia as adequate to cover pain at rest and with activity.

Box 10-4 Steps to Providing Effective Opioid Analgesia Postoperatively

- Choose appropriate agent.
- Choose suitable route of administration.
- Estimate appropriate dose.
- Estimate dosing interval.
- Assess for effect and side effects. Adjust above parameters.
- Consider concomitant administration of other analgesics in a multimodal fashion.

Table 10-3   Approximate Equianalgesic Doses of Opioids

Opioid	Equianalgesic dose in mg	
	Parenteral	**Oral**
Agonist		
Morphine	10	30
Meperidine	100	300
Oxycodone	15	20–30
Fentanyl	0.1	NA
Hydromorphone	1.5	7.5
Methadone	10	20
Codeine	130	200
Dextropropoxyphene	65 (for mild pain)	130
Tramadol	100	
Partial agonist		
Buprenorphine	0.4	0.4 (sublingual)

When small IV boluses of morphine (e.g., 1 or 2 mg every 3 to 5 minutes) or another equivalent opioid are titrated in the PACU initially, subsequent doses can be adjusted according to the patient's response, level of pain, or possible side effects. The age, rather than the weight, of the patient should be used as a better predictor of opioid requirements. In opioid naive patients, using PCA morphine for postoperative pain relief after major surgery, the first 24 hours' requirements were shown to approximate the relationship.

Morphine requirements for the first 24 hours after major surgery = 100 – age.

Elderly patients require lower doses of opioids, and the duration of analgesia is usually longer. In children, however, weight is the most important determinant.

Nevertheless, considering the significant inter-individual variability, further adjustments may be necessary based on the initial clinical responses. For this reason, continuous observation and reassessment is mandatory.

When intramuscular or subcutaneous doses have to be used, suggested starting doses of morphine range, according to age, from 7.5 to 12.5 mg in 20- to 39-year-old patients, to 5 to 10 mg in 40- to 59-year-old patients, 2.5 to 7.5 mg in 60- to 69-year-old patients, 2.5 to 5 mg in 70- to 85-year-old patients, and 2 to 3 mg in patients older than 85.

The "Number-Needed-to-Treat" (NNT) Concept

This concept shows the effort required to achieve a particular therapeutic effect using pharmacologic or other methods. NNT describes the difference between active treatment and the control (i.e., placebo) and is described by the equation: 1/(proportion of patients with at least 50% pain relief with analgesic – proportion of patients with at least 50% pain relief with placebo). The best NNT is obviously 1, when every patient who receives treatment benefits and no patient given the placebo does benefit. However, there are very few circumstances in which a treatment is close to 100% effective and the control or placebo completely ineffective, so NNTs of 2 to 5 are considered satisfactory in showing effective analgesia. For adverse effects, the Number-Needed-to-Harm is used, which should be as large as possible.

NNTs have been used for comparisons among different analgesics. The efficacy of a single IM dose of 10 mg of morphine for moderate to severe postoperative pain, expressed in NNT, is 3. This means that one out of every 3 patients achieved more than 50% pain relief with 10 mg of morphine, which they would not have achieved with the placebo. This NNT (3) for 10 mg of IM morphine compares with other agents as shown in Table 10-4.

Side Effects of Opioids in the Postoperative Setting

These include respiratory depression, hypoxia, dysphoria, sedation, pruritus, nausea, vomiting, gastrointestinal slowing and constipation, and urinary retention. Most side effects are dose-dependent and respond to dose reduction. Otherwise, pharmacologic treatment is necessary, using specific agents, such as antiemetics to control nausea and vomiting (Box 10-5).

Table 10-4   Comparison of Analgesics for Moderate to Severe Postoperative Pain Using NNT

Analgesic (oral, except morphine)	Dose (mg)	NNT	95% confidence interval
Morphine (intramuscular)	10	2.9	2.6–3.6
Ibuprofen	400	2.7	2.5–3.0
Diclofenac	50	2.3	2.0–2.7
Naproxen	440	2.3	2.0–2.9
Ketorolac	10	2.5	2.2–3.0
Aspirin	600 to 650	4.4	4.0–4.9
Acetaminophen	1000	4.6	3.9–5.4
Acetaminophen plus codeine	600 to 650 + 60	3.1	2.6–3.9
Acetaminophen plus codeine	1000 + 60	1.9	N/A
Acetaminophen plus dextropropoxyphene	650 + 60	4.4	3.5–5.6
Tramadol	100	4.8	N/A

Box 10-5   Side Effects of Opioids

- Respiratory depression
- Hypoxia
- Dysphoria
- Sedation
- Pruritus
- Nausea, vomiting
- Gastrointestinal slowing and constipation
- Urinary retention
- Neuroexcitatory effects
- Opioid-induced hyperalgesia

Respiratory depression can be prevented with careful titration and individualization of the doses. Long-acting opioids or high doses are more likely to produce depression. Unrelieved pain tends to antagonize the opioid induced respiratory depression, while residual anesthetics, benzodiazepines, antihistamines, and many sedating antiemetics tend to increase its incidence. Patients with major upper abdominal or thoracic surgery, electrolyte abnormalities, hypovolemia, renal or liver dysfunction, raised intracranial pressure, or sleep apnea are more susceptible to respiratory depression and its sequelae (Box 10-6).

While a decrease in respiratory rate has been proven to be a late and unreliable sign in predicting respiratory depression, sedation is a better indicator and should be monitored and charted in those receiving postoperative opioids, in addition to other parameters, using a special sedation scale:

0 = no sedation
1 = mild, occasionally drowsy, easy to rouse
2 = moderate, frequently or constantly drowsy, easy to rouse
3 = severe, somnolent, difficult to rouse
S = normal sleep

Box 10-6   Patients More Susceptible to Opioid-Induced Respiratory Depression and Its Sequelae

- Patients with major upper abdominal surgery
- Patients with thoracic surgery
- Electrolyte abnormalities
- Hypovolemia
- Renal or liver dysfunction
- Raised intracranial pressure
- Morbid obesity or sleep apnea

Specific protocols, trained personnel, drugs (e.g., naloxone), and equipment should be readily available to treat impending respiratory depression.

Opioids can also produce episodic hypoxemia, in addition to hypoventilation, due to intermittent upper airway obstruction. Regardless of the mechanism, the opioid induced hypoxemia in association with the postoperative lung changes can lead to profound decreases in hemoglobin oxygen saturation postoperatively. Because of the risk of hypoxemia in the postoperative period, supplemental oxygen has been recommended for at least the first 2 or 3 postoperative days after major surgery as well as in elderly or high-risk patients.

Other risks are associated with the neuroexcitatory effects of normeperidine (an active metabolite of meperidine). For this reason, meperidine should not be used for more than 72 hours postoperatively, or in patients with renal failure, and should be better avoided in PCA. Furthermore, the pharmacologic properties of this drug (i.e., negative inotropic effect, atropine-like effect, histamine release) would discourage its selection as a first choice analgesic agent. Chronic morphine administration, impaired renal function, and age greater than 70 years have also all been associated with hyperalgesia and neuro-excitotoxicity from the morphine-3-glucuronide metabolite.

In hypovolemic patients opioids may cause hypotension via reducing a previously raised sympathetic tone that frequently accompanies pain. Vasodilation as a result of histamine release may also cause hypotension with some agents, such as morphine or meperidine.

Of particular concern are finally the inhibitory effects on the gastrointestinal function, which, together with the nausea and vomiting, may delay the oral intake of fluids and enteral feedings. This problem has been attempted to be attenuated by reducing the opioid doses using the concomitant administration of other analgesics (e.g., multimodal analgesia).

Routes of Administration of Opioids Postoperatively

Possible routes of administration will vary through the postoperative period and depend on many varying factors. Oral administration is effective provided the patient can swallow the drug into a functional gastrointestinal tract, such as after minor or ambulatory surgery. Intramuscular or subcutaneous injections may result in inadequate analgesia, if absorption of the injected drug is reduced as a result of poor peripheral perfusion (from sympathetically-induced vasoconstriction, hypovolemia, or hypothermia), while delayed absorption when perfusion returns may cause problems. The IV route permits a rapid, predictable, and immediately observable response, but needs meticulous attention and use of special nursing care in the wards. The sublingual route (i.e., buprenorphine) bypasses hepatic first-pass metabolism, while novel techniques using transnasal or transmucosal fentanyl have been described. Neuraxial administration will be described in the appropriate section.

Finally, intraarticular administration of morphine can produce analgesia after arthroscopic surgery.

Weak Opioids and Compound Preparations

Weak opioids include codeine, dihydrocodeine, dextropropoxyphene, and tramadol. These may be combined with acetaminophen in oral preparations and are frequently prescribed for moderate pain, such as after day-case or ambulatory surgery.

Patient-Controlled Analgesia

Intermittent IM injections of opioids result in large fluctuations, producing peaks and troughs in plasma drug concentration between drug injections. Drug concentration at the peaks will exceed limits associated with analgesia (i.e., the therapeutic window) and produce sedation or respiratory depression. Drug concentrations at the troughs may have fallen below the lower limit for analgesia, and the pain escalates in very high levels. A delay between the request and the next drug administration will allow pain to increase even higher, to intolerable levels. In IV PCA, a computer-controlled pump is used to administer small intermittent boluses of a drug via IV, on demand, by the patient. The bolus dose is preset and a lockout period is built into the system, during which the pump is refractory to further patient demands. This eliminates the large plasma fluctuations and maintains a tighter pain control by tending to keep drug concentrations within the analgesic window. Sedation or somnolence will prevent the patient from activating the pump, while escalation of pain from a previously tolerable level will result in activation and subsequent analgesia using a much smaller dose than in IM injection. Built-in safety algorithms prevent overdosing. Thus, PCA overcomes the wide variability in patients' analgesic requirements and allows individualization of analgesia. Studies have shown that PCA results in greater patient satisfaction and improves ventilation when compared to conventional analgesia. Patients most likely to benefit are:

- Those who've had major surgery and cannot be fed by mouth.
- Those with marked incident pain, such as during physiotherapy or dressing changes.
- Those with contraindications to IM injections (from coagulopathy).
- Those strongly motivated and appropriately educated.

In addition, side effects are reduced when PCA is managed by an Acute Pain Service versus a "nonpain" specialist physician. It is imperative that the patient should be visited frequently, assessed, and the settings be readjusted as needed. Most PCA devices allow interrogation and assessment of the history of use over a time period. Attempts to activate the device by pressing the activation button and episodes of actual administration of an analgesic bolus are being recorded and displayed. A high discrepancy between unsuccessful attempts and actual bolus administrations is indicative of not optimally managed pain.

PCA pumps offer the following options to be selected or preprogrammed before use (Table 10-5, Box 10-7):
1. Opioid selection.
2. Opioid concentration. This needs to be accurately entered for the pump to deliver the proper dose.
3. Loading dose. Those in pain, while the pump is being set up, should be given the selected opioid IV

Box 10-7 PCA Pump Programming Parameters

- Opioid concentration
- Loading dose before PCA initiation
- Bolus dose
- Lockout interval
- Continuous background infusion (not always necessary)
- Maximum dose limit

Table 10-5 Common Initial Values for IV PCA Settings

Setting	Value	Comment
Loading dose	Variable	Titrate for each patient before starting PCA.
Concentration	Variable	Standardized for each drug.
Bolus dose	Morphine 1–2 mg	Consider reducing to half in patients over 70 years of age.
	Fentanyl 20 µg	
	Hydromorphone 0.2 mg	Meperidine should be better avoided, particularly in more than 48 hours.
	Meperidine 10 mg	
Lockout interval	5–10 minutes	
Background infusion	Start with no background infusion	Patients with severe pain at night, or opioid tolerance may need background infusion. Use with caution.
1-hour maximum limit	10 mg morphine or equivalent	Varies according to age and prior opioid use.

in incremental doses (e.g., morphine 1 to 2 mg every 3 to 5 min.), until satisfactory analgesia is achieved.

4. Bolus dose. This is the dose to be given on demand by the patient, if this is requested outside the lockout interval.

5. Lockout interval. This limits the dosing interval. Large discrepancies between numbers of demands and numbers of boluses actually given indicate inadequate pain control.

6. Continuous background infusion. This is not always necessary because it may lead to unwanted effects. If chosen, hourly infusion rate should be approximately one quarter of the anticipated hourly opioid requirement.

7. Maximum dose limit. Setting a 1-hour maximum dose limit may safeguard against mishaps and alert against unsatisfied analgesia needs.

Nonopioid Analgesics
Nonsteroidal Anti-Inflammatory Drugs (NSAIDs)

These medications are more suitable for providing analgesia after outpatient, ambulatory surgery, in addition to being part of multimodal analgesia after more serious surgery. They can be the drugs of first choice after minor surgery.

NSAIDs are very effective against mild to moderate pain, such as after minor or moderate surgery. On the contrary, they are not very powerful as sole agents against severe pain that accompanies major procedures or trauma. Nevertheless, they can improve opioid analgesia; they have a significant opioid-sparing effect and can be useful in reducing opioid doses and side effects when used concurrently. Most NSAIDs are available in oral and rectal forms, and some can be given parenterally.

Because of certain side effects NSAIDs cannot be used in all patients. NSAIDs interfere with platelets, increase bleeding time, and some studies have shown increased blood loss. Appropriate perioperative use of NSAIDs has been successful and uncomplicated in several millions of patients worldwide. Nevertheless, ketorolac has been implicated in cases of sudden renal dysfunction, so vigilance is required. Risk factors include concomitant use of nephrotoxic antibiotics (e.g., aminoglycosides), raised intraabdominal pressure (e.g., laparoscopy), hypovolemia, and age more than 65 years. Risk of acute renal failure also increases after 5 days of therapy with ketorolac. Other side effects include gastrointestinal complaints and bleeding, aspirin-induced asthma, and precipitation of heart failure in susceptible patients. Drug interactions have also been reported with other drugs that include warfarin, oral hypoglycemics, phenytoin, digoxin, antibiotics, and antihypertensives.

Selective cyclooxygenase-2 inhibitors are effective analgesics for chronic pain, with fewer gastrointestinal side effects (but similar renal and liver toxicity); how-ever, more research is needed to prove their safety and efficacy for acute postoperative pain.

NSAID Doses. It is better to choose short-acting NSAIDs for postoperative analgesia so that cessation of the drug in case of ensuing side effects will abate them quickly. Ketorolac constitutes a reasonable choice, provided dosage recommendations are followed. Table 10-6 lists the agents and dosing characteristics.

Acetaminophen

Acetaminophen (paracetamol) is effective for mild to moderate pain (NNT = 4.6 for 1000 mg), and as an adjunct to opioids for more severe pain (NNT = 2 for 1000 mg with codeine 60 mg). Recommended doses for adults with no underlying renal or liver problems are 500 to 1000 mg, orally or rectally, every 3 to 6 hours, with a maximum daily dose of 6 gr in divided doses for acute pain, and 4 gr a day for chronic pain. Acetaminophen can significantly reduce postoperative opioid requirements up to 50%. A parenteral formulation is in use in Europe, and has been shown to be effective for postoperative analgesia. Liver disease and glucose-6-phosphate dehydrogenase deficiency are contraindications, but overall acetaminophen is safer than NSAIDs (Box 10-8).

Other Analgesics

Various other analgesics have been used alone or in combination for pain relief during the postoperative period.

Eutectic mixture of local anesthetics cream of lidocaine 2.5% and prilocaine 2.5% may provide comfort after superficial cutaneous procedures. The same agent, applied perioperatively around the operated area, has been shown to reduce postoperative analgesic requirements as well as the incidence and intensity of chronic pain in women undergoing breast surgery for cancer.

Inhalation of 50% nitrous oxide in oxygen (i.e., Entonox) has been used in the United Kingdom for analgesia in the wards, especially upon brief painful procedures (e.g., dressing changes, drain tube removal).

Because of the pivotal role of the NMDA receptor in mediating the central sensitization, drugs acting as NMDA antagonists have been under trial. Ketamine may be used by low-dose infusion in cases of difficult pain relief with opioids, but its usefulness is limited by psychotomimetic effects. Nevertheless, parenteral infusions of 0.25 mg/kg/hr may be helpful in selected cases. Dextromethorphan, another NMDA blocker with a better safety profile when combined with opioids, is under investigation.

The novel anticonvulsant and antihyperalgesic agent, gabapentin, has also been shown to be effective in reducing postoperative pain in certain settings as well as the transition to chronic pain.

Table 10-6 NSAIDs Dosing Characteristics

Drug	Dose (mg)	Dosing interval (h)	Maximum daily dose (mg)	Time to peak plasma concentration (h)	Elimination half-life (h)
ORAL FORMULATIONS					
Salicylates					
Aspirin	300-600	4	3600	1-2	0.25
Diflunisal	250-500	12	1000	2-4	8-12
Acetic Acids					
Indomethacin	50-100	6-12	200	1-2	6
Diclofenac	25-50	8-12	150	2-4	7
Sulindac	100-200	12	400		
Ketorolac (<65 yrs)	10	4-6	40	1	4-6
Ketorolac (>65 yrs)	10	6-8	30		
Propionic Acids					
Ibuprofen	200-800	6-8	2400	0.5-1.5	2-2.5
Ketoprofen	100	12-24	200	0.5-2	1.5
Naproxen	250-500	12	1000	1-2	15
Oxicams					
Piroxicam	10-20	24	20	2-4	53
Tenoxicam	10-20	24	20	1-2.6	72
Anthranilic Acids					
Mefenamic acid	500	8	1500	2-4	3-4
Parenteral Formulations					
Ketorolac (<65 yrs)	10-30	4-6	90	1	4-6
Ketorolac (>65 yrs)	10-15	4-6	60		

REGIONAL ANESTHETIC OR INVASIVE ANALGESIC TECHNIQUES

When used for postoperative pain management these techniques have advantages that include:
- Excellent analgesia at rest and upon movement and coughing.
- Some techniques may reduce postoperative morbidity and improve overall outcome.
- Most blocks are simple and rapidly effective.
- Duration may be prolonged by the use of catheters.

Box 10-8 Acetaminophen

- effective for mild to moderate pain
- useful adjunct to opioids for more severe pain
- 500 to 1000 mg, orally or rectally, every 3 to 6 hours
- liver disease and glucose-6-phosphate dehydrogenase deficiency are contraindications
- safer than NSAIDs

- Minimal systemic side effects from recommended doses.
- Avoidance of the side effects of opioids and NSAIDs.

Disadvantages include:
- Injections may not be well-accepted by patients.
- Limited duration of local anesthetics may require catheter placement.
- Sensory blockade from local anesthetics may result in trauma, and motor blockade may be unpleasant or undesirable.
- Intense analgesia may mask signs of painful complications (such as pain indicating compartment syndrome, peritonitis, or angina).
- Sympathetic blockade and hypotension may result from neuraxial local anesthetics (spinal or epidural).
- Risk of neurologic damage (very rare).

When regional techniques are considered for analgesia, they should be discussed with the patient and surgeon before surgery. Patient refusal or lack of understanding are strong contraindications as well as sepsis at the injection site (or systemic) and coagulopathy. Preexisting neurologic deficits should be documented meticulously. Regional anesthetic or invasive analgesic techniques include the following.

Wound Infiltration with Local Anesthetics

This is a well-established technique for analgesia after minor surgery or pediatric surgery performed under anesthesia. The benefits are less certain after major surgery, but even there infiltration with local anesthetic allows a small reduction in postoperative opioid requirements or pain scores. Benefits are more prominent when large volumes are infiltrated in deeper structures (e.g., fasciae, peritoneum) versus just subcutaneously.

Regional Techniques

"Single shot" techniques may provide many hours of postoperative analgesia, while the effects can be prolonged using catheters for repeated or continuous local anesthetic administrations. Commonly performed peripheral nerve blocks for postoperative analgesia include ilioinguinal, iliohypogastric, and genitofemoral nerve block (for inguinal and femoral hernia), dorsal nerve of penis blocks (for circumcision), femoral nerve block (for procedures on the front of the thigh above the patella or postknee arthroscopy analgesia), lateral femoral cutaneous block (for superficial procedures on the lateral thigh), sciatic or popliteal nerve blocks (for various lower extremity operations), ankle block (for foot surgery), digital block (for digit surgery), and intercostal blocks (for surgery involving chest or abdominal wall). These blocks can produce one-sided, lasting analgesia, with no hemodynamic instability, no urinary reten-

tion, thus expediting outpatient recovery. In addition, blockade of various plexuses may provide analgesia over a wide dermatomal range. These include the superficial cervical plexus block (for analgesia over the anterior neck, for example, after thyroid or carotid surgery), interscalene brachial plexus block (for the upper arm and shoulder), supraclavicular block (for the elbow and arm), axillary block (for the lower arm and hand), and the lumbar plexus block (for surgery in the thigh). Paravertebral blocks also can be useful after thoracotomy or breast surgery. Their main benefit, over the intercostal nerve block, is that they also block the posterior primary rami, which innervate the dorsal structures of the torso. They also do not cause bilateral sympathetic block, and result in less hypotension compared to epidurals (Box 10-9).

Continuous regional analgesia techniques have been used, employing special catheters placed at the nerves or plexuses to be blocked. Continuous brachial plexus blocks via an axillary approach can be achieved, using continuous infusions of bupivacaine 0.25%, at 0.2 to 0.4 mg/kg/hr, for a patient undergoing upper extremity orthopedic or vascular procedures. Other continuous techniques include the continuous femoral nerve block after total knee replacement and the continuous interscalene block after major shoulder surgery.

INTRATHECAL AND EPIDURAL ANALGESIA

Intrathecal Analgesia

Intrathecal local anesthetics, although they provide excellent conditions for surgery, do not last to cover the

---

Box 10-9 Common Peripheral Nerve Blocks for Postoperative Analgesia

Nerve blocks:
- Ilioinguinal, iliohypogastric and genitofemoral nerve block (for inguinal and femoral hernia repair)
- Dorsal nerve of penis blocks (for circumcision)
- Femoral nerve block (for procedures on the front of the thigh or knee)
- Lateral femoral cutaneous block (for superficial procedures on the lateral thigh)
- Sciatic or popliteal nerve blocks (for various lower extremity operations)
- Ankle block (for foot surgery)
- Digital block (for digit surgery)
- Intercostal blocks (for surgery involving chest or abdominal wall)

Plexus blocks:
- Superficial cervical plexus block (for analgesia over the anterior neck)
- Interscalene brachial plexus block (for the upper arm and shoulder)
- Supraclavicular block (for the elbow and arm)
- Axillary block (for the lower arm and hand)
- Lumbar plexus block (for surgery in the thigh)
- Paravertebral blocks (after thoracotomy or breast surgery)

postoperative period as well. Intrathecal opioids, given as a single dose together with the injected local anesthetics, may provide long-lasting analgesia, but the duration of pain relief may be unpredictable and variable. Fentanyl may produce analgesia for 1 to 6 hours, while morphine's effect ranges from 4 to 24 hours. Side effects, also variable and dose-dependent, include nausea, itching, sedation, urinary retention, and respiratory depression that may be delayed in the case of the morphine.

Epidural Analgesia

Epidural analgesia, with local anesthetics and/or opioids administered via a catheter, is utilized as a method of providing substantially improved pain relief and easier rehabilitation, with a possibly improved outcome. This applies to gains from easier mobilization, reduction of cardiac complications, improvement in respiratory function with fewer respiratory complications, earlier return and improved bowel motility after abdominal surgery, improved vascular graft patency, reduced deep venous thrombosis rate, and shorter hospitalizations.

Patients who can benefit the most from epidural analgesia are those subjected to surgical procedures such as cesarean section, thoracotomy, aortic aneurysm repair or major vascular surgery of lower extremities, total knee replacement, limb amputation, large upper abdominal surgery (such as pancreatectomy, open cholecystectomy, nephrectomy, liver surgery, stomach surgery), major lower abdominal surgery (involving small bowel, mesentery, colon, radical prostate, total abdominal hysterectomy), or thoracic trauma with rib fractures. Patients who may benefit are also those suffering from coexisting medical conditions, such as advanced respiratory disease or myocardial ischemia. Finally, although the evidence is equivocal, epidural analgesia has been used to prevent the transition to chronic pain after amputation (Box 10-10).

Local anesthetics and opioids, administered together, have a synergistic rather than additive effect allowing dose reduction and limitation of side effects. The risks are those of an epidural technique (i.e., infection, hematoma, abscess), those of the local anesthetic (i.e., cardiac and central nervous system), and those of the opioid (i.e., "early" or "late" respiratory depression, urinary retention, itching, nausea). The wrong drugs or doses can be given. There is an increased need for urinary catheterization. The risk of persistent neurologic sequelae after an epidural ranges from about 1 in 5000 to 1 in 100,000.

These medications can be administered intermittently, but most commonly a continuous administration technique is employed, using an infusion pump, while supplemental bolus doses are prescribed for breakthrough pain. A patient-controlled epidural analgesia technique is also available, wherein patients treat their pain by self-administering doses of analgesics via a programmed pump.

With regard to the required doses for analgesia, there is a significant variability amongst individuals, necessitating individualized treatment plans and careful titration. The first step in individualizing pain relief is to establish realistic treatment goals. The goal of titration is to use the smallest analgesic dose that provides satisfactory pain relief with the fewest adverse effects. In the presence of inadequate analgesia during epidural analgesia, the entire line of administration from the infusion pump to the patient's epidural catheter site should be checked first. Inadequate pain relief may be due to a number of mechanical and technical factors, including a disconnection of the catheter from the infusion pump tubing, an empty drug reservoir, a kinked catheter, a malfunctioning pump or tubing, or the epidural catheter may have been inadvertently pulled out. A neurologic assessment is also necessary to indicate the level of the block. Finally, a test dose of a small dose of lidocaine (2 to 3 ml of a 1.5% to 2% solution, with or without epinephrine), after negative aspiration, may confirm the presence of a functional catheter and the extent of a sensory block.

Epidural and intrathecal techniques can be safely applied in patients hospitalized on general hospital wards, provided that appropriate monitoring can be applied, an anesthesiologist is available to treat complications at all

---

Box 10-10   Patients Who Would Most Benefit from Epidural Analgesia

Patients who have had one or more of the following:
- Cesarean section
- Thoracotomy
- Aortic aneurysm repair or major vascular surgery of lower extremities
- Total knee replacement
- Limb amputation
- Major upper abdominal surgery (such as pancreatectomy, open cholecystectomy, nephrectomy, liver surgery, stomach surgery)
- Major lower abdominal surgery (involving small bowel, mesentery, colon, radical prostate, total abdominal hysterectomy)
- Thoracic trauma with rib fractures
- Advanced respiratory disease or myocardial ischemia

times, nursing staff follow certain policies and can detect side effects promptly, the epidural site is checked regularly, and, finally, pain scores, sedation, respiratory parameters, sensory, and motor block as well as hemodynamic signs are monitored frequently.

Agents Used in Neuraxial Analgesic Techniques

Local Anesthetics

Their effect is not limited to nociceptive blockade only, but side effects may occur related to sympathetic blockade (e.g., hypotension), motor blockade (e.g., weakness, inability to ambulate), urinary retention, or the systemic absorption and toxicity of the local anesthetics. The sympathetic blockade may be beneficial whenever an increase of the regional blood supply is desirable. Nevertheless, administered at reduced concentrations together with opioid agents can enhance quality of postoperative analgesia, at reduced risk of side effects. Suitable agents for epidural administration include bupivacaine at concentrations 0.0625% to 0.25%, or ropivacaine 0.05% to 0.2%.

Neuraxial Opioids

The presence of opioid receptors in the spinal cord is the basis of intrathecal or epidural injection of opioids in order to produce selective analgesia, without any significant sympathetic or motor blockade. This provides a significant advantage over the sole use of local anesthetics, the use of which is limited by the aforementioned, undesirable effects. Meperidine, however, has a direct local anesthetic effect that may lead to sensory and motor block when administered in the neuraxis.

Intrathecal administration of an opioid provides faster onset of action and allows the use of much smaller doses than the epidural route. The kinetics and characteristics of action of an epidurally administered opioid depend on its physicochemical characteristics, the most important of which is the lipid solubility; this determines the rate and extent of systemic absorption via the blood vasculature, local binding to fat, transfer across the membranes into the cerebrospinal fluid (CSF), and subsequent migration to other spinal or supraspinal segments. Lipophilic drugs, such as sufentanil or fentanyl, show a rapid and extensive systemic uptake with significant concentrations detected in the plasma within minutes after the injection. On the other hand, as a result of the enhanced binding at the neural segments at the level of the administration, the more lipophilic opioids have a faster onset of a more localized, intense, and short-lasting analgesia. A supraspinal

effect resulting from the systemically absorbed drug may enhance the direct antinociceptive effect at the spinal level, or according to some speculations, may predominate in the analgesic action. Fast systemic uptake may also lead to early respiratory depression.

On the contrary, the more hydrophilic drugs such as morphine show less systemic uptake and slowly cross the membranes passing into the CSF, where they migrate over time. This may produce a slower onset of a long lasting analgesia, which is not limited only to the levels of administration, but extends over time to include other spinal segments.

Side Effects of Neuraxial Opioids

These can be more severe after intrathecal rather than epidural administration (Box 10-11). They include:

1. Respiratory depression. This is the most serious side effect. It can be early, occurring within an hour after injection of lipophilic opioids, resulting from the fast systemic uptake. In the case of the hydrophilic drugs, however, it can be of delayed occurrence, as a result of the cephalad migration. Elderly, debilitated, or high-risk patients, those receiving concomitantly opioids or other depressants from the systemic route, those receiving higher doses of mainly hydrophilic opioids from the intrathecal rather than the epidural route, are at a much higher risk of developing respiratory depression. This may occur unexpectedly, even in the absence of a premonitory decrease of the respiratory rate, while a progressive decline in the mental status may provide a better imminent warning sign. Infusion of naloxone, carefully titrated, may reverse the respiratory depression, leaving the analgesia intact.

2. Nausea and vomiting.

Box 10-11   Side Effects of Neuraxially-Administered Agents

Local anesthetics:
• Sympathetic blockade (hypotension)
• Motor blockade (weakness, inability to ambulate)
• Urinary retention
• Systemic absorption and toxicity

Opioids:
• Respiratory depression
• Nausea and vomiting
• Pruritus
• Urinary retention
• Herpetic infections in pregnant patients

3. Pruritus, not necessarily related to histamine release, may be a neuroexcitatory effect. It is dose dependent and naloxone infusion, titrated from small rates, may reduce it without reversing analgesia. Small doses of propofol have been also shown to be effective.

4. Urinary retention, may develop insidiously, may produce bladder overdistention, and is also responsive to naloxone.

5. Neuraxial opioids may potentially reactivate herpetic infections in pregnant patients, something that may lead to transmission of the virus to the infant. Their use should be discouraged in parturients with a relevant history.

Clinical Use of Neuraxial Opioids

As mentioned previously, epidurally (or intrathecally) administered opioids diffuse and act at receptors in the dorsal horns, thus producing selective analgesia. They have a synergistic analgesic action with the local anesthetics, allowing doses (and side effects) to be reduced.

The physicochemical properties of different opioids reflect differences in the clinical analgesia and the profile of the side effects.

Hydrophilic opioids (e.g., morphine) have a longer residence time in the CSF and exhibit cephalad migration over time. This results in prolonged analgesia, but also potential for delayed respiratory depression 12 to 24 hours after a single dose. Furthermore, because of the distribution in the CSF and migration to distant segments, the analgesia is more extensive. The epidural catheter tip does not need to be close to the source of nociceptive input, and lumbar administration may provide effective analgesia in thoracic levels or the lower extremities. Morphine can be used in a continuous infusion (at concentrations 50 to 100 μg/ml), or in single intermittent boluses (5 mg for patients up to 50 years old and up to 3 mg for those older than 60). Onset time is 30 minutes, peak effect is in 60 to 90 minutes, and duration of action is up to 12 hours or more.

Lipophilic opioids, like fentanyl, migrate less and exhibit stronger binding at the neural segments close to the site of administration, thus producing more segmental analgesia of shorter duration. Onset time is 5 minutes, peak 20 minutes, and duration lasts 2 to 3 hours. Because of the short duration, fentanyl is more suitable for continuous epidural infusion at a rate 0.5 to 1 μg/kg/hr; significant plasma concentrations may result in early analgesia from systemic absorption, and early respiratory depression.

The side effects of epidural opioids are respiratory depression, nausea and vomiting, urinary retention, and pruritus. Naloxone, carefully titrated starting from very low doses, may suppress those side effects while leaving the analgesic effect intact.

Nonopioid Spinal Analgesics

These include:

- Neuraxial α$_2$ agonists (e.g., clonidine) that may synergistically enhance the opioid-induced analgesia, or prolong the duration of local anesthetics. They may also have analgesic effects as sole agents. Clonidine does not produce respiratory depression or nausea, but may cause hypotension, bradycardia, and sedation.

- γ-Aminobutyric acid agonists. Midazolam, neuraxially administered, has analgesic properties, but is still under investigation for clinical applications. The potential analgesic effects of baclofen as a neuraxial analgesic have not yet fully assessed.

- Neostigmine has analgesic effects when administered intrathecally. The main side effect is nausea and vomiting.

- Intrathecal NSAIDs, amitriptyline, as well as specific N-type calcium channel blockers (e.g., SNX-111), are under investigation with regards to use for postoperative analgesia.

Nonpharmacologic Methods for Acute Pain

Cognitive-behavioral treatment includes preparatory information, relaxation, imagery, hypnosis, and biofeedback. Physical therapeutic modalities include guided mobilization, application of superficial heat or cold, massage, TENS, and acupuncture. TENS therapy has been considered effective in a variety of postoperative situations including major abdominal or orthopedic surgery. Other studies suggest that acupuncture reduces pain and analgesic consumption following dental or abdominal surgery.

MULTIMODAL ANALGESIA

Multimodal analgesia employs various combinations of drugs, administered by the same or different routes, in order to improve the quality of analgesia with a reduction in side effects. NSAIDs, acetaminophen, local anesthetics, and other nonopioid analgesics can be used in combinations resulting in improved pain relief at rest, better pain relief during movement, easier mobilization, and earlier gastrointestinal recovery. For example, administration of an NSAID, such as ketorolac or ibuprofen, in combination with epidural opioids and local anesthetics, will provide additional analgesia at lower doses of all three analgesics, thereby reducing adverse effects of each.

By minimizing the opioid requirements, multimodal analgesia may produce effective analgesia upon movement allowing early ambulation. Furthermore, early enteral nutrition can be resumed faster by avoiding opioid-related side effects. The value of multimodal analgesia has been also proven in the day surgical patients, where dose reduction and improved analgesia allows earlier ambulation and fewer side effects.

PREEMPTIVE ANALGESIA

Preemptive analgesia aims to reduce pain by interventions applied before the noxious stimulation. Analgesics and/or local anesthetics prior to surgery may have prolonged effects that outlast their presence by preventing the central sensitization. However, evidence in humans has been equivocal, apparently because afferent nociceptive activity continues for quite a long time after surgery secondary to trauma and the inflammatory responses of the injured tissues. Nevertheless, more aggressive, rationally designed approaches to the management of early postoperative pain may reduce the transition to chronic pain.

POSTOPERATIVE ANALGESIA IN SPECIAL SETTINGS

Special considerations apply in day-surgery patients. Options for pain control include local anesthetics (by wound infiltration or nerve blocks), NSAIDS (they can be more effective than certain opioids), and short-acting opioids (the side effects of which may delay discharge from hospital). A significant percentage of day-case patients (10% to 20%) may experience moderate to severe pain following return at home that may affect activity or lead to unplanned hospitalizations. This can be prevented by adequate discharge planning and education about the use of medications at home.

ACUTE PAIN IN CHILDREN

Children of all ages, including neonates, definitely experience pain and its adverse sequelae. Principles of acute pain management should follow the same principles as in adults based on regular proper assessments (special scales have been devised), individualization of management plans, suitable prevention, and attempts to restore function. Multimodal analgesic techniques can be particularly useful in children as well as the conventional techniques, taking into consideration the differing needs, physiologic development, pharmacokinetics, pharmacodynamics, and specific side effects of the agents used. Morphine, for severe pain, can be used in doses 0.1 to 0.2 mg/kg, and repeated until analgesia is achieved. PCA can be used in children above 5 years of age, with boluses 0.02 mg/kg, lockout periods 5 minutes, and background infusions 4 µg/kg/h. Monitoring standards should be the same as in the adults. Acetaminophen is frequently used in doses 15 mg/kg every 5 hours orally, or rectally. NSAIDs can be used in the older children, but neonates show decreased clearance. Finally, local anesthesia can provide excellent analgesia, with the caudal technique being the most commonly used block for children. The use of epidural analgesia is also becoming more and more common in this population.

SUGGESTED READING

Abram S: Preemptive analgesia. Seminars in Anesthesia 16:263, 1997.

American Pain Society. Principles of Analgesic Use in the Treatment of Acute Pain and Cancer Pain, 4th ed. 1999.

Brennan TJ: Acute Pain Management. ASA Refresher Course Lectures, 2002, p 113.

Cook TM: Postoperative pain management. In Stannard CF, Booth S (eds): Pain. Churchill-Livingstone, 1998, p 131.

Fassoulaki A, Patris K, Sarantopoulos C, Hogan Q: The analgesic effect of gabapentin and mexiletine after breast surgery for cancer. Anesth Analg 95:985, 2003.

Fassoulaki A, Sarantopoulos C, Melemeni A, Hogan Q: EMLA reduces acute and chronic pain after breast surgery for cancer. Regional Anesthesia and Pain Medicine 25:350, 2000.

Fassoulaki A, Sarantopoulos C, Melemeni A, Hogan Q: Regional Blockade and Mexiletine: The effect on pain after cancer breast surgery. Regional Anesthesia and Pain Medicine 26:223, 2001.

Fassoulaki A, Triga A, Melemeni A, Sarantopoulos C: Multimodal analgesia with gabapentin and local anesthetics prevents acute and chronic pain after breast surgery for cancer. Anesth Analg 101:1427–1432, 2005.

Kehlet H, Dahl B: The value of multimodal or balanced analgesia in postoperative pain treatment. Anesth Analg 77:1048, 1993.

Kehlet H, Holte K: Effect of postoperative analgesia on surgical outcome. Br J Anaesth 87:62, 2001.

Lubenow TR, Ivankovich AD, McCarthy RJ: Management of acute postoperative pain. In Barash PG, Cullen BF, Stoelting RK: Clinical Anesthesia, 3rd ed. Lippincott-Raven, 1997, p 1339.

Moiniche S, Kehlet H, Dahl JB: A qualitative and quantitative systematic review of preemptive analgesia for postoperative pain relief. The role of timing of analgesia. Anesthesiology 96:725, 2002.

Moller AM, Smith AF, Pedersen T: Evidence-based medicine and the Cochrane Collaboration in anaesthesia. Br J Anaesth 84:655, 2000.

Rauck RL: Acute postoperative and posttraumatic pain management. In Miller RD, Abram SE (eds): Atlas of Anesthesia, Vol. VI. Churchill-Livingstone, 1998, p 41.

Sarantopoulos C, Fassoulaki A: Sufentanil does not preempt pain after abdominal hysterectomy. Pain 65:273, 1996.

Smith G, Power I, Cousins MJ: Acute pain—is there scientific evidence on which to base treatment? Br J Anaesth 82:817, 1999.

Wu CL: Perioperative regional anesthesia and patient outcomes. In American Society of Regional Anesthesia and Pain Medicine, 27th Annual Meeting Syllabus, 2002, p 37.

National Health and Medical Research Council, Commonwealth of Australia. Acute Pain Management: Scientific Evidence. Canberra, 1999. Available from: www.health.gov.au/nhmrc/publications/pdf/cp57.pdf

CHAPTER 11

Pediatric Pain

JAYA L. VARADARAJAN
STEVEN J. WEISMAN

INTRODUCTION

Pain in children is a complex constellation of unpleasant sensory, emotional, and perceptual experiences with associated autonomic, psychological, emotional, and behavioral responses. In newborns, infants, and older children, who are developmentally or verbally challenged, pain cannot be described in these terms, as the definition requires self-report. As a result, pain in children has gone unrecognized, misunderstood, and often undertreated, sometimes even neglected completely. The treatment and alleviation of pain are basic human rights that exist regardless of age and mandate treatment.

Pediatric pain management has blossomed into a specialty in recent years as more physicians are becoming aware of the need to adequately treat pain in infants and children. An organized system for management of acute and chronic pain in children was traditionally lacking in previous years. It has been known for many years that pediatric patients are more likely to have their pain treated less aggressively than their adult counterparts. The reasons for this possibly include lack of awareness on the part of the public, misinformation and lack of knowledge among physicians, and the inherent difficulty in assessing pain in an age group that may not be fully capable of verbally communicating with caregivers. Although accurate assessment of pain in children continues to be a challenge, there is a heightened awareness of the magnitude of this problem among physicians.

The development of nociception in infants was not well understood until very recently. It was known that the infant nervous system was immature and myelination of nerve tracts necessary for afferent impulse transmission incomplete; but we now know that the anatomic requirements for pain processing are in place prior to birth, as early as 22 to 24 weeks of gestation, so the fetus is capable of experiencing pain. Following the publication of a landmark article by Anand and Hickey in 1987, it is now globally accepted that the neonatal nervous system is capable of processing nociceptive input and neonates feel pain.[1] These investigators also demonstrated that infants whose pain was well-controlled intraoperatively with narcotics did well postoperatively.

Research in newborn animals has shown that failure to control pain results in a 'rewiring' of the pathways responsible for pain transmission in the dorsal horn of the spinal cord and results in increased pain perception for future pain insults. Surgical pain results in not only an immediate nociceptive response, but also results in changes in the activation pathways of nociception that eventually lead to hypersensitivity, hyperalgesia, and allodynia. Studies in rat models have demonstrated larger nociceptive receptor fields and immature descending inhibitory systems. There is also evidence that repeated nociceptive stimuli result in lowering of sensory thresholds and thermal hyperalgesia. A study of a rat model of chronic inflammation demonstrated neural remodeling in the spinal cord in the form of increased sprouting of primary sensory fibers with caudal extension and hyperexcitability of dorsal horn neurons. Increased and abnormal pain behaviors were seen later in the adult animals.

We are still unclear as to the extent of suffering felt by neonates, how much of the pain experience they remember, the effect of a painful experience on their development, and the impact of early pain experiences on their response to future pain. What we do know is that there is a lack of descending modulation in the spinal cord in neonates with a resultant lowered threshold to mechanical and thermal stimuli coupled with exaggerated hormonal, metabolic, and immune responses. This makes it all the more important that we are aggressive in treating pain in infants and children. Numerous studies have shown that the stress response can be blunted, pain can be adequately treated, and that there are multiple modalities available that are both safe and effective. Therefore, inadequate pain control in the intraoperative or postoperative period and poor management of chronic pain problems is no longer acceptable. Untreated pain in children from any cause can have long-term effects. In fact, not only do children experience pain, but also they are particularly vulnerable to the consequences of inadequate treatment.

ASSESSMENT OF PAIN IN CHILDREN

Pain assessment remains one of the biggest challenges in pediatric pain management. It is not possible to use a standard approach to every patient, since children present a range of differences in age and cognitive development. Also, the intensity of pain as experienced by the child is not often proportional to the objective degree of injury. Children have a more intense physical and emotional reaction to pain than adults. There is no other field where the need to tailor one's approach to the individual patient assumes more importance.

The modalities used to measure pain in children include physiologic, behavioral, and self-report measures. Physiologic parameters indicate the presence of pain through changes in physiologic variables that are assumed to be associated with pain. These include heart rate, blood pressure, respiratory rate, oxygen saturation, transcutaneous O_2 or CO_2 tensions, vagal tone, intracranial pressure, palmar sweating, serum cortisol, catecholamine, growth hormone and endorphin levels. Of these, the first three are the variables that can be practically measured clinically on a daily basis. Behavioral measures such as the quality and frequency of a child's cry, facial expressions, body positions, motor activity, changes in eating or sleeping habits, or cognitive functioning are very useful in assessing the level of pain in a child. The Children's Hospital of Eastern Ontario Pain Scale; Neonatal Infant Pain Scale; and Face, Legs, Activity, Cry, Consolability (FLACC) as well as many other observational scales have been validated for use in infants and children. Self-reports are communications of the experience of pain and are numeric measures such as the Visual Analog Scale, the Wong-Baker, Bieri or Oucher Faces scales, pain thermometer, poker chip tool, pain ladders, drawings, or maps. They do not address or reflect nociception directly. Although no self-report scale is ideal for all applications in all age groups, many are acceptable for use in children over 3 years of age. In children, the numeric rating scale (pain rated from 0 to 10) may be more reliable than the visual analog scale (10-cm line). However, it is reliable only in children who understand the concept of number and order (generally more than 7 years old). The facial expression scales make minimal cognitive and linguistic demands and may be used in children over the age of 3 years. Regardless of which self-report scale is used, it is important to explain the scale clearly and consistently to the child and encourage measurement rather than be strict about scaling quantities. It is also important to remember that children may not equate the end-points on different scales so all caregivers should use the same scale when talking to a child (Table 11-1).

Cognitively or physically impaired children are at greater risk for undertreatment of pain because they have underlying medical problems that are often painful and repeatedly need procedures that cause pain. Behavioral idiosyncrasies that may mask expression of pain in this population do not make the situation easier. Many behaviors that are otherwise typical pain indicators are inconsistent and difficult to interpret in these children because

Table 11-1	Developmental Sequence of Children's Understanding of Pain
0-3 mo	No apparent understanding of pain; memory of pain likely, but not conclusively demonstrated; responses appear reflexive and are perceptually dominated
3-6 mo	Pain response supplemented by sadness and anger response
6-18 mo	Developing fear of painful situations; words common for pain (e.g., owie, ouchie, boo-boo); localization of pain develops
18-24 mo	Use of the word "hurt" to describe pain; beginning to use noncognitive coping strategies
24-36 mo	Begins to describe pain and attribute an external cause to the pain
36-60 mo	Can give a gross indication of the intensity of the pain and beginning to use more descriptive adjectives and attach emotional terms such as "sad" or "mad" to the pain
5-7 yr	Can more clearly differentiate levels of pain intensity; beginning to use cognitive coping strategies
7-10 yr	Can explain why a pain hurts
>11	Can explain the value of pain

of physical problems. The parents and caregivers are usually an extremely good resource for pain assessment. Some of the commonly used composite scales, such as FLACC, have been validated in this patient population. The common causes for pain in the developmentally-delayed child include gastroesophageal problems, muscle spasm, constipation, and postoperative pain.

ACUTE PAIN IN CHILDREN

Acute pain refers to pain associated with a brief episode of tissue injury or inflammation such as that caused by surgery, burns, trauma, or procedures. In most cases the intensity of the pain diminishes steadily with time over a period of days to weeks. However, it produces changes in both the peripheral and central nervous system (CNS) that can result in the evolution of chronic pain. Some of the most common causes of acute pain in healthy children include procedures such as immunizations and blood draws. In children with associated illnesses, children are often subjected to peripheral venous line placements, central line placements, lumbar punctures, and bone-marrow aspirations. The consequences of not treating acute pain can be catastrophic. The unchecked release of stress hormones may exacerbate injury, prevent wound healing, lead to infection, prolong hospitalization, and even lead to death. The risks are greatest in the sickest and frailest of patients. Hence, there should be no reservation in treating a critically sick child or newborn with analgesics. In older children, adequate postoperative analgesia allows earlier ambulation, prevents atelectasis, and facilitates earlier recovery. There are also psychological consequences to the undertreatment of pain. Children who are subjected to painful procedures without adequate analgesia anticipate the next experience with an even greater degree of fear and anxiety. It is therefore extremely important that the first experience be made as pain-free as possible. We can take advantage of the child's cognitive development, coping

skill set, and intellectual ability to acknowledge the fact that the procedure is painful and, using these characteristics, we can offer support during the procedure. Denying or minimizing the pain is not beneficial for anyone involved. We are not always given the opportunity to address postoperative pain management at a preoperative, especially in this day of outpatient surgeries. However, it is essential that a thorough discussion, prior to the surgical procedure, takes place with the parent and child.

NONPHARMACOLOGIC MEASURES

These techniques help reduce anxiety and pain and may even reduce the requirement for opioids or other analgesics. Topical cooling or warmth is useful in some children. Oral sucrose, administered 60 seconds before a procedure, has been used for infants receiving heel pricks and immunizations and has been found to be safe and effective. Comfort measures such as swaddling and non-nutritive sucking, on a pacifier, for instance, have been known to reduce crying in infants. Transcutaneous electrical nerve stimulation (TENS) has been used for various types of procedural pain. Cognitive-behavioral techniques including meditation, biofeedback, guided imagery, hypnosis, and relaxation techniques, although being more common in chronic pain management, have been found to be useful for acute problems as well. Most of these techniques can be taught to children as young as 3 to 4 years of age. Acupuncture has become popular for management of incidental pain and other conditions associated with pain including postoperative nausea and vomiting.

CUTANEOUS

Topical administration of local anesthetics is widely used for pain associated with needle pricks, IV line placements, lumbar punctures, laceration repairs, and procedures on superficial skin lesions. Eutectic mixture of local anesthetics (EMLA) containing lidocaine and prilocaine can be used for cutaneous anesthesia. It needs to be in contact with the skin under an occlusive dressing for at least an hour prior to any procedure to provide sufficient cutaneous analgesia. This limits its use. In addition, there is the need to prepare multiple sites in the case of difficult IV placements. There is also the risk of methemoglobinemia from the prilocaine moiety. Prilocaine can also cause vasoconstriction and make blood collection from a heel prick more difficult. Liposomal lidocaine (LMX4) is also available for cutaneous anesthesia. It requires a 30-minute application and is associated with less vasoconstriction, but equivalent anesthesia. Outside of the United States, amethocaine (tetracaine) gel is available, and it appears to have similar onset and efficacy to LMX4.

Iontophoretic transcutaneous delivery of lidocaine has been used effectively for IV-line placement with analgesia being achieved in about 10 minutes. This methodology of transdermal delivery employs an external electric field to facilitate movement of ionizable drugs through the skin. The other drugs that can be delivered iontophoretically include corticosteroids, morphine, and fentanyl. The tingling sensation associated with the electric current may be uncomfortable for some patients and cutaneous burns from the electrical devices have been reported. A new system using superficial application of a yttrium aluminum garnet laser to remove the outermost layer of skin stratum corneum is also available (Epiture Easy Touch, Norwood Abbey Ltd). If liposomal lidocaine is then applied to the treated skin, anesthesia occurs in 5 to 10 minutes.

NONSTEROIDAL ANTI-INFLAMMATORY DRUGS

Aspirin (acetylsalicylic acid) is the oldest nonopioid analgesic. It is analgesic, anti-inflammatory, and antipyretic. Aspirin inhibits prostaglandin synthesis and release in an irreversible fashion. It also binds to platelets thus inhibiting their function in an irreversible fashion. Toxic effects are seen with large doses or repeated doses, gastrointestinal upset being the most common. Its use as an antipyretic has been associated with the development of Reye's syndrome with liver damage and CNS symptoms, which is the reason it is not widely used today in children. Its elimination is significantly slower in neonates compared to adults. However, it still does have a role in the management of mild to moderate pain such as in juvenile rheumatoid arthritis, where both analgesic and anti-inflammatory properties are desired.

Acetaminophen (e.g., Tylenol, Paracetamol) is an analgesic and antipyretic similar to aspirin. It blocks prostaglandin synthesis by inhibiting cyclooxygenase (COX) in the CNS, reduces substance P induced hyperal-gesia, and modulates spinal-cord production of hyperalgesic nitric oxide. It does not inhibit prostaglandin synthesis in other tissues. It is a weak analgesic, most appropriate for mild pain or as an adjunct in the treatment of moderate to severe pain. However, it has minimal anti-inflammatory and virtually no antiplatelet effect in doses traditionally used. Analgesic plasma concentrations of acetaminophen are not known, but concentrations of 10 to 20 μg/ml are thought to be antipyretic. Dosages of acetaminophen, either orally or rectally, vary from 15 to 40 mg/kg. However, recent data suggest that therapeutic analgesic levels for postoperative pain are more easily attained with doses in the range of 30 to 60 mg/kg. Antipyretic effects are more easily attained at lower doses. Although the responses are dose-dependent, it is limited by a ceiling effect. Acetaminophen is metabolized, even in the newborn liver with immature function, so it is safe to use in neonates. The elimination rate is similar in neonates, children, and adults. Repeated use of large doses in the range of 150 mg/kg per oral dose has been associated with liver damage. Plasma concentrations of 150 to 200 μg/ml are considered an indication for starting rescue therapy. The prodrug, propacetamol, is available in intravenous form in Europe.

Other nonsteroidal anti-inflammatory drugs (NSAIDs) are used widely in postoperative pain, inflammatory pain, such as juvenile rheumatoid arthritis, various bone, joint, and muscle pains, back pain, headache, dental pain, menstrual pain, and sickle cell vaso-occlusive crisis pain. These drugs exhibit an opioid-sparing effect, which results in reduced opioid-related side effects. They are also used as antipyretics. Indomethacin is used for closure of the patent ductus arteriosus in newborn or premature infants. Indomethacin and diclofenac have also been used in nocturnal enuresis. These drugs inhibit peripheral COX and decrease the metabolism of arachidonic acid to prostaglandins. They are more potent analgesics than acetaminophen, especially with mild postoperative pain. The nonsteroidals used in children include indomethacin, ibuprofen, diclofenac, piroxicam, and ketorolac with little evidence for one being better than the other in analgesic effectiveness. The two isoenzymes of COX are COX-1, which is constitutive, and COX-2, which is induced in trauma and inflammation. The common NSAIDs actively inhibit both COX enzymes. The selective COX-2 inhibitors—celecoxib and valdecoxib—are now being used more frequently, although neither has been approved for use in children.

The choice of an NSAID is dictated largely by convenience of administration, with ketorolac being the only one available in intravenous form. It is thus used largely for intraoperative and postoperative pain. Several injectable COX-2 inhibitors are also in development. NSAIDs are generally safe, with no central depressant effects, and are very effective in treating postoperative pain in outpatient surgery. However, one needs to be aware that gastrointestinal (GI) bleeding, bronchoconstriction, interstitial nephritis, with reduced renal blood flow and renal failure, have been reported with their use. They are associated with decreased platelet function and hence should be used with caution in surgeries where bleeding is a concern either intraoperatively or postoperatively (e.g., tonsillectomy). Routine use should be avoided in children who are at risk for GI bleeding or renal dysfunction. COX-2 inhibitors cause less gastrointestinal toxicity and have no effect on platelet function, but renal toxicity can still occur. When combined with opioids, in a multimodal treatment plan, they are useful in the treatment of severe long-lasting pain such as cancer pain.

OPIOID ANALGESICS

These remain the key component of analgesia for both acute and chronic moderate to severe pain. Ideally, they should be employed as part of a "balanced" or multimodal analgesic plan that includes an NSAID, and/or a local anesthetic (in the case of postoperative pain). All opioids are capable of treating pain regardless of intensity, if the dose is adjusted appropriately.

Oral Opioids

Oral opioids can be used in the later postoperative period in children who have had major surgeries, especially orthopedic procedures. The dosing of oral opioids should not be empirical, but instead based on both conversion of intravenous opioid requirements and on the patient's side effects. In children expected to have greater than 1 week of severe postoperative pain, a combination of sustained release and immediate release opioids may be helpful. It is imperative that the child and parents understand that this is not a permanent medication and the object is to get the child through a prolonged recovery period. Appropriate weaning schedules should be provided to the family and other alternative medications for the future discussed.

Codeine is an oral opioid commonly used as an antitussive and for mild to moderate pain. It has good oral bioavailability and is metabolized by the liver to morphine. This conversion is dependent on the enzyme P-450 2D6 that may be either absent or diminished in 5% to 10% of the population. These individuals have a decreased or absent analgesic response to codeine. The incidence of nausea with codeine is very high. It is commonly used in combination with acetaminophen, which potentiates its analgesic effect and allows use of a lesser dose of codeine (Table 11-2).

Oxycodone, hydrocodone, morphine, and hydromorphone are the other oral opioids commonly prescribed. They have excellent oral bioavailability, and oxycodone and hydrocodone are available in fixed combination with acetaminophen or ibuprofen. One must be cognizant of the fact that the total daily dose does not exceed the hepatotoxic dose of acetaminophen, which is about 90 mg/kg/day. Oxycodone is also available in slow-release form as OxyContin. Although its use in children is off-label, it is being used extensively for postoperative pain in major surgeries such as spine fusions or Nuss-procedures and also in chronic pain conditions such as sickle cell disease. Morphine is also available in various slow release preparations. A long-acting form of hydromorphone (Palladone) was taken off the market a few months after its introduction.

Table 11-2 Oral Opioid Dosing Guidelines

Drug	Equianalgesic dose	Intravenous/oral ratio	Usual starting oral dose
Morphine	10 mg	1:6 (single dose) 1:3 (chronic dosing)	Immediate release 0.3 mg/kg every 3-4 hr Sustained release (every 8-12 hr) 20-35 kg: 10-15 mg 35-50 kg: 15-30 mg >50 kg: 30-45 mg
Codeine	60 mg	N/A	Child <50 kg: 0.5-1.0 mg/kg every 3-4 hr Child >50 kg: 30-60 mg every 3-4 hr
Oxycodone	10 mg	N/A	Child <50 kg: 0.1-0.2 mg/kg every 3-4 hr Child >50 kg: 5-10 mg every 3-4 hr
Hydromorphone	2 mg	1:5	0.04-0.08 mg every 3-4 hr
Methadone	5 mg	1:2	0.2 mg/kg every 4-8 hr If excessive sedation occurs, lengthen dosing interval
Meperidine (pethidine)	100 mg	1:4	Child <50 kg: 2-3 mg/kg every 3-4 hr Child >50 kg: 100-150 mg every 3-4 hr Avoid chronic use

Intravenous Opioids

Intravenous opioids have a place in management of acute pain in the hospital setting. They can be administered as a continuous infusion, following standardized protocols, which in some cases may be preferable to intermittent dosing. They ensure prompt and consistent management of pain in the immediate postoperative period. The integration of a pain management plan into the overall perioperative plan is a key component. Continuous infusions of morphine or fentanyl are generally used in infants and children who are too young to derive maximum benefit from patient-controlled analgesia systems.

Morphine

Morphine is the gold standard for analgesia and that to which all other opioids are compared. Premature and term newborns have a reduced clearance and prolonged elimination half-life for morphine. In opioid-naïve infants, dosages used should be one-quarter to one-half of doses recommended for children, thus allowing room

to escalate slowly if needed. By the time the infant is 3 to 6 months of age, the pharmacokinetics are similar to that of older children and adults (Table 11-3).

Fentanyl

Fentanyl is favored for short procedures because of its rapid onset and brief duration of action. It is approximately 50 to 100 times more potent than morphine. It has a prolonged elimination half-life and diminished clearance in premature infants and newborns. In infants over 3 months of age, it has been reported that clearance is actually double that in older children and adults.[2] Since fentanyl metabolism depends on hepatic blood flow, it should be used cautiously in infants with elevated intra-abdominal pressure, both before, during, and after surgery. Its ability to block nociceptive stimuli with concomitant hemodynamic stability has made it the drug of choice for trauma, cardiac surgery, and critically ill children. Alfentanil is approximately 5 to 10 times less potent than fentanyl and has a very short duration of action. Sufentanil is a derivative that is approximately 10 times more potent than fentanyl.

Table 11-3   Intravenous Opioid Dosing Guidelines

Drug	Equianalgesic dose	Usual starting intravenous dose	Comments
Morphine	1.0 mg	Bolus: Children 0.1 mg/kg every 2-3 hr Infants 0.025-0.050 mg/kg every 2-3 hr Infusion: Children 0.03-0.05 mg/kg/hr Infants 0.015-0.03 mg/kg/hr	First choice in most settings
Hydromorphone	0.20 mg	Bolus: Children 0.02 mg/kg every 2-3 hr Infants 0.005-0.010 mg/kg every 2-3 hr Infusion: Children 0.006 mg/kg/hr Infants 0.003 mg/kg/hr	Similar to morphine, more potent
Fentanyl	0.01 mg (10 µg)	Bolus: Children 0.5-1.0 µg/kg every 1-2 hr Infants 0.25-0.50 µg/kg every 1-2 hr Infusion: Children 2-4 µg/kg/hr Infants 0.5-0-1.0 ug/kg/hr	Minimal hemodynamic effects Short duration with single boluses, useful for brief procedures
Methadone	1.0 mg	Bolus: Children 0.1 mg/kg every 4-8 hr Infants 0.025-0.050 mg/kg every 4-12 hr (extend interval and reduce dosing dramatically if sedation occurs)	May accumulate; requires careful titration to avoid delayed sedation Useful for prolonged action with episodic boluses if infusions are not feasible
Meperidine (pethidine)	10 mg	Bolus: Children 0.8-1.0 mg/kg every 2-3 hr Infants 0.4 mg/kg every 2-3 hr	Avoid if other opioids are available. Metabolite normeperidine may cause seizures. Uniquely useful in low doses (0.1 mg/kg) for postanesthesia rigors and shivering

Continuous infusions are commonly used in cardiac surgery and major orthopedic procedures. Remifentanil is approximately 10 times more potent than fentanyl and has an extremely short half-life necessitating continuous infusion. It can result in hyperalgesia, leading to dramatically increased requirements for postoperative opioids. Fentanyl or sufentanil may also be administered intranasally to provide sedation and analgesia within 10 minutes of administration. The fentanyl lozenge (oral transmucosal fentanyl citrate) is a nontraumatic and effective way to administer premedication in difficult children. It is also available to treat breakthrough cancer pain. Transmucosal absorption results in a rapid increase in plasma fentanyl concentration. Recently, a unique iontophoretic delivery system was developed for use with fentanyl in an adhesive patch form as a patient controlled analgesia unit.

Hydromorphone

Hydromorphone is a derivative of morphine and has 5 times the potency of morphine with a similar elimination half-life. It is thought to be less sedating than morphine, with fewer systemic side effects, which occur at doses higher than equianalgesic or clinically effective doses. It is an excellent alternative, when opioid rotation is desired in the tolerant patient, in patients with renal impairment, or those with intolerable side effects from morphine.

Meperidine

Meperidine (Demerol) is a synthetic opioid that is about 10 times less potent than morphine. It is not routinely used in children because of its propensity to cause seizures and hallucinations due to accumulation of the long-lasting metabolite normeperidine. A much smaller dose is used for the control of shivering in the postoperative setting.

Methadone

Methadone is primarily used in weaning opioids in tolerant children. However, it is being used more frequently for management of postoperative and intractable pain. It has an extremely long elimination half-life, close to 18 hours in children, with a very long duration of effective analgesia. It behaves like a slow-release preparation. Its principal metabolite is morphine. A major advantage is its very high bioavailability in the range of 80% to 90%, making it easy to convert intravenous dosing regimens to oral doses. There is some evidence that methadone also exhibits N-methyl-d-aspartate (NMDA) receptor inhibition which results in delayed onset of opioid tolerance.

Patient-Controlled Analgesia (PCA)

PCA has a definite place in pediatric pain management, especially in postsurgical and cancer-related pain.

The advantages are better patient acceptance, inherent safety, and good efficacy. There is evidence that PCA affords better pain control than intermittent nurse-administered bolus dosing. Preemptive pain management has special advantages in children because assessing pain is difficult and some children cannot or will not ask for analgesia. For this reason children benefit greatly from the continuous administration of analgesics. The use of fixed doses of medication in a "prn" manner can lead to episodes or cycles of pain followed by "rescue dosing" that causes excessive sedation and other opioid side effects. A basal infusion provides low-dose background analgesia, which is especially useful at night when the patient is asleep. However, the dosing of the basal infusion should be based on standard accepted parameters also taking into account associated medical problems. More frequent smaller doses of opioids, self-administered by the patient, lead to better analgesic titration. A short lock-out interval of 6 or 8 minutes allows the patient to "catch up" after he has been asleep for a few hours. There is also an overall reduction in opioid use and side effects when the patient is involved in his pain control. The child's control over his pain management has significant psychological benefits and allows him or her to anticipate increased physical activity (e.g., physical therapy) and cooperate effectively. We use PCAs in children as young as 5 years of age with excellent results. In younger or developmentally-delayed children, we have nurses or parents control the bolus doses. The basal infusion then is at a higher level with a longer lock-out time for individual doses, thus making the caregiver's job a little easier. Problems can arise when caregivers are overenthusiastic in pushing the PCA button in opioid-naïve sleeping children with the good intention of sparing them pain on awakening. This can lead to serious consequences, and it is critical to educate parents and caregivers on the working of the pump to ensure that they do not press the button if the child is asleep. In addition, any patient on PCA by proxy must be on continuous pulse oximetry monitoring. Morphine, hydromorphone, meperidine, and fentanyl are the drugs administered with PCA.

Although the adult literature does not support the use of background infusions, we feel that having a basal infusion significantly improves the quality of pain relief in children. As noted above, a new fixed-dose (40 µg/dose up to every 10 minutes) iontophoretic PCA fentanyl device is available. It does not require intravenous access and the system provides rapid titration of fentanyl, almost similar to intravenous administration (Table 11-4).

Successful use of continuous opioid therapy with or without PCA is dependent largely on the successful management of side effects and appropriate dose adjustments when pain is not well-controlled. The common side effects include nausea, vomiting, pruritus, urinary retention, dysphoria, constipation, and somnolence. All infants and children who are receiving continuous opi-

Table 11-4 PCA Doses

	PCA dose mg/kg/dose	PCA hourly max. mg/kg	Basal rate mg/kg/hr	RN-administered PCA bolus mg/kg (this is above basal/doses administered)
Morphine	0.01 to 0.03	0.1	0.01 to 0.03	0.05 to 0.1
Hydromorphone	0.002 to 0.006	0.02	0.002 to 0.006	0.01 to 0.02
Fentanyl	0.005 to 0.002	0.0035–0.005	0.001 to 0.004	0.001 to 0.002
	(0.5–02 µg/kg/dose)	(3.5–5 µg/kg/hr)	(1–4 µg/kg/hr)	(1–2 µg/kg)

oids should be monitored for respiratory rate, arousability, and oxygen saturation while on the medication. One needs to maintain a high index of suspicion in order to identify problems in an efficient manner. Inadequate pain control may necessitate changes in the basal infusion, intermittent dosing, or both.

OTHER DRUGS

Tramadol

Tramadol, a synthetic analog of codeine, is unique in that it provides analgesia by both opioid and nonopioid actions. It has a moderate interaction at the mu opioid receptor and its metabolite (O-desmethyl tramadol) binds to opioid receptors with an even greater affinity than the parent compound contributing to its analgesic action. Centrally, it inhibits reuptake of serotonin and norepinephrine and may also provide analgesia by an α-2 agonist effect. In addition, it may also have a selective spinal action as evidenced by its use for epidural blockade where it has been shown to prolong the duration of local anesthetics. Its use has not been associated with side effects that are commonly seen with other opioids or NSAIDs and it does not have a ceiling effect. Tolerance, psychological dependence, and euphoric effects have also not been reported in long-term clinical trials. It is, however, metabolized by the P-450 hepatic enzyme system, which may result in significant drug interactions [i.e., with tricyclic antidepressants (TCAs), antipsychotics, ketamine, digoxin, lithium, MAO inhibitors]. Tramadol has also been associated with increased risk of seizures, especially in patients who are on drugs that inhibit hepatic metabolism. The use of tramadol has been reported as an adjunct to caudal analgesia and in isolation for acute and subacute postoperative pain management.

Clonidine

Clonidine is an α-2 agonist that has traditionally been used for management of hypertension, attention deficit disorder, migraine prophylaxis, and Tourette's syndrome. Given orally prior to surgery, it has been shown to decrease postoperative opioid requirements. When part of a regimen for epidural or caudal blocks with local anesthetics and narcotics, it prolongs the duration of analgesia and significantly reduces narcotic requirements as well. Intrathecal administration has also been shown to help with intractable muscle spasms in spinal-cord injury patients. Transdermal clonidine has been used for continued analgesia in the postoperative period. It can cause hypotension, bradycardia, and sedation, but the pruritus, urinary retention, and respiratory depression commonly seen with opioids is not an issue. Clonidine should be used cautiously in neonates, infants, and children who are susceptible to the development of apnea.

Ketamine

Ketamine is a phencyclidine derivative with amnestic, sedative, and analgesic properties. It has been used for procedural sedation, as an anesthetic induction agent, especially in patients with congenital heart disease, as an adjunct for postoperative analgesia, and in chronic pain management. It produces its effects with minimal cardiovascular and respiratory perturbations. Ketamine antagonizes the NMDA-receptor and appears to interfere with the development of hyperalgesia and spinal-cord wind-up. Animal studies have demonstrated cross-tolerance between opiates and ketamine. Intrathecal ketamine has been used in Europe for its local anesthetic properties and as an additive to epidural or caudal analgesia. Concomitant administration of a benzodiazepine and antisialagogue is recommended to counteract the emergence delirium, nightmares, and increased salivation that are seen with its use.

Capsaicin

Capsaicin is the chemical substance in hot chili peppers that causes their spiciness and heat. It has been used for management of chronic pain states associated with a burning sensation and mechanical allodynia. Acute application to the skin results in a stinging, burning sensation interpreted as pain, but chronic application leads to depletion of substance P from cutaneous C fibers leading to their ultimate degeneration and a degree of analgesia. The problems associated with the acute application clearly limit use of capsaicin in the younger pediatric population, but it has been used in older children. Capsaicin has been effectively used for the treatment of cancer-related mucositis if it is administered as a candied lozenge.

Regional Techniques

Regional techniques in children include a variety of both peripheral and central blocks that are used for intraoperative and postoperative pain control. Regional blocks are generally performed with the child anesthetized. When performed at the onset of the procedure, immediately after anesthetic induction, regional blocks in children do set up fast enough so that they form a large component of anesthetic management. This results in reduced use of narcotics and volatile anesthetics and the side effects thereof. The variations in positioning as a result of anesthesia and securing the airway, sometimes less well-defined landmarks, and the proximity of nerves to vascular structures, make regional anesthesia in children slightly more challenging for the anesthesiologist.

The local anesthetics used in children are those used in adults. Ilioinguinal block is performed for surgeries in the lower abdomen and inguinal area. It is relatively easy to perform and has a very good success rate. Axillary block is performed for surgeries in the forearm and hand. An indwelling catheter can be left in place for postoperative dosing and infusion. Interscalene blocks are useful for shoulder surgery and also have the advantage of being able to leave in a catheter for continued postoperative pain relief. Bier blocks can also been performed. Femoral block and fascia iliaca blocks are performed for surgery of the lower extremity. The fascia iliaca block can effectively replace the 3-in-1 block with a single injection technique. It is important to be vigilant about the total dose of local anesthetic used in regional blocks for children (Table 11-5).

Epidural Analgesia

Epidural analgesia provides superior pain control and better respiratory mechanics after major thoracic, abdominal, and pelvic procedures. Epidural analgesia hastens recovery, reduces complications, and facilitates mobilization of the patient. By combining general anesthesia with epidural analgesia, especially in neonates, prolonged postoperative ventilation can be avoided. Epidural analgesia is also associated with a lower incidence of postoperative respiratory depression and cardiovascular complications in comparison to intravenous opioids in all age groups. In addition, patients managed with epidural analgesia have an earlier discharge from the ICU and shorter hospital stays.

Single shot caudal epidural blocks are the most commonly performed blocks in children for both intra- and postoperative management. They are simple, easy to perform, reliable and, for the most part, safe. They are useful for a variety of outpatient urologic, orthopedic, and general surgical procedures below the T4 dermatomal level including hernias, hydroceles, hypospadias, and lower extremity procedures. The sacrum of a child is flat and in most cases, the bony landmarks are easily seen and palpable. The wide sacral hiatus overlying the uncalcified sacrococcygeal ligament provides easy, direct access to the caudal epidural space. Needle insertion at this level has a reduced risk of causing direct spinal-cord trauma, as the dural sac ends between the S-1 and S-3 level. However, one should always examine the area looking for dimples, hair patches, pigmented lesions, or fistulous tracks that could be indicators of spinal anomalies. Since the caudal block is usually combined with general anesthesia, the focus of drug choice is duration of action rather than rapidity of onset. Therefore, longer acting

Table 11-5 Dosing Guidelines for Local Anesthetics			
Drug	Single bolus (mg/kg) plain	Continuous with epi*(1:200,000)	Infusion (mg/kg/hr)
BIRTH TO 6-12 MONTHS			
Lidocaine	4	5	0.8
Bupivacaine/Ropivacaine	1.5–2.0	2	0.2
Chloroprocaine	30	30	30
1 YR AND OLDER			
Lidocaine	5	7	1.6
Bupivacaine/Ropivacaine	2	2.5	0.4
Chloroprocaine	30	30	30

Epi, epinephrine.

drugs like bupivacaine or ropivacaine are the common choice. Single shot caudal analgesia with bupivicaine can last as long as 6 to 8 hours. Epinephrine 5 µg/ml is often added to the solution to serve as a marker of intravascular injection, producing ST segment elevation and T-wave changes within 20 seconds of administration. Opioids and/or clonidine can be safely added to the local anesthetic to prolong the analgesia. One must be cautious, however, about discharging patients after they receive any peridural opioids. Liposomally-encapsulated morphine for slow-release epidural administration has recently been approved for use in adults. There are no data yet available on pharmacokinetics or safety in children (Table 11-6).

Epidurals are especially effective when the catheter tip is at the dermatomal site of incision. This involves either lumbar or thoracic placement, but they can also be introduced caudally and threaded up to the site of surgery, even thoracic, with or without fluoroscopic guidance. Radiographs, in the case of radio-opaque catheters, can identify the position of the catheter tip or a water-soluble dye can be used to identify the location. More recently, there have been descriptions of catheters advanced from a caudal location with a low current nerve stimulator used to detect the tip by the presence of muscle twitches.

Thoracic placement is slightly more challenging than lumbar or caudal. The spinal cord is larger in this region and can be injured by a needle inserted too deeply. The spinous processes are longer, slant sharply downward, and the interspaces are narrower. A paramedian approach rather than midline is sometimes necessary. An 18 or 20 gauge Tuohy or Crawford needle is commonly used and the epidural space can be identified by a "loss of resistance" technique using normal saline. Air should be avoided in children to avoid the risk of air embolism from inadvertent intravenous injection in the presence of a patent foramen ovale, ventricular septal defect (VSD), or atrial septal defect (ASD). Test dosing for intravascular placement differs from that performed in awake adults in that there is a large reliance on heart rate and ST segment changes on the electrocardiogram (EKG). Epinephrine at a dose of 0.5 µg/kg should be employed with local

anesthetic. In spite of meticulous caution, up to 10% of the time, there can be a false negative response to intravascular injection. Therefore, continuous monitoring is essential and incremental dosing of the treatment dose assumes great importance. The most common drugs used are a mixture of local anesthetics and opioids, with clonidine being added more commonly. This has been shown to prolong local anesthetic action and reduce the use of opioid and local anesthetic, as mentioned earlier. Some use levobupivacaine or ropivacaine, which are said to provide lower risk of cardiovascular compromise from inadvertent intravascular injection. When the catheter tip is at the dermatome of surgery, fentanyl is often the opioid of choice. When it is further from the site of operation, such as a lumbar catheter for a thoracotomy incision, water-soluble opioids such as morphine or hydromorphone are used to have the desired spread. Epidural infusions can be set up as epidural PCAs, where the patient can get additional doses for breakthrough pain that occurs as a result of coughing, voiding, nursing care, or activity. It is essential to educate the patient and family about the longer time needed for an epidural bolus to take effect compared to an intravenous bolus of the same drug. Patients receiving epidural or caudal opioids should be monitored in the hospital with continuous pulse-oximetry and watched for signs of impending respiratory depression. Adjuvant NSAIDs, such as ketorolac, can be safely used if the nature of the surgery and medical condition permits.

Epidurals in children are uniformly performed in the anesthetized state because of issues with cooperation and safety. This has continued to be a controversial issue, as it takes away the safety feature of an awake-patient reporting pain on accidental encountering of the spinal cord or nerves. However, one needs to balance the risk of injury in an awake, scared, and/or thrashing child with the possibly rare risk, in experienced hands, of nerve injury. The pediatric anesthesia community maintains that there is considerable experience with the placement of epidural catheters in sleeping patients with no case reports of permanent neurologic complications as a result of this practice even with catheters placed in the lumbar or thoracic regions (Table 11-7).

Contraindications for placement of epidural catheters are similar to those for adults and include intrinsic coagulopathy, anticoagulant use, sepsis, progressive neurologic disease, bony abnormalities, infection at the site of insertion, and patient/parent refusal. Infection from epidural catheters used for postoperative pain is rare. Relative contraindications to the use of patient-controlled epidural analgesia include physical inability to use the button, cognitive inability to understand how to use it, and lastly the patient's (or parent's) desire to not assume responsibility for pain control.

Table 11-6	Volumes of Local Anesthetic (0.25% Bupivacaine or 0.2% Ropivacaine) for Single-Dose Caudal Block

Volume (mL/kg)	Dermatomal level
0.5	Sacral (T10-T12)
0.75	T-12 (inguinal)(T8-T10)
1	Lower thoracic (T6-T8)
1.25	Mild to high thoracic (T4-T6)

Table 11-7 Epidural Doses

A. INFANTS <6 MONTHS OR PATIENTS AT RISK FOR RESPIRATORY DEPRESSION

Solution	Epidural loading doses	Epidural dose ml/kg/hr	PCEA dose µg/kg/dose	Onset minutes	Duration hours	After epidural is discontinued, may		
						Discontinue monitors in __ hrs	Discontinue Foley in __ hrs	Give IV or PO analgesics
10µg/ml Morphine + 1/16% Bupivacaine	10-30µg/kg + 0.3-0.5ml/kg (0.25%)	0.1-0.3	NA	20-30	6-12	4	4	As soon as patient experiences discomfort
3µg/ml Hydromorphone + 1/16% Bupivacaine	1-3µg/kg + 0.3-0.5ml/kg (0.25%)	0.1-0.3	NA	15	4-6	4	4	As soon as patient experiences discomfort
1µg/ml Fentanyl + 1/16% Bupivacaine	0.5-1µg/kg + 0.3-0.5ml/kg (0.25%)	0.1-0.2 (neonates; <6 mo age; tip at site)	NA	10	2-3	4	4	Immediately

B. INFANTS, CHILDREN, AND ADOLESCENTS >6 MONTHS

Solution	Epidural loading doses	Epidural dose ml/kg/hr	PCEA dose µg/kg/dose	Onset minutes	Duration hours	After epidural is discontinued, may		
						Discontinue monitors in __ hrs	Discontinue Foley in __ hrs	Give IV or PO analgesics
20µg/ml Morphine + 1/16% Bupivacaine	25-50µg/kg + 0.5-1ml/kg (0.25%)	0.1-0.4	1/6-1/4 hourly rate	20	6-12	12	4	As soon as patient experiences discomfort
5-10µg/ml Hydromorphone + 1/16% Bupivacaine	5-10µg/kg + 0.5-1ml/kg (0.25%)	0.1-0.4	1/6-1/4 hourly rate	15	4-6	4	2-4	As soon as patient experiences discomfort
2µg/ml Fentanyl + 1/16% Bupivacaine	1-2µg/kg + 0.5-1ml/kg (0.25%)	0.1-0.4	1.6-1/4 hourly rate	10	2-3	0-2	0-2	Immediately

*BUPIVICAINE DOSE MAXIMUM 0.2 MG/KG/HR IN NEWBORNS; 0.4 MG/KG/HR IN OLDER INFANTS/CHILDREN.
*Thoracic epidurals should be at the lower end of these ranges (0.1-0.15 cc/kg/hr maximum).
*Morphine dose is usually between 3-5 µg/kg/hr. May be increased if patient is not sedated.
*Ropivacaine may be substituted for bupivacaine. Consider loading with 0.2% and using 0.1% for infusions.
*Clonidine may be added to any of the above solutions. Consider using 1 µg/ml and reducing your opioid dose by 50%. Also consider loading with 1-2 µg/kg and reducing the original opioid load by 50%. AVOID CLONIDINE IN NEONATES (APNEA).
*FOR PATIENTS WHO ARE NOT WELL-CONTROLLED, consider a bolus equal to the volume of 1-hour infusion and then increase the rate by 20%. If there is a question of whether the epidural is working, test with 3-5 mg/kg lidocaine (0.5-1%). If no block, discontinue epidural and change pain therapy. Avoid testing with bupivacaine (0.25%).

Spinal Blockade

Spinal blockade is not commonly performed in children. The benefit of avoiding a general anesthetic and using the spinal as the sole modality is often not possible, as children are unlikely to cooperate in the wakeful state with placement of a spinal needle. The only exception to this is the expremature infant who is less than 46 to 62 weeks postconceptual age who is to undergo surgery below the umbilicus (e.g., inguinal hernia repair). In this age group, because of the high risk of postoperative apnea following a general anesthetic, spinal anesthesia with hyperbaric tetracaine or bupivacaine is the anesthetic of choice. It is also indicated when it would be prudent to avoid general anesthesia for other reasons, such as respiratory illness, the presence of a mediastinal mass, or progressive muscular disease. The incidence of postdural puncture headache in children is unknown. Spinals are contraindicated in newborns with inadequate coagulation secondary to congenital or acquired bleeding disorders because of the risk of spinal hemorrhage. Difficult airways and unstable hemodynamic status are relative contraindications. In very unusual circumstances, catheters can be placed intrathecally for treatment of longer-term pain syndromes.

Regional anesthesia can be a very useful adjunct to general anesthesia for many children. Its risks and benefits need to be carefully weighed before attempting it, especially given the more complicated nature of the technique in smaller children. However, the skillful anesthesiologist can offer most techniques used in adults to infants and children to facilitate effective pain relief.

CHRONIC PAIN IN CHILDREN

Chronic persistent pain refers to conditions of persistent or nearly constant pain over a period of 3 months or more. The incidence of chronic pain in children has been conservatively estimated to be 10% to 15% of the population. The absence of objective signs of sympathetic nervous system arousal with chronic pain, in contrast to acute pain, may lead the inexperienced physician to discount the complaints of the child. There is no neurophysiologic or chemical test that can measure chronic pain; one needs to take the patient's story at face value. These patients can be very challenging and often, as opposed to adults, the etiology is unclear. The common ailments are headaches, myofascial pain, abdominal pain, chronic regional pain syndrome (CRPS), cancer pain, phantom limb pain, and spasticity pain.

Chronic recurrent pain refers to repetitive painful episodes alternating with pain-free intervals. This is seen in arthritis or sickle cell disease, where pain recurs from either repeated joint inflammation or episodes of vaso-occlusion with distal ischemia or infarction. These types of pain are mechanistically similar to repetitive acute pain. However, their repetitive nature may lead to psychological sequelae similar to chronic pain. Pain may also persist from abnormal excitability in the peripheral or CNS in the absence of ongoing tissue injury. This is also not uncommon in children.

Children with chronic pain have significant alterations in their lifestyles, poor school attendance, inability to identify with peers, and social withdrawal. The child's pain condition has a significant impact on the functioning of the entire family. Most pediatricians have limited experience in treating children with chronic pain and "doctor shopping" may be something the family has resorted to in order to end their journey.

Unlike acute pain, which signals a specific nociceptive event and is self-limited, chronic pain may start out as an acute event but continues beyond the normal expected time of recovery. Also chronic pain in children is the result of integration of biologic processes with contribution from psychological factors, sociocultural factors, individual development, and family dynamics. In order to evaluate and treat chronic pediatric pain effectively and efficiently, a multidisciplinary team-oriented approach is most successful. Such programs incorporate physicians, nurses, pain psychologists, psychiatrists, physical therapists, social workers, and occupational therapists into a treatment team. The physician needs to acknowledge the multidimensional nature of the patient's pain and his or her pain experience and treat it from the various angles that each member of the multidisciplinary team brings to the group.

Drugs Used in Chronic Pain

Tricyclic Antidepressants

TCAs inhibit reuptake of serotonin and norepinephrine, thus facilitating inhibitory neurotransmitter activity at the level of the spinal cord. They have also been shown to block both Na^+- and Ca^{++}-gated channels and to inhibit the NMDA-receptors contributing to analgesia. They have been used in a variety of chronic pain conditions, including neuropathic pain, abdominal pain, migraines, and myofascial pain. The onset of analgesic effect is much quicker than the onset of antidepressant effect. Amitriptyline and nortriptyline are commonly used TCAs. Because of their anticholinergic side effects, they should be started at a low dose and titrated to affect over a period of several weeks. The target is usually 0.5 to 1mg/kg/day. They both facilitate sleep and should be given before bed, but persistent morning somnolence is not uncommon, especially with amitriptyline. All TCAs may prolong the QTc interval and cause tachyarrhythmia in patients with known prolonged QTc syndrome, especially desipramine and imipramine. We routinely obtain a baseline EKG in all patients prior to starting a TCA. Nortriptyline has a better side-effect profile than amitriptyline especially with regard to the antimuscarinic and sedative effects. If the patient is also on other drugs such as selective serotonin reuptake inhibitors (SSRIs) or tramadol, periodic measurement of TCA level is also warranted as these drugs are all metabolized by the same p450-hepatic pathways. The use of antidepressant agents is further complicated by the recent warnings from the Food and Drug Administration about the possible association of increased suicidality in teenagers being treated with these drugs for depression. In the event that these drugs are incorporated into the treatment plan, weekly follow-up is required during the first month of treatment with monthly visits thereafter.

Selective Serotonin Reuptake Inhibitors

Most SSRIs are less effective as analgesics than TCAs with the exception of venlafaxine. This drug is chemically similar to tramadol. The antinociceptive effect is believed to be mediated by the κ, δ, and α-2 adrenergic receptors suggesting a potential use in the management of various chronic pain syndromes, but further studies in humans are needed to establish indications and dosing guidelines. Many patients with chronic pain also have either primary or secondary anxiety or depressive symptoms. Therefore, the addition of an SSRI may be quite beneficial. SSRIs could result in clinically relevant drug interactions when administered with other drugs metabolized by the cytochrome P-450 system. They are most significant with agents that have a narrow therapeutic index such as TCAs, benzodiazepines, theophylline, antiepileptics, some narcotics (e.g., codeine, hydro-codone, oxy-codone, tramadol), and antiarrhythmics. As for TCAs, when a patient is started on an SSRI, close follow-up is required.

Anticonvulsants

Carbamazepine, one of the oldest anticonvulsant drugs used, is no longer a first-line drug especially when the child has hematologic or hepatic dysfunction. Sodium valproate or divalproex sodium is used for neuropathic pain states and migraines, but is used specifically if mood-stabilization is also a goal. Patients on these agents need to have regular assessment of their hematologic and liver profiles. Gabapentin was originally used for childhood seizures, but has slowly replaced most other agents in the management of neuropathic pain states. Its clinical use has, however, far outpaced published data in children and it has become a first-line drug at most centers. Topiramate is also being used, although most studies have been exclusively done in adults.

Chronic Pain Conditions

Musculoskeletal Pain

Musculoskeletal pain is a common complaint in children, attributable largely to overuse, trauma, normal skeletal growth, and growing pains. This is effectively treated with NSAIDs, massage, muscle stretches, and reassurance. It is important, in these children, to make sure that they do not suffer from other major illnesses as a cause of this pain. However, extensive work-up is often not warranted. Once major illness has been ruled out, the management centers around lifestyle changes, including sleep and diet, exercise, and structuring of social activities. Aerobic exercises and strength training have a localized effect, but also have a more generalized beneficial effect on mood, sleep, appetite, and general well-being. There is a subset of patients that have musculoskeletal pain from specific disease processes. These include orthopedic conditions such as Perthes disease, slipped capital femoral epiphyses, Osgood-Schlatter disease, congenital hip dysplasia, infectious diseases such as osteomyelitis, septic arthritis, Lyme disease, and inflam-

matory conditions such as rheumatic fever, systemic lupus erythematosus, arthritis, and arthropathies. The majority of these conditions are treated symptomatically with heat or cold, splints, adaptive devices, physical therapy, acetaminophen, and NSAIDs, along with specific treatment as indicated by the underlying condition.

Myofascial Pain Syndromes/Fibromyalgia

Back pain in children is unlikely to be related to the common causes of low back pain in adults, namely discogenic pain or arthropathy. Children with scoliosis will rarely have back pain that needs to be treated aggressively with NSAIDs or opioids. Myofascial pain involving single or multiple muscle groups is the more common cause in the otherwise healthy pediatric population, especially in the adolescent and early adult years. This is characterized by widespread pain, trigger points on examination, referred pain, generalized fatigue, sleep-related problems, mood disturbances, and may be associated with headaches and abdominal pain. The incidence reported has been between 1% and 6% of the population. Temporomandibular joint dysfunction with myofascial pain is a common disorder in children. For the more common myofascial syndromes, localized heat application, regular aerobic exercise, physical conditioning, improved sleep hygiene, cognitive-behavioral techniques, massage therapy, muscle relaxants, NSAIDs, and low-dose TCAs have been known to afford success, improving both pain and sleep disturbances. Acupuncture on a regular basis has been successful in children with myofascial pain and fibromyalgia.

Neuropathic Pain

Neuropathic pain is seen in peripheral neuropathies, central pain syndromes, and complex regional pain syndromes. Neuropathic pain in children can be very challenging to treat and often requires therapy with both conventional analgesics and adjuvant drugs. It is the result of injury to or degeneration of peripheral nerves or the pain pathways in the CNS with the normal inhibitors of pain and descending modulators of nociception not being fully functional. Pain is typically perceived as being burning in nature with associated allodynia, hyperalgesia, and hyperpathia. Since the injury is not to the peripheral nociceptors, but rather to the pathways proximal to them, the target tissue has an abnormal sensory potential, often refractory to conventional analgesics. Since there is very little evidence-based research about neuropathic pain in children, current treatment strategies are extrapolated from accepted strategies used in adults. TCAs are well-established in the treatment of many neuropathic conditions such as diabetic neuropathy or postherpetic neuralgia. TCAs have consistently been shown to be the single most efficacious class of alternative analgesics for neuropathic pain and are often the first choice over anticonvulsants. Neurontin, however, is now the most widely used drug and is started at a dose of 10 mg/kg, escalating slowly to 50 mg/kg 3 times a day. Pediatric experience with drugs such as topiramate, lamotrigine, and pregabalin is very limited.

Intravenous lidocaine infusions are used by some centers. Blood levels of lidocaine should be checked frequently to maintain a blood level 2 to 5 µg/ml. Mexiletine, an oral analog of lidocaine, is used to treat peripheral neuropathies but its use might be limited by gastrointestinal side effects. Although opioids are traditionally considered ineffective for neuropathic pain, they may have a place in neuropathic pain related to cancer or phantom pain.

Chronic Regional Pain Syndrome Type I

CRPS Type I, previously called Reflex Sympathetic Dystrophy, refers to a syndrome of persistent neuropathic pain associated with nondermatomal autonomic dysfunction. It differs significantly in children from adults in that there appears to be a predominance of lower extremity involvement and association with trivial injuries such as minor sprains or twists related to contact and competitive sports such as baseball, soccer, gymnastics, and dance. The clinical findings include temperature and color changes, allodynia, cyanosis, edema, and eventually dystrophic and osteoporotic changes. The current International Association for the Study of Pain (IASP) diagnostic criteria include: At least two neuropathic pain descriptors (e.g., burning, dysesthesia, paresthesia, mechanical allodynia, cold hyperalgesia), at least two physical signs of autonomic dysfunction (e.g., cyanosis, mottling, hyperhydrosis, edema), and a decreased temperature of at least greater than 3°C in the affected limb. The cause of pain in CRPS Type I is not completely understood, but is believed to be related to abnormal discharges in sympathetic afferent nerves along with nociceptive effects produced by the incidental trauma.

There is evidence that CRPS Type I in children is benign and will respond to physical therapy. The prognosis for recovery is generally good if treatment is initiated early enough. Approaches to treatment have been varied, but the primary objective is mobilization of the involved limb actively and passively in regular, aggressive physical therapy. This is crucial to strengthen and restore muscle and joint function. All other modes of treatment are primarily supportive measures to facilitate the primary objective, thus restoring normal function and preventing limb atrophy. Our bias is that a combined regimen of physical therapy, including TENS and medical management with TCAs (e.g., amitriptyline, antiepileptics, gabapentin) along with cognitive-behavioral pain management techniques, is superior to interventional approaches in children. There are reports of reduced pain and improved functioning after intensive physical therapy and cognitive behavioral therapy (CBT) without sympathetic blockade. Anesthesia-monitored deep sedation with propofol has been used to allow manipulation of the affected extremity in children who are unable to tolerate physical therapy. Neural blockade does have a role in facilitating physical therapy and desensitization in older children. Both individual and family psychotherapy plays a key role in restoring issues in the family that interfere with recovery. Except for the small fraction of patients who respond to over-the-counter analgesics and increased physical activity of the affected extremity, CRPS Type I is definitely a disease that is best managed at a multidisciplinary pediatric pain management center.

Headache

Headache in children has various etiologies. The incidence is around 10% to 20% in children less than 10 years of age. The common causes of headache in children are migraine, tension-type headaches, psychogenic headaches, and those related to refractive errors, dental braces, sinusitis, sleep apnea, viral illnesses, and temporomandibular joint dysfunction. Migraine headaches become more common around puberty in both boys and girls. Approximately 60% of children who suffer from migraine headaches will continue to suffer as adults. The incidence of tension-type headaches usually increases from early school-age into adolescence. Children sometimes have the fear that they could have a brain tumor and, certainly, any headache with signs of elevated intracranial pressures or focal neurologic signs warrants further investigation and imaging. Most children seen in chronic pain clinics will have had extensive prior neuroimaging to rule out brain tumors, vascular, or other structural anomalies. Headache treatment may be preventative or abortive and includes acetaminophen, NSAIDs, TCAs, SSRIs, β-blockers, anticonvulsants, and abortive drugs such as triptans and ergotamines. Opioids may be very rarely indicated. Nonpharmacologic treatment is invaluable in the management of pediatric headaches. This includes biofeedback, relaxation techniques, cognitive reframing, and a variety of standard psychotherapeutic interventions. Acupuncture and TENS may also be an option.

Abdominal Pain

Abdominal pain is a common complaint in school-age children and a common cause of school absenteeism. Recurrent abdominal pain is defined as pain occurring at least once a month for 3 consecutive months, accompanied by pain-free periods, and severe enough to interfere with a child's normal activities. The pain is usually periumbilical, varied in duration and severity, and may be associated with nausea, vomiting, changes in food intake, and disturbances in sleep and bowel movements. It is often difficult to find a specific cause for the pain and most patients presenting to a pain clinic have undergone a battery of tests including imaging and endoscopies by GI specialists before being referred. Some children have associated headaches. Needless to say, it is important to exclude potentially dangerous organic causes such as ulcers, lactose intolerance, ulcerative colitis, Crohn's disease, and infection. It is then important to communicate to the patient and family that, although an organic cause cannot be found, the pain physician believes that the pain is real and will try his utmost to manage it. Management is multidisciplinary, incorporating dietary changes to avoid constipation and possible lactose intolerance, sleep hygiene, learning of biofeedback, coping skills and relaxation techniques, and medications such as NSAIDs, COX-2 inhibitors, TCAs, tramadol, or SSRIs. Regional blocks should be performed only if there is a definite organic cause for pain. Lytic blocks are almost never performed in children, unless for cancer-related pain in a child with limited life expectancy. Pelvic pain is seen in older adolescents and can be secondary to endometriosis, pelvic inflammatory disease, ovarian cysts, musculoskeletal injury, psoas abscesses, or constipation. It is often useful to have female patients be seen by a gynecologist to rule out pathology and try other hormonal means of treatment. Treatment then is similar to that outlined above.

Cancer Pain

The management of cancer pain in children is extremely challenging. Almost all children who suffer from cancer will experience pain during the course of diagnosis, treatment, and end of life. The pain in these children can be classified into four broad categories: (a) cancer-related pain (e.g., bone pain, somatic pain, neuropathic pain, terminal care); (b) treatment-related pain from chemotherapy, radiation, infection, phantom limb pain; (c) procedure-related pain; and (d) pain unrelated to the cancer (e.g., headache, trauma, or other medical issues such as appendicitis, which are incidental). Often the pain from procedures and treatment is worse than the pain from the cancer itself. An integrated team approach with oncologists, psychologists, pain management specialists, and palliative care specialists is crucial in the successful management. Appropriate psychological intervention and an appreciation of the child's understanding of his or her illness also plays a major role. It is also important to understand the family's reaction to the situation, their support systems, and their coping mechanisms. A huge challenge is broaching of the subject of palliative care. Families often are reluctant to make the transition from active curative therapy to palliation. They are also unsure as to how they would explain this to the dying child. Social workers, nurses, and child-life workers may prove to be an invaluable asset in working with the families.

Pharmacologic management by the World Health Organization analgesic ladder is effective for many children with cancer. At presentation or during the course of disease treatment, severe pain should be aggressively managed with early use of opioid analgesics. It is appropriate to select the analgesic agent that seems best matched to the severity of the patient's pain and then climb the ladder as needed rather than starting at the bottom. In addition, some cancer pain can be opioid resistant (e.g., spinal cord or nerve root compression from an intraspinal tumor). In these cases, adjuvant analgesics such as TCAs or gabapentin are indicated, although these agents were not part of the original schema. A regimen of round-the-clock sustained release opioids along with short-acting immediate release agents for breakthrough pain is a good start. Dosages may be adjusted based on response. Patients unable to tolerate oral opioids can be managed with intravenous dosing, usually employing PCA. Fentanyl lozenges and transdermal fentanyl preparations are also well-accepted by children. Rarely, children with terminal cancer may benefit from neuroaxial opioids delivered via an epidural or intrathecal catheter. Implanted pumps are not the norm in management of these patients, largely due to the rapidly progressive nature of their diseases. Invasive procedures such as celiac plexus blockade or neurosurgical ablations are even less commonly used. Opioid requirements in terminal malignancy may be extremely variable, partly depending on the nature of the malignancy and extent of metastases. The key to success is incorporation of a plan at the outset for management of side effects, such as constipation, sedation, pruritus and nausea. Neuropathic pain secondary to metastasis or chemotherapy requires management with TCAs, gabapentin, or TENS units. Antihistamines, corticosteroids, and skeletal muscle relaxants are the other adjuvant drugs that are used in conjunction with the traditional analgesics.

Sickle Cell Disease

Sickle cell disease pain can be a very difficult problem to treat. It is a hemoglobinopathy characterized by recurrent acute and chronic pain, related to red cell sickling and obstruction of the microvasculature with embolism, inflammation, and infarction of organ tissue. Painful vaso-occlusive crises are heralded by pain in the extremities, long bones, chest, and abdomen leading to frequent hospitalizations for pain management with intravenous opioids. The severity and intensity of pain in an individual patient can be very variable, but it can also vary from one patient to the next. A standard protocol for all sickle cell patients is unlikely to be helpful. There is always the risk of undertreatment or inappropriate treatment. Sickle cell disease pain forms a continuum from acute to chronic. The superimposition of unpredictable acute pain crises on top of chronic pain complicates the pain assessment and management in these patients. Many of these patients manage their baseline constant pain with

NSAIDs, opioids, and other modalities such as hydration. They often require hospitalization to manage the more severe pain of the vaso-occlusive crises. These patients may be opioid-tolerant because of their baseline home-opioid use, and this is an important factor to consider when dosing their IV opioids. In addition, the severe nature of their pain results in high opioid requirements. Once a patient's IV-opioid requirement is known and their crisis is improving, it is often possible to convert to a sustained release oral opioid with immediate release medication for breakthrough pain. If kidney function is normal, it is beneficial to use adjuncts such as ketorolac or another NSAID. Epidurals have been used for management of acute painful crises, especially in patients that are intolerant of opioids. It is important that the patient with sickle cell disease also learn cognitive-behavioral pain management techniques since this is an illness characterized by painful episodes in a chronic fashion. A thorough evaluation of the biologic and psychological aspects of the patient and his family and support system needs to be made. Emotional support, chronic blood transfusions, hydroxyurea along with NSAIDs, TCAs, gabapentin, and use of both short- and long-acting opioids are the cornerstones of therapy in this difficult population.

Nonpharmacologic Measures in Chronic Pain

Cognitive-behavioral approaches such as hypnosis, muscle relaxation, breathing exercises, TENS, biofeedback, group therapy, and acupuncture can augment any of all of the pharmacologic interventions.

Children are very responsive to pain-reducing strategies that involve their imagination and sense of play. Children less than 6 years of age can be distracted with blowing bubbles or playing other games. Older children engage well in external or abstract interventions such as guided imagery, distraction, and transformation, counting, and breathing techniques. These techniques help the child intervene at the level of thinking, thus modifying the feelings experienced and behaviors displayed by the child. Hypnosis has been found to be helpful in reducing procedural distress, either by causing amnesia of the events surrounding the hypnotic trance or by inhibiting transmission of pain signals at the level of the dorsal horn. Progressive muscle relaxation helps children recognize and reduce tension associated with pain and decrease anxiety and discomfort. Learning to decrease body tension is an acquired skill. Relaxation training requires initial instruction by a psychologist or therapist, but also mandates frequent practice to be successful. It has been demonstrated to be effective in the treatment of migraine and tension headaches. Biofeedback consists of the measurement and control of a physiologic response not nor-

mally thought to be under voluntary control. α-Electroencephalogram, muscle electromyography, skin temperature, and temporal pulse feedback are used to provide immediate information, allowing a child to observe and modify the level of body tension. These techniques have been found to be useful for management of migraine and chronic headaches, abdominal pain and procedure pain, and as a tool to teach relaxation. Children are quick learners and are more open-minded than adults about being able to self-regulate, thus they are ideal candidates for biofeedback. The short attention span of some children, tendency to engage in other activities during a session, and anxiety about the equipment could present a problem in some. Art and play has also been used to help children with a variety of pain problems to express themselves and reduce their fears. Problem solving, roleplaying, modeling, and behavioral reversal help children by reducing anxiety, teaching skills, and increasing their self-confidence in being able to consistently display a behavior.

TENS units generate a nonpainful stimulus at peripheral nerves through electrodes applied to the skin and facilitate the closing off of gates for pain transmission. They may stimulate the body to produce endorphins that act as natural painkillers. TENS is useful in the management of many pain problems, including acute pain after chest surgery, knee pain, and cancer pain. It is relatively inexpensive, easy to use, and has no serious side effects or complications. As in adults, TENS is contraindicated in children with pacemakers and over the carotid arteries and eyes. Traditionally, it has been used only in children old enough and cognitively mature enough to communicate. Children may be afraid of the unit, and the skill of the therapist plays a major role in the success of its use.

Ultrasound to subcutaneous tissues is another modality that can be used in older children who can comprehend its functioning. It is contraindicated in younger children where the growth plates may not have closed.

Hydrotherapy, including warm or tepid whirlpools and contrast baths, are often well-accepted by children because of the buoyancy afforded by the water and the enjoyable sensation it provides in addition to helping with pain. Exercise in water can be quite helpful in the musculoskeletal disorders.

Acupuncture is rapidly becoming one of the most commonly used forms of complementary medicine for various pain problems. The mechanism may be similar to TENS. Stimulation of small pain fibers may inhibit spinal transmission of other pain signals. There is evidence that through stimulation of the acupuncture energy channels, intrinsic opioid pathways are activated, leading to profound analgesia. Acupuncture has been used successfully in tennis elbow, myofascial pain, dental pain, postoperative and chemotherapeutic pain, headaches, endometriosis, abdominal pain, and CRPS Type I. Despite their needle-phobia, children do seem to do well with acupuncture.

In any child with chronic pain, it is important to rule out other psychiatric illnesses such as depression, obsessive compulsive disorder, suicidal ideation, conversion disorders, and post-traumatic stress disorder, following sexual or physical abuse. Munchausen syndrome is a rare occurrence. A small subgroup may experience pain as a manifestation of psychiatric disease—a diagnosis of somatoform pain disorder should always be backed by positive psychiatric findings and should not be a diagnosis of exclusion. For some children, reinforcement of the sick role perpetuates pain behaviors and amplifies the intensity of the pain experience. It is important to remember that certain aspects of chronic pain could become a learned behavior.

Although chronic pain in children does not have much of an economic impact on society, it is a major social problem, since it has an impact on school attendance and exacts an enormous toll in suffering by the child and his or her family. Recurrent school absenteeism is similar to adult work disability syndrome. The management should include, in addition to possible pharmacologic interventions, physical and occupational therapy, CBT, and individual and family counseling. Patients should be counseled on the importance of good nutrition, sleep habits, and exercise. Home tutoring programs and the additional attention these children obtain with the adjustments made in the home, possibly with one parent choosing to stay home to attend to the child in constant pain, may unintentionally reinforce the illness in the mind of the child. Major goals need to be established to improve psychological functioning, provide support for the entire family, and establish communication with the child's school. Efforts should be focused on making the pain tolerable so that it is possible for the child to return to school. Initially it may have to be on a part-time basis and returning to participation in family and social activities may follow. The patient and family need to understand that the accomplishment of these goals may take months.

CONCLUSION

Pain is a complex, multidimensional phenomenon. The historic undertreatment of pediatric pain reflects the attitudes and values that surrounded the specialty. Pain management has always been an essential component of care provided by a pediatric anesthesiologist. It is not surprising, therefore, that pediatric anesthesiologists are at the forefront for improving pain management resources in children's hospitals. Many children's hospitals have now developed acute, chronic, and combined programs for management of pain in children. Compassion has always been the hallmark of the care provided for children. Both from a humanitarian and physiologic standpoint, pain management should now be considered an integral part of their medical care as well.

REFERENCES

1. Anand K, Sippell W, et al: Randomized trial of fentanyl anesthesia in preterm neonates undergoing surgery: effects on the stress response. Lancet i:243-248, 1987.

2. Singleton MA, Rosen JI, et al: Plasma concentrations of fentanyl in infants, children, and adults. Canadian Journal of Anesthesia 34:152-155, 1987.

SUGGESTED READING

Anand KJ, Hickey PR: Pain and its effects in the human neonate and fetus. N Engl J Med 317(21):1321-1329, 1987.

Anderson BJ, Holford NH: Rectal acetaminophen pharmacokinetics. Anesthesiology 88(4):1131-1133, 1998.

Bray RJ, Woodhams AM, et al: Morphine consumption and respiratory depression in children receiving postoperative analgesia from continuous morphine infusion or patient controlled analgesia. Paediatric Anaesthesia. 6(2):129-134, 1996.

Doyle E, Robinson D, et al: Comparison of patient-controlled analgesia with and without a background infusion after lower abdominal surgery in children. Br J Anaesth 71(5):670-673, 1993.

Eccleston C, Morley S, et al: Systematic review of randomised controlled trials of psychological therapy for chronic pain in children and adolescents, with a subset meta-analysis of pain relief. Pain 99(1-2):157-165, 2002.

Eccleston C, Yorke L, et al: Psychological therapies for the management of chronic and recurrent pain in children and adolescents. Cochrane Database Syst Rev(1):CD003968, 2003.

Eichenfield L, Funk A, et al: A clinical study to evaluate the efficacy of ELA-Max (4% Liposomal Lidocaine) as compared with eutectic mixture of local anesthetics cream for pain reduction of venipuncture in children. Pediatrics 109(6): 1093-1099, 2002.

Finkel JC, Rose JB, et al: An evaluation of the efficacy and tolerability of oral tramadol hydrochloride tablets for the treatment of postsurgical pain in children. Anesth Analg 94(6):1469-1473, 2002.

Fitzgerald M: The sprouting of saphenous nerve terminals in the spinal cord following early postnatal sciatic nerve section in the rat. J Comp Neurol 240(4):407-413, 1985.

Fitzgerald M, Jennings E: The postnatal development of spinal sensory processing. Proc Natl Acad Sci USA 96(14): 7719-7722, 1999.

Franck LS, Greenberg CS, et al: Pain assessment in infants and children. Pediatr Clin North Am 47(3):487-512, 2000.

Howard RF: Current status of pain management in children. Jama 290(18):2464-2469, 2003.

Kashikar-Zuck S, Goldschneider KR, et al: Depression and functional disability in chronic pediatric pain. Clin J Pain 17(4): 341-349, 2001.

Koppel RA, Coleman KM, et al: The efficacy of EMLA versus ELA-Max for pain relief in medium-depth chemical peeling: a clinical and histopathologic evaluation. Dermatol Surg 26(1):61-64, 2000.

Krane, EJ, Dalens BJ, et al: The safety of epidurals placed during general anesthesia. Reg Anesth Pain Med 23(5):433-438, 1998.

Lesko SM, Mitchell AA: The safety of acetaminophen and ibuprofen among children younger than two years old. Pediatrics 104(4):e39, 1999.

Palermo TM: Impact of recurrent and chronic pain on child and family daily functioning: a critical review of the literature. J Dev Behav Pediatr 21(1):58-69, 2000.

Perquin CW, Hazebroek-Kampschreur AA, et al: Pain in children and adolescents: a common experience. Pain 87(1):51-58, 2000.

Peters JW, Hoekstra Bandell IE, et al: Patient controlled analgesia in children and adolescents: a randomized controlled trial. Paediatric Anaesthesia. 9(3):235-241, 1999.

Rose JB, Finkel JC, et al: Oral tramadol for the treatment of pain of 7-30 days' duration in children. Anesth Analg 96(1):78-81, 2003.

Ruda MA, Ling QD, et al: Altered nociceptive neuronal circuits after neonatal peripheral inflammation. Science 289(5479): 628-631, 2000.

Schechter NL, Berde CB, et al: Pain in infants, children, and adolescents. Philadelphia, Lippincott Williams & Wilkins, 2003.

Taddio A, Ohlsson A, et al: A systematic review of lidocaine-prilocaine cream (EMLA) in the treatment of acute pain in neonates. Pediatrics 101(2):E1, 1998.

CHAPTER 12

Management of Neuropathic Pain

CONSTANTINE SARANTOPOULOS

INTRODUCTION

The term *neuropathic pain* describes a heterogeneous category of chronic, painful conditions that arise as a result of traumatic lesions, diseases, or dysfunction of the normal afferent neural pathways. The clinical characteristics vary, and include delayed onset of pain after nervous system lesions, various spontaneous and evoked manifestations of pain, various "burning" and/or "shooting" sensations, pain in an area of sensory loss, and unpleasant dysesthesias.

Neuropathic pain is traditionally categorized on the basis of the underlying cause or on the anatomic location of the precipitating lesion. The underlying causes of painful neuropathy are variable and include metabolic diseases (e.g., diabetes mellitus, uremia), herpes zoster and HIV infections, drugs or chemicals (i.e., alcohol, chemotherapeutics, and anti-HIV drugs), immune deficiencies, malignant diseases, traumata and ischemic states. The anatomic sites of lesions causing neuropathic pain may be located in a range from the primary afferent nerve fibers in the periphery, to the highest cortical centers, but peripheral neuropathic pain constitutes the most prevalent category (Box 12-1).

Despite some advances in understanding its pathophysiology, neuropathic pain still remains a significant clinical challenge. Patients suffering from neuropathic pain do not respond well to conventional analgesics, such as opioids or nonsteroidal, anti-inflammatory analgesics. Nevertheless, in an attempt to control the manifestations of neuropathic pain and the associated chronic pain behavior, other pharmacologic agents have been tried and introduced in clinical practice. The adoption of these agents, which include tricyclic antidepressants and antiepileptic drugs, has been based on results from preclinical investigations as well as several clinical studies.

The specific cellular and molecular mechanisms underlying neuropathic pain have not been completely elucidated, with regards to etiologic significance for each. However, it seems that membrane hyperexcitability in those neurons that have lost their normal anatomic integrity, or their regular synaptic, physiologic, or electrical patterns seem to be a common denominator for many, if not all types, of neuropathic pains. Many of the manifestations of neuropathic pain seem to be provoked by alterations in the peripheral nervous system. Following nerve injury, the damaged peripheral nerves become more excitable, with regard to their ability to

Box 12-1 Common Causes of Painful Neuropathic Pain

- Metabolic diseases (e.g., diabetes, mellitus, uremia)
- Herpes zoster and HIV infections
- Drugs or chemicals (i.e., alcohol, chemotherapeutics, and anti-HIV drugs)
- Immune deficiencies
- Malignant diseases
- Trauma
- Radiation
- Ischemic states

generate action potentials, and this leads to spontaneous, ongoing, ectopic electrical activity. The dorsal root ganglia have been also recognized as an important focus of significant aberrant electrical activity as well. Thus, increased excitability of primary afferents results into a marked increase in the afferent nociceptive traffic from the peripheral fibers to the dorsal horns, producing central sensitization. Despite the lack of definition of specific mechanisms, a correlation between spontaneous firing and injury-induced pain has been reported in humans and in animal models. With regards to the physiologic basis of this aberrant activity, substantial evidence exists for alterations in the expression of ion channels on peripheral afferents following nerve injury, a fact that also provides the basis for specific therapeutic interventions.

GENERAL PRINCIPLES OF TREATMENT

All patients suffering from neuropathic pain are not the same, and those with the same apparent cause may present with different clinical manifestations, different cognitive and behavioral responses, and different degrees of social adaptation. Lack of understanding of all the mechanisms, at all levels, renders selection of treat-

Box 12-2 Principles of Neuropathic Pain Management

- A biopsychosocial approach is appropriate.
- Management should be individualized.
- Multimodal therapy is necessary in most cases.
- Consider concurrent rather than sequential application of multimodal treatments.
- Therapies based on evidence or subjected to critical appraisal should be chosen first.
- Disability and psychological dysfunction need special attention.

ments more difficult, but some general principles of management can be followed (Box 12-2):

1. A biopsychosocial approach rather than a classical "disease" model is more appropriate. According to the latter model, diseases or nosologic entities are viewed mechanistically as pathogenetically induced by definite causative agents, manifested by certain symptomatologies, and amenable to specific treatments aiming to reverse the pathogenetic processes. This prevailing view seems to be effective in most fields of the traditional medicine, but not in chronic-pain management. Most manifestations of neuropathic pain should be viewed as mainly behavioral, and so far no reliable method has been accepted to objectively measure or assess pain. Pain behavior is a consequence of a variety of interacting factors, wherein a series of psychological, family, and social factors, acting as positive or negative reinforcers, tend to establish certain behavioral patterns, through which patients interact with the health professionals. Secondary benefits (professional, legal, financial) may also play a predominant role determining a particular patient's responses. Finally, therapeutic interventions aiming to restore function may be more appropriate than those just targeting a certain behavioral vocalization of pain. In this context, adopting a bio-psychosocial model is more appropriate; this, in addition to treating pain as a symptom, should focus on patient education and restoration of function at all levels (physical, psychological, within the family, and social).

2. Management should be individualized. Best outcomes can only be achieved only when data from clinical evidence are integrated with a thorough assessment of the individual patient, so that problems as well as desired outcomes are clearly defined.

3. Patient participation in decision making and management is essential. This requires an appropriately informed patient, with regard to realistic expectations, advantages/disadvantages/side effects of proposed treatment modalities as well as to the availability of alternative options.

4. Multimodal therapy is necessary in most cases. Because of the complexity of the underlying pathophysiology of neuropathic pain, different treatments aimed at specific sites and mechanisms involved in the pain processes may be necessary. Other symptoms, in addition to pain, may require treatment as well (e.g., motor weakness, insomnia, depression, anxiety, constipation, nausea). Furthermore, concurrent application of different modalities, through additive or synergistic actions, may allow dose reduction, improve efficacy, and minimize side effects. The latter is important in order to enhance patients' compliance, which is relatively poor in many cases of chronic pain.

5. Concurrent rather than sequential application of multimodal treatments should be used.

6. Therapies based on evidence or subjected to critical appraisal should be chosen first.

7. Disability and psychological dysfunction need special attention. In many instances functional impairment (either physical or psychological) constitutes the predominant problem, and remains disguised under the verbal or gestural behavior that characterizes chronic neuropathic pain.

PRACTICAL MANAGEMENT

Prevention of Certain Types of Neuropathic Pain

Early interventions have been proposed to prevent the development of types of neuropathic pain, but the techniques remain still under dispute. The techniques of "preemptive analgesia" may not work so well in the clinical, as they do in the experimental setting, apparently because of the complexity of the pathophysiology of pain in the latter. Various treatment modalities have been either proposed or proven to reduce progression of acute painful conditions to chronicity.

Topical application of eutectic mixture of local anesthetics (EMLA) cream around the breast, during the early perioperative period of breast surgery for cancer, may reduce the incidence of the postmastectomy pain several months later. Perioperative epidural infusions of local anesthetics, opioids, and adjuvants, such as clonidine, have been used to prevent the development of postamputation pains (phantom pain and stump pain), but studies are equivocal. Apparently, pre-existing and long-lasting nociception, coexisting conditions, such as ischemia and chronic neuropathy, extensive involvement of somatic areas may override the short-term protective benefit of perioperative analgesics.

Sympathetic blocks within 2 months of an attack of acute herpes zoster may reduce the incidence of postherpetic neuralgia, although the suggestion has not been based on a controlled-randomized study.

Evaluation of Patients with Neuropathic Pain

Many patients, before they reach the pain clinic, have already been extensively evaluated, so it is often desirable to withhold further fruitless searches for a "cause" of the pain. Nevertheless, in all cases a thorough medical history is taken and physical examination is conducted, and the subjective experience of pain and functional disability is quantified. Special questionnaires have facilitated objective assessment of patients (e.g., McGill Pain Questionnaire).

The diagnosis of neuropathic pain is based on the history and the physical examination. There may be a history of a metabolic disease causing neuropathy (e.g., diabetes, uremia, hypothyroidism, amyloidosis), infection (e.g., herpes zoster, HIV infection), intoxication (e.g., alcohol, mercury, arsenic), malignancy (e.g., cancer, myeloma), radiation therapy, use of certain drugs (e.g., Adriamycin, vincristine, cis-platinum, drugs against HIV infection, amiodarone), ischemic conditions, or conditions associated with nerve injury or entrapment. Pain can be spontaneous or evoked, continuous or paroxysmal, but a quality of "burning," "stabbing," "lancinating," or an "electric shock-like" nature may distinguish it from a nociceptive etiology. Furthermore, the description of pain may predict subsequent response to analgesics. "Shooting," paroxysmal symptoms may be more likely to respond to anticonvulsants, while tricyclic antidepressants should be tried first for symptoms of a continuous, "burning" quality. Allodynia and hyperalgesia may be present as well as sensory changes or unpleasant abnormal sensations (dysesthesias). Tapping of neuromas, at an amputation stump or an injury site, may produce evoked painful sensations in a radiating electric-shock-like sensation (Tinel's sign). Usually, in neuropathic pain, the experience of pain is accompanied by significant emotional dysfunction and mental distress. At the time when patients are referred to the pain clinic several treatments may have been tried and have failed.

Additional studies are sometimes requested only if they are going to clarify incomplete diagnoses or guide the therapeutic interventions. Intravenous drug tests (e.g., lidocaine, phentolamine, fentanyl) are occasionally used to aid diagnosis, response, and selection of treatment. Diagnostic nerve blocks are also used but, because of the high incidence of false positive and false negative responses, the results should be interpreted with caution. The placebo effect accounts for many false positive results. Nerve blocks may also be poor prognostic indicators of the response to surgical or chemical neuroablative procedures. Laboratory investigations, depending on each individual case they may range from simple blood or urine tests, to electrophysiologic studies (electromyography and nerve conduction studies) and to imaging studies (e.g., MRI of the spine, computerized tomography, nuclear scans).

Diagnostic nerve blocks can be employed based on the principles that if "painful" afferent traffic originates from a certain neural pathway, pain may be reproduced by the needle placement close to that structure, relieved completely by selective administration of local anesthetics, and the duration or relief would match the duration of action of the injected drug. Prognostic blocks assess the degree of responsiveness to planned treatment modalities, such as neuroablative techniques or implanted devices. Both types of blocks are very difficult to interpret because of the complex neural anatomy and pathophysiology of chronic pain, systemic absorption, and effects of drugs used as well as the high prevalence of placebo phenomena in chronic patients.

Treatment Plans

These will be determined by various factors, including a thorough understanding of the treatment goals. This will further depend on a definition of the desirable outcome for each particular patient. Treatment plans should primarily focus on functional improvement, reduction of symptoms and suffering, limitation of environmental reinforcers of pain behavior, minimization of dependence on the health-care system, and return to work. The usual therapeutic approach is multimodal, based on pharmacologic agents, and also includes physical therapy, graduated exercise programs, encouragement of activity as well as cognitive, behavioral, and supportive measures to provide functional restoration despite continuing pain. Nerve blocks and interventions may also be part of this management.

PHARMACOLOGIC MANAGEMENT OF NEUROPATHIC PAIN

Although the treatment of the neuropathic pain can be difficult, optimum treatment can be achieved by understanding therapeutic options, the mainstay of which is pharmacotherapy. Selection of treatments can be facilitated by evidence-based data from clinical trials, but in many cases, because of relative lack of such data, by trial and error.

Three major classes of medications are used in the treatment of neuropathic pain: tricyclic antidepressants (TCAs), "membrane-stabilizing drugs" (anticonvulsants/sodium channel blockers), and other agents [clonidine, capsaicin, nonsteroidal anti-inflammatory drugs (NSAIDs), and rarely opioids which may be effective in some cases as "nonspecific" analgesics]. Individual responses to different agents, doses, and serum levels are highly variable. The results of pharmacologic therapy can be enhanced by other treatments, which include specific invasive procedures as well as physical modalities, transcutaneous nerve stimulation (TENS), biofeedback, occupational therapy, relaxation, etc.

The available current critical literature supports mainly the use of TCAs, some anticonvulsants (i.e., gabapentin, carbamazepine), topical or systemic local anesthetics (i.e., lidocaine, mexiletine), and clonidine for peripheral neuropathic pain. There is also support for the use of IV regional blocks with bretylium and ketanserin, corticosteroids, and clonidine for the complex regional pain syndromes. Capsaicin seems to also have a significant effect for both disorders.

Opioids in Neuropathic Pain

The long-term use of opioids in patients with neuropathic pain, although expanding, remains highly controversial. There is no definitive consensus so far that opioids are beneficial for patients with chronic pain, except those suffering from pain due to cancer.

Traditionally, neuropathic pain is considered to be insensitive to opioids. It has been shown that damage to primary afferent nerves results in decreased expression of opioid receptors not only on peripheral sensory nerves, but on spinal neurons in the pain pathways as well, thus reducing the efficacy of opioid agents. In addition, other substances may reduce the efficacy of opioids, such as the neuropeptide cholecystokinin (CCK). Opioid and CCK receptors are coexpressed in the same spinal neurons, and activation of the former increases release of CCK neuropeptide, which then reduces the effectiveness of opioid agonists in a feedback manner. Thus, multiple mechanisms, including decreased opioid receptors and increased CCK-induced inhibition of opioids, make opioids ineffective in treating neuropathic pain.

A lot of times, a major affective component is present and a learned pain behavior facilitated by an interaction of environmental or social reinforcers is the main problem. Opioids may act as reinforcers themselves and help perpetuate further similar maladaptive learned pain behavioral patterns by enhancing endogenous neural reward systems. Opioids may encourage passivity and make certain patients less compliant with the entire rehabilitation program, but may facilitate activity in others (unfortunately, very few). Overall, there is a lack of an adequate number of well-conducted surveys of long-term opioid administration to suggest that they can be effective, safe, and nonaddictive in patients with neuropathic pain. Thus, the long-term use of opioids in the management of neuropathic pain should be avoided. Nevertheless, meticulously selected patients suffering from intractable neuropathic pain may be considered potential candidates for a trial, provided that an agreement has been established that even in the case of subsequent long-term use, evidence of treatment failure will result in discontinuation of the treatment. In this context, agents with a weak N-methyl-D-aspartate (NMDA) inhibitory effect, such as methadone and propoxyphene, may have a theoretic advantage over other agents.

Tricyclic Antidepressants

TCAs are effective for both peripheral and central neuropathic pain. Clinical studies have documented their efficacy over placebo in several conditions (i.e., diabetic neuropathy, postherpetic neuralgia, atypical facial pain, central neuropathic pain). However, 5% of patients may have to stop treatment because of major adverse effects. Selective Serotonin Reuptake Inhibitors (SSRIs) and atypical antidepressants are not effective as analgesics, but are associated with fewer major adverse reactions.

The analgesic effect depends on enhancement of endogenous noradrenergic and serotoninergic inhibitory mechanisms, but some of them may weakly inhibit the NMDA-receptor and the aberrant sodium channels that proliferate on injured neurons as well. The analgesic effect is separate from the antidepressant effect and occurs with much lower doses. Agents with both noradrenergic and serotoninergic effect (amitriptyline) appear to be more efficient than other antidepressants. Actually, most evidence from well-conducted, controlled, randomized studies has proven the superiority of amitriptyline versus the non-tricyclic compounds. Amitriptyline, despite a potential for side effects especially at the higher doses, still remains the gold standard. Doses can be started at 10 or 25 mg at bedtime and titrated up to higher doses (150 mg) according to clinical response. Side effects include anticholinergic effects and possible arrhythmogenicity. In case of intolerable anticholinergic side effects or excessive drowsiness, nortriptyline or desipramine can be reasonable alternatives. In patients suffering from sleep disorders due to pain and/or depression, more sedating antidepressants (amitriptyline or doxepin) should be selected first (Box 12-3).

Anticonvulsants/Sodium Channel Blockers

Besides the TCAs, anticonvulsants and sodium channel blockers are the other commonly used group of drugs for the treatment of neuropathic pain. The neuronal hyperexcitability and corresponding membrane channel changes in injured neurons have many features in common with the cellular changes in certain forms of epilepsy. This has led to the use of anticonvulsant drugs for the treatment of neuropathic pain. Carbamazepine and phenytoin were the first anticonvulsants to be used in controlled clinical trials. Studies have shown these agents to relieve painful diabetic neuropathy and paroxysmal attacks in trigeminal neuralgia. Nevertheless, their use was complicated by pharmacokinetic shortcomings and frequent adverse side effects.

Empirically, pain with a paroxysmal "lancinating" or "shooting" nature is more likely to respond to anticonvulsants, while a constant, "burning" quality may predict better responsiveness to TCAs; many times both types of drugs are given concomitantly. Anticonvulsants have been found helpful in the management of trigeminal neuralgia, diabetic neuropathy, in migraines as well as in a number of other painful conditions. Drowsiness, dizziness, and disturbance in gait are common adverse effects.

Recently, the novel antiepileptic agent gabapentin proved to be especially effective at relieving allodynia and hyperalgesia in animal models. Furthermore, it has been shown to be efficacious in numerous small clinical studies and case reports in a wide variety of neuropathic pain syndromes as well as other types of pain. Specifically, this agent has been clearly demonstrated to be effective for the treatment of neuropathic pain in diabetic neuropathy, postherpetic neuralgia, trigeminal neuralgia, painful neuropathy from HIV infection, cancer, complex regional pain syndromes, pain after mastectomy, etc. This supportive evidence, combined with the drug's favorable side-effect profile in various patient groups (including the elderly) and lack of drug interactions, renders it an attractive agent for clinical practice. Slow titration is a key-point for a successful treatment. Usual doses start at 300 mg, at bedtime, slowly titrated up to 900 mg or 1200 mg 3 times a day. There is significant variability, with some patients obtaining relief with serum levels below the "therapeutic" range for epilepsy, whereas others require "toxic" serum levels before pain relief is obtained (without intolerable side effects) (Box 12-4).

Agents with inhibitory effects at the sodium channels have proved efficacious in several neuropathic pain states. Aberrant sodium channel frequently accompany several types of nerve injury and may account for the electrical excitability in such states. Lidocaine, administered systemically from the intravenous route, or topically in the form of 5% ointment or skin patches, is frequently employed in the management of several neuropathic conditions, including postherpetic neuralgia. Mexiletine, an oral analogue of lidocaine, can also be

---

Box 12-3 TCAs as Analgesics in Neuropathic Pain

- Amitriptyline: the "gold" standard
- Switch to nortriptyline or desipramine in case of intolerable drowsiness or anticholinergic side effects
- Amitriptyline or doxepin helpful for insomnia

Box 12-4 Anticonvulsants and Sodium Channel Blockers in Neuropathic Pain

- Gabapentin: first-line drug. Caution in the elderly and renal patients.
- Lidocaine, administered systemically or topically.
- Mexiletine, oral analogue of lidocaine, (frequent gastrointestinal side effects).
- Lamotrigine or topiramate, as third-line choices.

used in the management of peripheral neuropathies, but its use can be limited by frequent gastrointestinal side effects. Pain and allodynia from peripheral nerve injury, diabetic neuropathy, postherpetic or trigeminal neuralgia, and dysesthetic pain following spinal-cord injury or peripheral nerve injury can be relieved from systemic lidocaine or mexiletine. Lidocaine can be used intravenously in a preliminary trial, in doses 3 to 5 mg/kg over 30 to 45 minutes (provided precautions against toxicity are taken), in order to assess responsiveness. If trial is successful, treatment with mexiletine up to 10 mg/kg daily, in 3 divided doses may follow. Many clinicians directly try mexiletine without prior trial. Adverse effects from intravenous lidocaine include light-headedness, somnolence, nausea, and perioral numbness. History of heart disease, conduction abnormalities, or certain arrhythmias is a contraindication. Mexiletine may produce significant gastrointestinal intolerance (e.g., nausea, vomiting, epigastric discomfort).

Other Agents

Clonidine can also effectively treat many patients with neuropathic pain. Finally, topical agents can be used and may be effective in subpopulations of patients, such as the capsaicin cream, and a mixture of the local anesthetics lidocaine and prilocaine (EMLA).

Capsaicin is an alkaloid derived from pepper, which can deplete substance P from primary afferent terminals. Topically applied capsaicin cream may be helpful (in addition to other analgesics) in pain from diabetic neuropathy and other conditions, but initial burning sensation, need for frequent applications, and prolonged use may limit compliance and success rates. It has been also used against post-mastectomy pain.

Quinine sulphate (200 to 300 mg/day) reduces episodes of nocturnal leg cramps, in the elderly, if taken regularly, but patients should be monitored for adverse effects (e.g., nausea, thrombocytopenia, leukopenia). Calcitonin has been used for phantom pains.

Muscle relaxants (e.g., baclofen, cyclobenzaprine), glucocorticoids, anxiolytics, and hypnotics as well as clonidine and sympatholytics are also used in special circumstances.

Neural Blockade

Anesthesiologists originally became involved in pain management because they perform nerve blocks, but not infrequently the rationale for attacks on the peripheral nociceptive "wiring" ignores the multidimensional complex central pathophysiology and behavioral dimensions of neuropathic pain.

Therapeutic blocks are used to reduce pain by diminishing afferent input from sources of pain on injured peripheral nerves. Local anesthetics, steroids, and other agents can be used for non-neurolytic blocks.

Local anesthetic blocks can provide pain relief significantly outlasting the known conduction block of the local anesthetic, but, even so, only in few patients the effect outlasts 1 month, and the repeated use of these blocks is not recommended. Nevertheless, they can be used as an aid to physical therapy, or to facilitate other similar therapeutic interventions (e.g., mobilization, exercise) from which more benefit is expected.

The substance n-butyl-p aminobenzoate, a congener of benzocaine, has been found recently to produce up to 6 months of sensory block, without motor involvement, and has been used in cancer patients, so far.

Corticosteroid injections reduce local inflammation from tissue or nerve damage, but they can also suppress spontaneous neuronal discharge in neuromas and produce conduction block upon C fibers. Sometimes they may provide long-lasting pain relief, but there is no compelling evidence that they are efficacious. According to studies[1,2] there is no proven benefit associated with their use, which may lead to potential side effects. Besides, it has been shown that a significant percentage of painful conditions may resolve over time without invasive interventions.

Neuroablative blocks are used to provide long-lasting relief by ablating the painful nerve, without increased risk of neuroma formation or deafferentation (which may occur after surgical transection). Radiofrequency thermocoagulation or cryogenic blocks have also been used with supposedly no or minimal risk of neuropathy. For example, branches of the trigeminal nerve can be blocked with local anesthetics to provide brief relief, but permanent neurolysis has the risk of neuralgia of deafferentation type. However, if pain responds well to frequent such blocks, radiofrequency lesions of the trigeminal ganglion can be subsequently used to relieve pain.

Cryoanalgesia provides a temporary but long-lasting anesthetic block. When nerve fibers progressively cool, temporary conduction block occurs. The incidence of neuroma formation and neuropathy after cryoanalgesia is minimal. This method is appropriate for painful conditions originating from small, well-localized, and rather superficial lesions of the peripheral nerves, such as neuromas and entrapment neuropathies, but cryoanalgesia should always be preceded by a diagnostic nerve block. There is no evidence with regard to efficacy, but it may be helpful in well-selected patients.

Radiofrequency lesioning uses heat generated by an ionic electrical field in the tissue, after insertion of a special needle probe close to the nerve. Radiofrequency lesioning is more applicable for analgesia of deeper situated nerve structures and has been effectively used for cervical and lumbar facet denervation, dorsal root ganglion lesion, gasserian ganglion ablation, and lumbar sympathetic chain ablation. It should always be preceded by a diagnostic nerve block. Lack of evidence from adequate number of randomized controlled studies constitutes a major limitation of the technique.

Prophylactic blocks are sometimes used to prevent acute nociception from causing development of chronic pain conditions. Early sympathetic blocks have been proposed to reduce the incidence of postherpetic neuralgia and regional techniques prior to amputation to decrease the incidence of phantom or stump pain.

Chemical neurolytic blocks are performed by using chemical neurolytics such as phenol or alcohol to ablate nerves in patients with cancer and limited life expectancy.

ADJUNCTIVE THERAPIES

Traditional adjunctive therapies include a wide range of physical, occupational, and educational interventions and can play an important role in the overall management. Their goals are to contribute to the pain relief, prevent disability, restore function, and educate the patient.

Many techniques are applied by physical therapists, including exercises, application of superficial or deep heat, cold, electrotherapy, splints and braces, laser, and ultrasound. Although the principles and clinical applications have been extensively described in textbooks, surprisingly few controlled trials investigating the efficacy and outcome of such approaches have been published.

According to the "Gate Theory," TENS may block pain transmission via selective activation of large fibers. TENS can be helpful in some patients with neuropathic pain, but few well-conducted studies exist to prove its effectiveness. Nevertheless, despite the lack of evidence, the simplicity and lack of serious side effects may indicate the application of the technique in many painful conditions.

Nevertheless, most clinical trials data and meta-analyses suggest that interventions that combine exercise and psycho-educational approaches can have a clinically significant impact on reducing pain and improving functional status for many conditions.

Spinal-Cord Stimulation for Neuropathic Painful Conditions

Spinal-cord stimulation (SCS) has been used in the United States for more than 30 years. Rationale for its use is that SCS provides pain relief by modulating the pain processing at the spinal-cord level. Although many theories exist on the mechanisms involved, the most widely accepted theory is based on the "gate control" activation of inhibitory pathways. Stimulating electrodes placed dorsally into the epidural space may activate many spinal pathways including the endogenous inhibitory systems. A direct conduction block of the afferent nociceptive input has also been hypothesized, but SCS allows normal perception of acute pain in humans. SCS may also improve circulation and tissue oxygenation in patients with arterial insufficiency, perhaps due to a functional sympathectomy.

Technically, electrodes are placed into the epidural space, followed by stimulation patterns adjusted as to elicit not-unpleasant paresthesiae covering the painful area. Then, a trial follows for a few days to few weeks later, and, if successful, a permanent generator is implanted subcutaneously and connected to the epidural leads. The number and type of electrodes implanted and the type of stimulation vary.

The efficacy of SCS has not been proven because available studies are limited from methodologic flaws and may have been biased from lack of randomization and blinding.

Patients with neuropathic pain localized in the extremities have been regarded classically as the most appropriate candidates for SCS. SCS has been tried in the following conditions:

- Failed back surgery with dominant radicular pain in the extremities and minimal mechanical axial back pain.
- Complex Regional Pain Syndromes (e.g., Reflex Sympathetic Dystrophy, causalgia).
- Peripheral neuropathies (SCS has been tried in brachial plexus neuropathic pain from trauma or radiation, diabetic neuropathies, or postherpetic neuralgia. It has also been used in multiple sclerosis patients).
- Phantom limb pain and stump pain.
- Ischemic extremity pain and peripheral arterial insufficiency.
- Angina (intractable angina not surgically correctable can be treated with SCS).

The biggest problem is infection that occurs in about 5% of the cases (i.e., superficial or deep soft tissue infection, or epidural abscess) (Box 12-5).

Deep brain stimulation has also been applied stereotactically by neurosurgeons in the thalamus or the

Box 12-5 Indications for Consideration of Spinal-Cord Stimulation

- Peripheral neuropathic pain localized in the extremities
- Failed back surgery with dominant radicular pain in the extremities
- Complex regional pain syndromes
- Phantom limb pain and stump pain
- Ischemic extremity pain and peripheral arterial insufficiency
- Intractable angina

periaqueductal gray, but the overall acceptance of the technique is low.

Alternative Therapies

Acupuncture has been suggested as a potentially valuable adjunctive therapy, but unfortunately, carefully designed, high-quality trials assessing its efficacy are rare.

Psychosocial Interventions

Anxiety, fear, depression, frustration, and other emotions may intensify the pain response. Psycho-educational interventions comprise a broad array of approaches that have been used to manage pain. They include:

- **Patient education:** lectures, demonstrations, pamphlets, newsletters, video presentations, and other techniques may improve adherence behavior and have positive impact on the outcome.
- **Cognitive-behavioral therapy/behavioral modification:** this refers to a variety of psychosocial approaches designed to enhance self-control and achieve the best possible level of physical and emotional function within the confines of the condition. Psychotherapy or group therapy can also be effective in selected patients.

SPECIFIC NEUROPATHIC PAIN CONDITIONS

Herpes Zoster and Postherpetic Neuralgia

Postherpetic neuralgia is pain persisting in the dermatomes affected by herpes zoster, after the resolution of the acute herpes zoster and the healing of the rash caused by the infection. Herpes zoster (shingles) is caused by the varicella-zoster virus, which infects the sensory ganglia and their area of innervation. It results in pain over the distribution of the affected nerve, together

with a vesicular rash over the same area. Pain may be of dysesthetic nature, accompanied by allodynia, hyperalgesia, and severe itching, but may precede the rash. Advanced age is a major risk factor. Acute episodes resolve, but pain may persist in a significant percentage of patients. Old age is a risk factor. Pain persists in 60% of those above 60 years at 1 month, and in 15% at 6 months up to 1 year after resolution.

Proper treatment during the acute phase will control pain and may prevent complications.

Antiviral agents are helpful. Famciclovir has been shown to reduce pain duration after acute herpes zoster and acyclovir to reduce prevalence of postherpetic pain. Idoxuridine may also provide short-term pain relief in acute zoster. NSAIDs and TCAs can be used during the acute phase, while mild opioids can be tried for refractory pain. Amitriptyline started during the acute episode may also prevent postherpetic neuralgia. High-dose steroids, added to antiviral agents, may speed healing of acute herpes zoster, but there is no evidence that may have preventive effects.

Subcutaneous infiltration with local anesthetics and steroids has also been used for treating acute pain, but there is no evidence about long-term effects. Early sympathetic blocks have been reported in a noncontrolled study to prevent postherpetic neuralgia, but this has not been confirmed. Nevertheless, they may be tried in the acute phase and repeated according to the patient's response. Somatic blocks can be also used for pain relief.

Pain from postherpetic neuralgia can be relieved by TCAs (e.g., amitriptyline, nortriptyline, desipramine), lidocaine patches applied topically, or topical capsaicin cream. Gabapentin has also been proven to be effective. However, evidence proving that TENS, benzodiazepines, antiviral agents, antiprostaglandins, and acupuncture are effective in the chronic setting is currently insufficient.

Complex Regional Pain Syndrome

Complex regional pain syndrome (CRPS) describes a syndrome of pain with allodynia and hyperalgesia, functional impairment, and vasomotor or sudomotor instability. CRPS Type I corresponds to the old term "reflex sympathetic dystrophy" (RSD), and CRPS Type II refers to "causalgia." These painful conditions may or may not be "sympathetically maintained," depending on the response to diagnostic sympathetic blockade. The presence of sympathetic hyperactivity can be demonstrated with greater or lesser ease in a certain percentage of these patients, but it does not constitute an etiologic association. A number of laboratory tests have been used to aid the diagnosis, but they are not very specific. Etiology remains unknown, despite a variety of speculations.

Clinical Presentation

There may or may not be a history of injury. Pain is present in more than 90% of cases, is of burning quality, not relieved by rest, and may be accompanied by hyperalgesia and allodynia. Pain does not follow any specific radicular or neural distribution, and sometimes it spreads to the entire extremity, or the ipsilateral body. Other findings are sudomotor and vasomotor changes, cyanosis or discoloration, edema, coldness, mottling, localized changes in sweating, pale, smooth and shiny skin, and changes in hair growth and nails. Severe cases are complicated by joint stiffness, contractures, atrophy, osteoporosis, and diminished use of the affected limb. Various tests have been suggested to facilitate diagnosis, including triple phase bone scan, thermography, sympathogalvanic testing, test of sweat gland function, but specificity is questionable. Sympathetic blocks may assess the degree of sympathetic involvement.

Treatment

Desensitization, gradual physical therapy, and occupational therapy constitute the mainstay of the treatment, with functional recovery being the primary goal. This can be facilitated by multidisciplinary treatment protocols utilizing various regional sympathetic or IV sympathetic blocks, analgesic medications (mainly NSAIDs, TCAs, and gabapentin), TENS, or SCS and psychological interventions. Early aggressive treatment yields the best results.

Diagnostic/prognostic sympathetic blocks may guide therapy: If sympathetic blockade relieves pain, further treatments should include more frequent blocks, ablative therapy with radiofrequency lesioning, neurolysis, or surgery (the results of which have not been validated by adequate studies), and systemic sympatholytics (e.g., clonidine, prazosin). Failure of sympathetic blockade would contraindicate continuation of such treatments.

Nevertheless, the evidence that sympathetic blocks cure RSD is not strong, and there is no proof that the sympathetic block, rather than a transition from disuse to use, facilitated from physical therapy, promotes rehabilitation and change.

Natural history is also unclear. It has been shown that despite early physicians' reports of excellent responses in most patients 2 to 3 months post-treatment, a year later, two-thirds of these patients were officially disabled. This may suggest complex pathophysiology, coexistence of behavioral factors, or simply that benefit of the treatment does not always persist. Early treatment may have the best results, but if there is any self-limitation in RSD (the one-third of cases who remain active) then early treatment may claim as cures those who would have improved anyhow. It is unknown if early treatment could cure those who would otherwise have had pain of long duration.

Central Pain

Central pain can result from spinal and supraspinal lesions, and the onset of pain may be delayed even by years after the original injury. Nearly all patients have some sensory abnormalities, and recognition of the syndrome may require testing for subtle sensory disturbances (especially temperature alterations). The goal of treatment in central pain is pain reduction rather than complete pain relief. Principles of treatment include:

1. Treatment of other concurrent underlying painful conditions.
2. Use of antidepressants (particularly TCAs: amitriptyline or nortriptyline) combined with psychosocial support. This is the "backbone" of treatment. Anticonvulsants may be also efficacious (particularly if the pain has lancinating, sharp or stabbing components).
3. If the above steps are not efficacious clonidine and/or mexiletine can be added and may be helpful.
4. Effective management of side effects of the above medications will often determine the success of the treatment, by facilitating acceptance and compliance of a certain potentially useful drug.
5. Techniques, such as the SCS (for the spinal-cord patients) or thalamic stimulation may be tried in selected patients with the most refractory pain.

Postamputation Pain Syndromes

The term includes chronic pain conditions that develop after limb amputations. Stump pain develops at the remaining stump of the amputated limb, and may or may not coexist with phantom pain. The latter is a painful sensation, which is felt in the absent part of the extremity.

Stump pain is frequently caused by a neuroma in the stump. This may produce a painful sensation elicited by careful palpation at the site of the stump. Other causes should also be sought, such as mechanical pressure from a nonproperly fitting prosthetic device, bone spurs, infection, etc. These should be treated appropriately. Sometimes surgical revision of the stump may be indicated to correct an underlying cause, such as to resect a neuroma.

Otherwise, nonspecific analgesic measures, such as medications (e.g., anticonvulsants, TCAs) or infiltrations with local anesthetics and/or steroids may be helpful.

Phantom pain usually occurs shortly after amputation, but may resolve spontaneously several months later. It should be distinguished from not-painful phantom sensations. It may also coexist with stump pain. Treatment includes pharmacotherapy (e.g., TCAs, anticonvulsants, calcitonin), trials of sympathetic blocks in case of the presence of causalgic characteristics, or, in intractable cases, SCS or dorsal root entry zone lesions.

REFERENCES

1. Koes BW, Scholten RJPM, Mens JMA, Bouter LM: Efficacy of epidural steroid injections for low-back pain and sciatica: a systematic review of randomized clinical trials. Pain 63:279–288, 1995.
2. Nelson DA: Dangers from intraspinal steroid injections. Arch Neurol 47:255, 1990.

SUGGESTED READING

Abram SE: Advances in chronic pain management since Gate Control. 1992 Bonica Lecture. Regional Anesthesia 18:66, 1993.

Abram SE: Pharmacology of pain control. In Brown DL (ed): Regional Anesthesia and Analgesia. Philadelphia, W.B. Saunders, 1996, p 671.

Abram SE, JD Haddox (eds): The pain clinic manual, 2nd ed. Philadelphia, Lippincott Williams & Wilkins, 2000.

Dickenson A: Spinal cord pharmacology of pain. Br J Anaesth 75:193, 1995.

Hogan Q, Abram SE: Diagnostic and prognostic neural blockade. In Cousins M, Bridenbaugh PO (eds): Neural Blockade in Clinical Anesthesia and Management of Pain. Philadelphia, Lippincott Williams & Wilkins, 1998, p 837.

Justins DM: Management strategies for chronic pain. Ann Rheum Dis. 55:588, 1996.

Kalso E, Tramer MR, Moore RA, McQuay HJ: Systemic local anaesthetic type drugs in chronic pain: a qualitative systematic review. Eur J Pain 2:3, 1998.

Kingrey WS: A critical review of controlled clinical trials for peripheral neuropathic pain and complex regional pain syndromes. Pain 73:123, 1997.

Koltzenburg M: The sympathetic nervous system and pain. In Dickenson A, Besson JM (eds): The Pharmacol-ogy of Pain. Berlin, Springer, 1997, p 61.

Krames ES: Mechanisms of action of spinal cord stimulation. In Waldman SD, Winnie AP (eds): Interventional Pain Management. Philadelphia, W.B. Saunders, 1996, p 407.

McQuay HJ. Carroll D, Jadad AR, et al: Anticonvulsant drugs for management of pain: a systematic review. BMJ 311:1047, 1995.

McQuay HJ, Moore RA: An Evidence-Based Resource for Pain Relief. Oxford, Oxford University Press, 1998.

McQuay HJ, Tramer M, Nye BA, et al: A systematic review of antidepressants in neuropathic pain. Pain 68:217, 1996.

Millan MJ: The induction of pain: an integrative review. Prog Neurobiol 57:1, 1999.

Moller AM, Smith AF, Pedersen T: Evidence-based medicine and the Cochrane collaboration in anaesthesia. Br J Anaesth 84:655, 2000.

Morley S, Eccleston C, Williams A: Systematic review and meta-analysis of randomized controlled trials of cognitive behavior therapy and behavior therapy for chronic pain in adults, excluding headache. Pain 80:1, 1999.

Onghena P, Van Houdenhove, B: Antidepressant-induced analgesia in chronic non-malignant pain: a meta-analysis of 39 placebo-controlled studies. Pain. 49:2051992.

Rang HP, Urban L: New molecules in analgesia. Br J Anaesth 75:145, 1995.

The Oxford Pain Internet Site. University of Oxford and the Nuffield Department of Anaesthetics, Oxford, UK. Available from: http://www.jr2.ox.ac.uk/bandolier/booth/painpag/index2.html. Accessed August 24, 2005.

Sandkuhler J: Neurobiology of spinal nociception: new concepts. Prog Brain Res 110:207, 1996.

Sorkin LS, Carlton SM: Spinal anatomy and pharmacology of afferent processing. In Yaksh TL, et al (eds): Anesthesia: Biologic Foundations. Philadelphia, Lippincott Williams & Wilkins, 1998, p 577.

Stucky CL, Gold MS, Zhang X: Mechanisms of Pain. PNAS 98:11845, 2001.

Xu XJ: Novel modulators in nociception. In Dickenson A, Besson JM (eds): The Pharmacology of Pain. Berlin, Springer, 1997, p 211.

Zhang WY, Li, Wan Po A: The effectiveness of topically applied capsaicin. A meta-analysis. Eur J Clin Pharmacol 46:517, 1994.

Back and Neck Pain

CARIDAD BRAVO-FERNANDEZ

INTRODUCTION

Next to the common cold, low back pain (LBP) is the most frequent complaint among those who seek medical advice. Neck pain is the next most common symptom. Back pain is experienced by as many as 80% of Americans. In 1994, the Agency for Health Care Policy and Research stated that "LBP problems affect virtually everyone at some time during their life" and that the problems "are the most common cause of disability."[1] LBP and neck pain pose a significant health impact. In addition to the healthcare costs involved, there is a heavy economic burden associated with the loss of days at work.

Although most practitioners believe that acute LBP episodes resolve within 1 month, there is a wide variation in the reported time course. Data from the Cochrane Library and the Danish Article Base shows that about 62% still experience some pain after 12 months and that 60% had experienced relapses at 6 months.[2] The percentage of relapses was higher in those with a prior history of LBP.

The lower lumbar area carries most of our body weight and is the most common site of LBP. The pain, which can arise from several tissue components, is associated with multiple mechanisms. Arriving at a prompt and accurate diagnosis is especially important in the case of fractures, malignancies, and other organic disease entities. Factors affecting LBP include:

- Age: greatest incidence between ages 30 and 50
- Height: > 6 feet tall
- Weight: obesity in the highest 1/4 of weight range
- Gender: females have more generalized back pain; males radiculopathy
- Tobacco use: slight increase in risk—1.5%
- Fitness: 9 times more likely in those less fit
- Occupation: risk with repetitive improper movement, vibration, heavy lifting
- Psychological: increased risk with job dissatisfaction

CLASSIFICATION

Neck and back pain can be classified, similar to other disease processes, into degenerative, inflammatory, metabolic, traumatic, infectious, neoplastic, and congenital. Often more than one etiology can be found to contribute to the generation of pain. The origin of the pain can be classified anatomically. The pain generator can be the bony structures with its joints and foramina, ligaments, discs, nerves, and muscles. Radiology findings are often used to make an anatomic diagnosis.

Pain can also be classified by the presenting symptom and its dermatomal distribution. Finally, back and neck pain can be classified according to its duration. Acute pain is described as lasting less than 3 months. Chronic pain is associated with symptoms that last more than 3 to 6 months.

ANATOMY

The spine is made of bony elements, joints, intervertebral discs, ligaments, muscles, and nerves. Pain can arise from any of these components in the spine. These components can cause neck and/or back pain.

SPINE PAIN

Most spine structures have been reported as sources of pain.[3] The International Association for the Study of Pain (IASP) defines spine pain by its location—cervical spine pain, thoracic spine pain, lumbar spine pain, and sacral spine pain.

Neck pain arises anywhere between the occiput and the first thoracic vertebral spinous process. The cervical nerves arise above their respective vertebrae. C1 has no cutaneous branches and C2 follows the sensory distribution of the occipital nerve.

Lumbar spine pain can arise anywhere from the T12 spinous process to the top of the sacrum. The lumbar nerves arise below the transverse process of each vertebra.

Sacral spine pain can arise from the "tip of the first sacral process to the sacrococcygeal joints." Laterally, it can include the superior and inferior iliac spines.

DEFINITIONS OF PAIN

Definitions of pain are important. *Somatic pain* is associated with impairment or altered function of skeletal joint and/or muscle structures with their related neural elements. It is usually described as aching and constant.

Axial pain is felt in or near the midline of the neck or back. It can be midline or paramedian or both.

Referred pain is perceived as occurring in an area of the body that is different from the location of the actual source of pain. A common example is pain arising from discs, ligaments, or joints of the spine that is referred to the extremities.

Radicular pain is associated with injury or irritation of a nerve root. Pain associated with radiculopathy may arise from mechanical stimulation of the nerve root, spontaneous activity arising from the injured root, or from denervation with distortion of central sensory processing. Radicular pain is perceived mainly in an extremity, follows a dermatomal pattern, and is usually "shooting" in quality. It is commonly, but not always, associated with motor, sensory, or reflex changes.

CAUSES OF NECK AND BACK PAIN

Arthritis, a systemic disease, results in inflammation of the joints. The pain is worsened by immobility. In the spine inflammation of the facet joints causes pain that worsens with lumbar and cervical extension and rotation. Osteoarthritis leads to bony spur formation from wear-and-tear with degeneration of the articular cartilage. Compression of the nerves as well as bone rubbing on bone leads to pain. "Facet syndrome" is a term applied to osteoarthritis that is caused by aging, injury, and overload of the facet joints. This can often be related to degeneration of the disc leading to joint problems (Box 13-1).

Spinal stenosis is a narrowing of the spinal canal. This narrowing can be segmental (a specific spine area) or widespread. Some individuals have a congenitally narrowed spinal canal. This can become worse where bony spurs, degenerated discs, or thickened ligamenta flava result in further narrowing. Spinal stenosis can be present in both younger (congenital) and older (degenerative) persons. As these structures begin to press on the spinal cord and/or nerve roots, symptoms of numbness, tingling, weakness, and pain can become evident. When the cervical area is involved, the symptoms can affect both arms and legs. Lumbar spinal stenosis often produces symptoms of neural claudication, consisting of leg pain, weakness, and numbness brought on by ambulation and relieved by rest. Symptoms are less severe when the patient leans forward using a walker or shopping cart.

Damaged or degenerated discs can cause discogenic pain. The outer one-third of the annulus fibrosis contains sensory innervation, and degeneration or tears in the annulus can produce pain. The pain may be localized to the lumbar area or referred to the buttock or lower extremities. Discogenic pain is aggravated when movement places stress on the disc. As we age, discs degenerate with loss of water content and its ability to absorb "shock." Tears occur in the annulus that can heal with

---

Box 13-1 Common Causes of Low Back and Neck Pain

Discogenic
Radiculopathy
Facet arthropathy
Sacroiliac arthropathy
Spondylolysis
Myofascial

scarring that can weaken the disc. With repeated tears and scars, the disc height decreases, shifting weight bearing to the facet joints, which leads to facet degeneration. Discography may help identify a specific disc as a pain generator.

Bulging discs are common and can be found as an "abnormality" on MRI. Disc bulging is related to degenerative changes in the annulus, particularly radial tears producing separation of layers of the annulus. Bulging discs may be associated with spinal stenosis, radicular pain, or discogenic pain.

A herniated disc is a displacement of the nucleus pulposus through the annulus. The extruded material can enter the spinal canal or the neural foramen. Herniated discs are most common in the lumbar spine because of the higher compressive forces there. Herniated discs are least common in the thoracic area. Disc herniation can produce mechanical compression of the spinal cord or nerve roots, causing pain and sensory loss in a dermatomal distribution as well as segmental weakness. The proteoglycans contained in the nucleus are extremely tissue irritating and can produce a chemical radiculitis. It is often possible to determine the nerve involved by the anatomic distribution of signs and symptoms. The term often used when the lower lumbar or sacral dermatomes are involved is sciatica. When the problem starts in the neck, the pain is perceived along the arm and hand. In either case, the physician should check for loss of sensation, strength, and deep tendon reflexes. When the entire spinal cord is involved, a myelopathy can affect extremities bilaterally. In the case of a cervical myelopathy, the symptoms can present in both upper and lower extremities as well as involved bowel and/or bladder symptoms.

Facet arthropathy develops in the synovial joints between vertebrae. The synovial fluid lubricates the joints and fills the joint capsule within the ligaments. These joints allow movement between vertebrae. As the discs degenerate with aging and desiccation, the relationship at these joints is altered. The degenerative changes of osteoarthritis can also cause pain. These changes in the lumbar area cause pain in the low back, often radiating into the buttocks and thighs. Lumbar facet pain is worsened by extension and rotation that puts pressure on the joints. In the neck area, facet pain is often referred to the shoulder and proximal upper extremity. There is often associated paraspinous tenderness with pain that radiates from the point of compression (Box 13-2).

Sacroiliac arthropathy results from inflammation or degeneration of the sacroiliac joint. Inflammation of the joint is common in psoriatic arthritis and ankylosing spondylitis. Degenerative arthritis of the joint is a common source of LBP. Sacroiliac pain is usually felt in the sacral region and often radiates to the buttock, thigh, or calf.

Box 13-2 Lumbar Facet Arthropathy

Signs and symptoms
    Axial LBP (with or without referred leg pain)
    Aggravation of pain with back extension
    Tenderness over spine, paravertebral muscles
Imaging studies
    Plain radiographs with oblique views
    CT scan
    MRI
    Bone scan with SPECT (tomography)
Facet injections
    Local anesthetic—diagnostic
    "Depo" corticosteroid—therapeutic
Medial branch blocks
    Local anesthetic—diagnostic/prognostic
    Radiofrequency lesion—therapeutic

In addition to the structures mentioned, muscles along the spine can be a source of pain. Muscles do help to support the spine at all levels. In the cervical area there are the semispinalis capitis, longissimus capitis, splenius capitis, obliques, scalenes, and the sternocleidomastoid. The lumbar area has the erector spinae, the multifidus, quadratus lumborum, psoas major, and rectus abdominus. These muscles allow us a variety of postures and flexibility of movement. However, when strained or sprained, they can be significant pain generators.

Myofascial pain is common and can be caused by overuse, improper posture, trauma, or sprains. The paraspinous muscles provide support and mobility to the spine. When the muscles are injured, they can produce chronic pain. Myofascial pain often occurs in conjunction with radiculopathy, facet arthropathy, or discogenic pain. On physical exam, trigger points can be found in tight muscle bands that cause characteristic radiating pain on palpation.

DIAGNOSIS

Diagnosis for neck or lower back pain can only be made after a history of the patient's complaint. Some of the information needed regarding the pain complaint:

- Time of onset
- Related trauma
- Location, intensity, and quality of the pain
- Radiation pattern
- Associated neurologic changes
- Factors that worsen or improve the pain
- Sleep-pattern alterations
- Bowel or bladder problems
- Previous surgery
- Treatments and results

PHYSICAL EXAMINATION

A thorough physical examination is necessary to help determine the source of the neck or back pain. The exam can be focused on the affected area—neck, shoulders, arms, low back, legs. The exam needs to include:

- **Gait.** Gait should be observed from anterior, posterior, and lateral views. An antalgic gait indicates increased pain with weight-bearing on the affected side. Patients with spinal stenosis are more comfortable leaning forward on a walker or shopping cart. A lateral pelvic tilt (Trendelenburg sign) may indicate weakness of the gluteus medius.
- **Balance and coordination.** The patient should be able to balance on one foot with the eyes closed for 15 seconds.
- **Range of motion and special tests—low back.** Check flexion, extension, lateral bending, and rotation. Limitation of low-back flexion because of pain may indicate disc herniation with either discogenic pain or radiculopathy. Pain on extension is more likely to indicate facet arthropathy. Shober's test allows for differentiation between hip and spine flexion. Marks are made on the midline of the spine 10 cm above and 5 cm below the level of the posterior superior iliac spines. Normally, elongation of the distance between the marks is at least 5 cm. Extension should shorten the distance by 2 cm.
  - Straight-leg raising (SLR) tests for low lumbar or sacral nerve root irritation. Significant radiculopathy often produces pain with less than 30-degree hip flexion. Radicular pain is aggravated by ankle dorsiflexion during the SLR maneuver (Gower's sign). Pain in the opposite leg during the SLR maneuver almost always indicates disc herniation. Lasègue's sign, also indicative of radiculopathy, involves flexing the hip and knee to 90 degrees in the supine position then slowly extending the knee. A variation of the maneuver involves knee extension with the patient seated. If the patient can extend the knee completely while sitting upright, the sciatic stretch sign is negative. If this test is negative but SLR is positive, one might suspect malingering or factitious disease.
  - FABER test (flexion, abduction, external rotation) also known as Patrick's test, involves flexing the knee and placing the heel on the opposite knee, then lowering the femur toward the table. Groin pain may indicate hip joint pathology, while sacral pain indicates sacroiliac joint pathology.
  - Leg-length discrepancies can cause or aggravate back pain. Measure the distance from the anterior superior iliac spine to the lateral malleolus on each side.

- Axial loading of the skull or rotation of the shoulders that produces LBP are considered signs of "non-organic" pain.
- **Range of motion and special tests—neck.** Check flexion, extension, lateral bending, and rotation. Axial compression on the vertex with the head tilted toward the affected side will often exacerbate the pain of cervical radiculopathy (Spurling's test). Distraction, or the application of upward pressure to the chin and occiput, may relieve radicular pain but may aggravate muscle pain. With both tests, pressure is gradually applied and is held for 30 seconds.
- **Tenderness.** Tenderness is elicited over common trigger points (scalene muscles, trapezius, rhomboids, and levator scapulae for neck and upper back pain, gluteus medius, piriformis, paravertebral muscles, and tensor fascia lata for LBP). Palpation of the shoulder, spinous processes, occiput, sacroiliac joint, hip joints, and trochanteric bursa should be done routinely. Overreaction to mild to moderate palpation, especially if accompanied by exaggerated vocalization or grimacing, may be indicative of "non-organic" pain.
- **Motor.** Test for all major upper and lower extremity muscle groups. If the patient can walk on his toes and heels, then L5 and S1 motor function is largely intact. Give-away weakness (sudden release of motor activity) indicates functional or nonorganic sources of pain. Another such sign is an abnormal Hoover test. The examiner places both hands under the supine patient's heels and asks the patient to perform a straight leg raise maneuver. Failure to press down on the opposite heel indicates malingering. Marked weakness that is inconsistent with other observations is another sign of malingering or factitious disease. An example would be marked weakness of plantar flexion in the presence of normal Achilles tendon reflexes or extreme quadriceps weakness in a patient who can stand without assistance.

  Test biceps, triceps, and brachioradialis reflexes in the upper extremity and Achilles and patellar reflexes for the lower extremity.
- **Sensory.** Test for touch, cold, two point discrimination, vibration, and proprioception. Look also for tactile and cold allodynia. Nondermatomal sensory changes may indicate nonorganic symptoms, but is sometimes seen in complex regional pain syndrome and other types of neuropathy (Box 13-3).

DIAGNOSTIC TESTS

Tests that can be useful diagnostically include plain radiographs, MRI scans, CAT scans, myelography, including CT myelograms, bone scans, electromyograms, and

Box 13-3 Physical Signs of Lumbosacral Radiculopathy

Affected Nerve Root	Sensory Loss	Weakness	Diminished Reflex
L-4	Low anterior thigh	Knee extension	Patellar
L-5	Lateral calf, dorsum foot Web space 1st, 2nd toe	Foot dorsiflexion	Tibialis posterior (not always present normally)
S-1	Posterior calf, lateral foot, heel	Foot plantar flexion	Achilles

discograms. Blood tests can be used to look for infection, arthritis, metabolic diseases, and certain cancers.

Plain radiographs can show loss of disc height, degenerative changes in facet and sacroiliac joints, spondylolysis (pars fracture), spondylolisthesis (anterior displacement of the vertebral body), scoliosis and kyphosis, and vertebral compression fractures. They can also demonstrate congenital and developmental abnormalities such as transitional vertebrae and spina bifida occulta, and Scheuermann's disease. Occasionally they will reveal malignant disease, metabolic disease, or infection. Flexion and extension views can help determine whether instability is present.

CT scans provide excellent imaging of bony structures of the spine. They are particularly helpful for demonstrating facet and sacroiliac degeneration and spinal stenosis. They can also demonstrate some soft-tissue abnormalities such as disc herniation.

MRI scans provide much better imaging of soft tissues than CT scans. Since they also demonstrate bony changes reasonably well, they have largely replaced CT scans for spine imaging. CT is mainly used when MRI is contraindicated by the presence of metallic implants. MRI is very sensitive in detecting degenerative disc changes. It is important to understand that the large majority of asymptomatic individuals over 60 and a substantial minority of younger patients exhibit MRI abnormalities. One cannot determine whether a particular MRI abnormality is painful. Findings are only helpful if there is a good correlation with symptoms. Even then there is no guarantee that the lesion demonstrated is the pain generator. MRIs are very effective at demonstrating infection, bony metastases, and vertebral fracture. They can also provide visualization of the spinal cord, nerve roots, epidural fat, and paravertebral soft tissues.

It must be noted that many, if not most, degenerative changes seen on spine imaging studies are painless. Most people who are over 50 years old as well as many people who are younger than 50, will have demonstrable degeneration of intervertebral discs, and facet joints. The great majority of these individuals are asymptomatic. Often the radiographic changes seen in symptomatic patients do not correlate to their complaints of pain. One must be cautious, therefore, in assuming that a radiographic abnormality is the explanation of a patient's pain.

Bone scans demonstrate increased uptake wherever there is osteoblastic activity, such as erosion through joint cartilage, bony fracture, or bone infection or tumor. Tomographic or single photon emission computed tomography (SPECT) bone scans can more accurately localize the site of increased bone turnover.

Electrodiagnostic testing, which includes electromyography and nerve-conduction studies, can demonstrate nerve pathology and differentiate between peripheral nerve and nerve root involvement as well as demonstrating upper motor neuron pathology, such as myelopathy. They can also demonstrate whether a neurologic abnormality is acute or long-standing.

Discography can reveal anatomic defects, such as annular tears during radiographic dye injection. Definition of these defects is most accurate when the technique is combined with CT scan. If mild pressurization of the disc during injection reproduces the patient's pain, this provides evidence that the injected disc is a source of clinical pain. This evidence is particularly convincing if similar injection of adjacent discs are relatively painless.

TREATMENT

Many treatment options are available. Choosing one depends on the underlying problem. Most back and neck pain problems do not need surgical intervention. The goal of treatment is to reduce pain, to avoid further degeneration or injury, and to return to activity. Rest, bedrest in particular, for more than 2 or 3 days can worsen pain and weaken muscles. A return to activity, even with some pain, is beneficial.

Physical Therapy

Physical therapy teaches patients to decrease stress on the neck and back while retaining function. It should be begun very early in the course of acute back and neck pain. No more than 2 to 3 days of bedrest should be prescribed after an injury, after which early mobilization should be initiated in order to maintain strength and flexibility. Loss of muscle strength, tone, and range of motion, or deconditioning, is a common cause of long-term disability.

Physical therapy can include many different types of activities. Stretching and strengthening are beneficial as well as an essential part of the treatment for myofascial pain disorders. Pool therapy (aquatic exercises) is particularly helpful or low-back problems, since this type of activity decreases pressure on the lumbar spine during exercise. Posture training is important in avoiding positions that contribute to back and neck pain. Traction can also unload disc compression and relieve pain. Traction and other modalities such as heat, ultrasound, ice, and transcutaneous electrical stimulation provide temporary relief, which is helpful insofar as it allows the patient to participate in therapeutic exercises.

For patients with radiculopathy associated with disc herniation, extension exercises, such as the McKenzie exercises, can reduce intradiscal pressure and decrease symptoms of nerve root irritation. Centralization of pain (i.e., relief of distal extremity symptoms) is a good prognostic indicator. Pain may increase in some patients with a large central disc protrusion or foraminal stenosis, and the exercises should be discontinued. Flexion exercises are helpful for patients with pain from facet arthropathy. Increased abdominal muscle tone tends to reduce stress on the facet joints. These exercises must be combined with aggressive weight-loss programs in obese patients, particularly those with significant abdominal fat deposition.

Lumbar corsets may be helpful early in the course of rehabilitation to control available range of motion. The patient should be weaned from their use early in order to prevent dependence on them and to reduce the risk of loss of range of motion and strength of supporting muscles.

Education is an important aspect of the rehabilitative process. Patients must be taught the importance of maintenance of strength and flexibility. They should also understand that a certain amount of pain is normal during the rehabilitation process and that pain does not equate with harm to the back or neck. This is particularly true for patients with long-standing pain whose disability and pain are often related to deconditioning and cognitive-behavioral changes rather than to spine pathology.

Medications

Medications can be used in the management of neck and/or LBP. These can be as easily available as over-the-counter (OTC) anti-inflammatories like aspirin, acetaminophen, ibuprofen, or naproxen. Other NSAIDs are available by prescription in higher potency formulations than the OTC medications. Cyclooxygenase 2 inhibitors and nonacetylated salicylates, such as choline magne-

sium trisalicylate, have fewer upper GI-tract and anti-platelet side effects.

Neuropathic pain may respond well to anti-convulsant medications such as gabapentin, oxcarbazepine, zonisamide, and topiramate. Many of the new drugs in this class have a wide margin of safety and appear to be at least as effective as older drugs such as carbamazepine, valproic acid, and phenytoin. Tricyclic antidepressants are efficacious in many types of neuropathic pain and may help with pain-related sleep deprivation. Weight gain is a common side effect and may be problematic in obese patients. If significant depression is present, treatment with serotonin selective reuptake inhibitor type antidepressants may be appropriate.

For muscle spasms, muscle relaxants can be helpful, but usually long-term use is not recommended. Baclofen, cyclobenzaprine, methocarbamol, metaxalone, and tizanidine are commonly used for muscle spasm associated with back or neck injury. Carisoprodol and diazepam are somewhat more sedating and more habituating and should not be used as first-line drugs.

During the early phases of acute back pain opioid analgesics are appropriate. The goal for opioid use should be improvement in function and increase in physical activity. Pain relief in conjunction with continued inactivity is unacceptable, and continued use of analgesics should be contingent on continued progress with rehabilitation. Side effects of opiates include sedation, constipation, nausea, sexual dysfunction, insomnia, and immunosuppression. A history of substance abuse is a relative contraindication.

Some patients with chronic pain may benefit from long-term analgesic use. Patients who experience substantial relief (i.e., major reduction in pain ratings) and continued improvement in function and physical activity without significant tolerance development may be candidates for long-term opioid use. On the other hand, patients who remain inactive, who require repeated dose escalation, and who experience only slight pain relief should not be maintained on these drugs. There is substantial evidence that long-term opioid use can produce sensitization of central pain projection systems and can contribute to disability in some individuals.

Smoking cessation should be encouraged in all patients who smoke. There is evidence that smoking interferes with disc nutrition and that smokers experience accelerated spine degeneration compared to non-smokers. There is also evidence that smokers are significantly less likely to respond to certain treatments such as spine surgery and epidural steroid injections.

Injections

Injections directed at the areas of the spine thought to be causing pain symptoms are used diagnostically and therapeutically. Diagnostic blocks are used to identify nerves and/or structures that are responsible for generating the pain sensation. Therapeutic injections are thought to provide relief by blocking pathological reflex activity, reducing central sensitization, stabilizing nerve membranes, and reducing inflammation.

Most injections utilize local anesthetics and/or steroids. Diagnostic blocks are done with local anesthetics alone. The local anesthetics most frequently used are lidocaine 1% to 2% and bupivacaine 0.25% to 0.5%. Lidocaine has a more rapid onset and shorter duration of effect. The steroid medications most often used are methylprednisolone acetate and triamcinolone diacetate, both of which are long-acting "depo" steroids. Generally, the maximum dose of methylprednisolone is 80 mg, and the maximum of triamcinolone is 50 mg. Combinations of local anesthetics and steroids provide rapid pain reduction followed by prolonged anti-inflammatory effects.

Epidural Steroid Injections

Epidural steroid injections are used in the cervical and/or lumbar spine. The block is used to reduce nerve root inflammation caused by mechanical compression or chemical irritation. It is used mainly for the relief of symptoms of nerve root irritation and is relatively ineffective for axial LBP. Efficacy is highest among patients whose pain is of relatively recent onset (i.e., less than 1 year). Success is lower among patients who have undergone previous back surgery, patients who are unemployed because of their back pain, and patients who smoke. Patients with spinal stenosis who experience symptoms of neural claudication are relatively unlikely to experience lasting benefit from epidural steroids. In general, conservative management of symptoms of lower extremity pain, weakness, and sensory changes brought on by walking is often ineffective, and surgical management may be required. Unfortunately, most patients with these symptoms are elderly and may not be good surgical candidates.

Prior to the initial injection, the patient should undergo a careful examination, documenting any preexisting neurological dysfunction, the presence of sciatic stretch signs (positive straight leg raising), areas of tenderness, and range of motion of the spine. The injection is generally performed as close as possible to the affected nerve root. However, cervical epidural injections are usually performed at C6-7 or C7-T1 because of the technical difficulty of introducing an epidural needle at higher interspaces. While many of these injections are done without fluoroscopic control, many practitioners are using fluoroscopy, particularly in patients who have had previous surgery or who have severe degenerative changes. Injection of non-ionic radio-opaque dye provides documentation of spread to the pathological neural structures.

Epidural injections are usually given at 2- to 4-week intervals in order to evaluate the response to each injection. Further epidural injections are given if there is a positive response. After a series of three injections, a waiting period of 6 months is usually allowed to pass before repeating the injections to avoid complications of steroids—immune suppression, fluid retention, altered glucose metabolism, cataract formation, stomach ulceration, osteoporosis, aseptic necrosis of major joints, etc. (Box 13-4).

Several approaches to the epidural space are used. The simplest technique is to use a standard translaminar approach without fluoroscopy. A loss of resistance technique using air or saline is the most common technique. A hanging drop technique can be used for cervical epidurals performed in the sitting position, but pathological changes related to the patient's condition may change the normal negative pressure.

If conditions that predispose to technical difficulty with the procedure are present, such as obesity, severe degenerative changes, previous surgery or scoliosis, it may be preferable to perform the procedure with fluoroscopic

---

Box 13-4   Epidural Steroid Injections

Indication: pain associated with radiculopathy
Steroid preparations
    Triamcinolone Diacetate 50 mg
    Methylprednisolone Acetate 80 mg
Injection site: close to level of pathology
    Translaminar
    Caudal
    Transforaminal
Frequency of injection
    Up to 3 injections over 6 weeks
    Repeat only if partial improvement from previous
      block
Contraindications
    Coagulopathy
    Active local or systemic infection
    History of adverse reaction to steroids
    Use with caution in diabetics
Adverse effects
    Adrenal suppression
    Cushingoid symptoms
    Sodium and fluid retention
    Hyperglycemia
    Immunosuppression
    Epidural abscess
    Accidental intrathecal injection
      Headache
      Aseptic meningitis
      Possibly arachnoiditis
      Septic meningitis

guidance. The use of fluoroscopy also allows for the identification of intravascular placement of the needle tip. The patient is positioned with the fluoroscope directed in a slight caudo-cranial direction. A slight paramedian approach is used since it is impossible for the patient to flex the spine and separate the spinous processes in the midline. The needle is directed toward the upper third of the interlaminar space, as close as possible to the midline. Documentation of the extent of spread of radiographic dye is done in the anteroposterior and lateral views prior to injection of local anesthetic and steroid. The lateral view is difficult to obtain with cervical epidurals because shoulders limit exposure of the lower cervical spine.

The caudal approach can be useful if a patient has so much degenerative disease that the translaminar approach is very difficult or impossible. If a patient has had prior surgery with lumbar scarring and with altered anatomy, a caudal can help deliver the medication solution to the lumbar space either through the needle or through a catheter. Placement of the needle into the caudal canal through the sacral hiatus is made much easier by the use of fluoroscopy in a lateral view. If radiographic dye does not spread to the affected nerve root(s) a radio-opaque catheter can be introduced into the caudal epidural space via a Tuohy or Hustead needle and advanced under direct vision to the desired area. If a spring-wire reinforced catheter is used, placing a slight bend in the catheter close to the tip allows the operator to direct or steer the tip more effectively. However, in previously operated patients scarring may prevent the catheter from reaching the desired location.

The transforaminal approach can be used if the affected nerve root can be identified definitely. In the lumbar spine, an oblique view is obtained, and the needle is advanced to a position just below the pedicle. For an S-1 approach, the needle is advanced into the S-1 foramen. For the cervical transforaminal injection, the patient is positioned supine with oblique positioning of the fluoroscope. The foramen is visualized and the needle tip is positioned at the posterior edge of the foramen, in contact with the superior articular process. It is particularly important to inject a small amount of dye to insure that there is no intravascular or intrathecal spread.

Drugs for Epidural Injection

A test dose of a local anesthetic will minimize the risk of intrathecal injection. Two to 3 ml of 1% lidocaine will usually produce a discernible sensory block within several minutes if injected intrathecally. If the test dose fails to produce a prompt response, it is assumed that the needle tip is not intrathecal, and the corticosteroid may then be injected. For translaminar injections, methylprednisolone acetate (Depo-Medrol) 80 mg or triamcinolone diacetate (Aristocort Intralesional) 50 mg is usually used. This may be injected alone or further diluted with preservative-free normal saline or additional local anesthetic.

For transforaminal injections, 1/4 to 1/2 of that dose is generally used. When the caudal approach is used, the full steroid dose is used, but is generally diluted in 5 to 15 ml normal saline or 0.5% lidocaine. Bupivacaine can be used instead of lidocaine, but recovery time is much greater if the block is more extensive than anticipated.

Radiographic dyes should be newer "nonionic" formulations that are safer for intrathecal administration. These agents, such as iopamidol (Isovue) and iohexol (Omnipaque), have lower osmolality than older agents. Severe allergic reactions are possible, however.

Risks

As with any intervention, there are risks in doing epidural injections. Perhaps the most common complication of any epidural is a dural puncture ("wet tap"). This occurs in 0.1% to 5% of all injections. A possible consequence is a postdural-puncture headache (positional HA) with nausea, vomiting, photophobia, and interference with activities of daily living. The HA usually resolves with bedrest, oral fluid loading, caffeine, and analgesics. If the HA persists, a "blood patch" can be done. Another even more infrequent risk is intravascular injection of local anesthetic containing solution. In addition to local anesthetic toxicity, there is a risk of embolization of particulate material if the "depo" steroid is injected intra-arterially. Injection into a radicular or vertebral artery can have devastating consequences.

Intrathecal injection can result in a "high spinal" requiring airway and circulatory management. There is some controversy regarding the possible neurotoxic effects of intrathecal injection of steroid suspensions. Benzyl alcohol (a component of multidose Depo-Medrol and Aristocort Intralesional preparations) have local anesthetic and neurotoxic properties. While epidural administration of these preparations has not been associated with neurological damage, there may be a potential for injury with intrathecal administration. Because of several case reports of adhesive arachnoiditis following multiple intrathecal injections of methylprednisolone acetate, there is some concern that this is a possible complication in patients with disc disease as well. While there is little evidence that arachnoiditis can result from a single intrathecal steroid injection, many physicians recommend abandoning the procedure for at least a week if a wet tap occurs. Aseptic meningitis has been reported after intrathecal steroid injection, but in all cases published so far, there were no lasting neurological consequences.

Since the corticosteroid preparations used for epidural injections contain particulate material, there is concern that injection into an artery can produce embolization and injury to tissues supplied by the artery. This is especially worrisome when performing cervical transforaminal injections, as embolization of a small radicular artery could produce spinal-cord infarction.

The use of fluoroscopy will minimize this risk. Nonionic radiographic dye injected during "live" fluoroscopy will demonstrate filling of blood vessels if the needle tip is intravascular.

Septic meningitis and epidural abscesses have been reported, most commonly in diabetic patients. Dural puncture most likely occurred in all septic meningitis cases.

Contraindications to epidural injections include patient refusal, anticoagulation, coagulopathy, sepsis, untreated tuberculosis, or localized infection near the injection site.

Other Injections

Facet injections are used to localize and to treat pain that is caused by degeneration and inflammation of the zygapophysial (facet) joint. The block can be done diagnostically using only local anesthetics. If pain relief is obtained, this confirms the joint as the pain generator. More prolonged pain relief can be obtained by injecting a small amount (about 1cc) of a steroid solution into the facet. The steroids help decrease the symptoms of joint arthritis.

Facet injections must be done using fluoroscopic guidance. In the lumbar region, an oblique view of the joint is obtained and the needle is directed toward the lower 1/3 of the joint, where the joint space is widest. Injection of 1/2 ml contrast will produce a facet arthrogram and will confirm injection into the joint capsule. Occasionally dye injection will reveal a synovial cyst, which can produce foraminal narrowing and radicular symptoms. Most practitioners do not use dye, as the total joint capacity is only 1 to 1.5 ml. Once the needle is in position, 20 mg methylprednisolone acetate or triamcinolone diacetate is injected along with 0.5 ml local anesthetic. Pain relief is sometimes very transient, lasting only the duration of the anesthetic. In some cases, however, pain relief may persist for 6 months or more.

Contraindications include patient refusal, infection over the site, and anticoagulation. Contrast should not be used in cases of previous allergic reactions. Complications are not common, but can include muscle spasms, infection, bleeding, and possible nerve irritation.

Medial branch nerve block involves local anesthetic blockade of the medial branch of the posterior primary division of each nerve root. The medial branch supplies sensory innervation of the facet joint. Each facet joint is supplied by fibers from the adjacent medial branch and from that of the level above. The block is done diagnostically to determine whether radiofrequency neurolysis will be effective. The nerve block, and the subsequent neurolytic procedure, is done at the upper medial edge of the transverse process. Denervation of the S-1 facet requires denervation at the upper medial border of the sacral ala and at the upper outer edge of the S-1 foramen.

Sacroiliac (SI) joint injections are done to diagnose and treat pain caused by degenerative or inflammatory conditions involving the SI joint. The joint consists of the superior, fibrous portion and the lower, cartilaginous portion. Injection of the cartilaginous portion of the joint is done under fluoroscopy. Once the posterior joint line is identified, a needle is placed in the lower portion of the joint, usually 1 to 2 centimeters cranial to the lowest end. Intraarticular placement can be confirmed using radiographic dye. This is followed by injection of 3 to 5 ml local anesthetic plus 20 to 40 mg methylprednisolone acetate or triamcinolone diacetate. Relief of pain helps to confirm the SI joint as a pain generator. As with facet arthropathy, pain relief lasting up to 6 months may occur. A technique for radiofrequency lesioning of the nerve supply to the joint has been described, but is less effective than techniques for facet denervation.

Trigger-point injections are used in the treatment of myofascial pain. This condition is associated with localized areas of tenderness located in tight muscle bands. These are generally found in typical muscle groups. The paraspinous muscles, levator scapulae, trapezius, rhomboids, and gluteals are commonly involved. The pain elicited from trigger points is frequently referred to distant sites, and can be confused with referred pain of spinal origin. The pain of trigger points can be relieved with injection of small amounts local anesthetic. Repeated injections combined with exercises that stretch the affected muscle groups may provide lasting improvement. When muscle pain is diffuse, as in fibromyalgia, injections of tender points are of little benefit.

There is insufficient data to determine which local anesthetic is most effective. Bupivacaine might not be the best choice, as it is more mycotoxic than other agents. There appears to be no benefit to injecting steroids in trigger points, and there may be some muscle degeneration as well as the well-known systemic effects associated with their use. In Oriental medicine tradition, dry needling of contracted muscle is used to release the tightness. At least one study has shown a high degree of correlation between acupuncture points and myofascial trigger points.[4]

REFERENCES

1. Yelin E: Cost of musculoskeletal diseases: impact of work disability and functional decline. J Rheumatol Suppl 68:8–11, 2003.

2. Hestbaek L, et al: Low back pain: what is the long-term course? A review of studies of general patient populations. Eur Spine J 12(2):149–165, 2003.

3. Bogduk N: Clinical Anatomy of the Lumbar Spine and Sacrum, 3rd ed. New York, Churchill-Livingstone, 1999, pp 187–188.

4. Chu J: The local mechanisms of acupuncture. Zhonghua Yi Xue Za Zhi (Taipei) 65(7):299–302, 2002.

SUGGESTED READING

Abram SE: The use of epidural steroid injections for the treatment of lumbar radiculopathy. Anesthesiology 91:1937-1941, 1999.

Abram SE, O'Connor TC: Complications associated with epidural steroid injections: a review. Regional Anesthesia 21:149-162, 1996.

Adams M, Bogduk N, Burton K, et al: The Biomechanics of Back Pain. Edinburgh, Churchill-Livingstone, 2002.

Bogduk N: The anatomical basis for spinal pain syndromes. J Manipulative Physiol Ther 18(9):603-5, 1995.

Frost H, et al: A fitness programme for patients with chronic LBP: 2-year follow-up of randomized controlled trial, Pain 75:273-279, 1998.

Harrison DE, et al: The sacroiliac joint: a review of anatomy and biomechanics with clinical implications. J Manipulative Physiol Ther 20(9):607-17, 1997.

Hopwood MB, Abram SE: Factors associated with failure of lumbar epidural steroids. Reg Anesth 18(4):238-43, 1993.

Karjalainen K, et al: Multidisciplinary biopsychosocial rehabilitation for neck and shoulder pain among working age adults: a systematic review within the framework of the Cochrane Collaboration Back Review Group. Spine 26(2):174-81, 2001.

Lehmann TR, et al: Predicting long-term disability in low-back injured workers presenting to a spine consultant. Spine 18(8):1103-12, 1993.

Rainville J, et al: LBP and cervical spine disorders. Orthop Clin North Am. 27(4):729-46, 1996.

Waddell G, et al: Clinical assessment and interpretation of abnormal illness behavior in LBP. Pain 39(1):41-53, 1989.

Complex Regional Pain Syndromes

STEPHEN E. ABRAM

INTRODUCTION

In order to define the Complex Regional Pain Syndromes, it is necessary to review the recent and current terminology. The previously accepted term reflex sympathetic dystrophy is now called Complex Regional Pain Syndrome type 1 (CRPS I) and the previously accepted term Causalgia is now called Complex Regional Pain Syndrome type 2 (CRPS II). One reason for the change in terminology is the fact that sympathetic nervous system contributions to these syndromes is not universal (i.e., some cases of CRPS I are not associated with sympathetically maintained pain).

CRPS I is a syndrome of extremity pain, usually burning in quality and involving the distal extremity, variably associated with sensory, motor, and autonomic nervous system dysfunction and with dystrophic changes involving skin, bone, and joints. It is most commonly initiated by trauma, often relatively minor, or surgery. CRPS II is a similar syndrome clinically, but by definition involves a major nerve trunk injury.

If it can be shown that increased sympathetic stimulation increases pain perception, or that a reduction in sympathetic nervous system activity decreases pain perception, then the patient with CRPS has sympathetically mediated pain. If a reduction in sympathetic activity fails to provide pain relief, then the patient has sympathetically independent pain.

EPIDEMIOLOGY

CRPS I usually follows a traumatic episode, the most common being wrist fractures and ankle injuries. Extremity surgery is a relatively common antecedent. Other inciting conditions include stroke, myocardial infarction, connective tissue diseases, limb immobilization, and malignancies. It is slightly more prevalent in women than men. The peak age distribution is around 50, although cases are described in children as well as in elderly patients. Psychological factors are obviously important in the development of symptoms in some patients. This is particularly true in cases involving children. A common scenario is the child who is a high achiever who is unable to meet parental expectation. The development of severe physical symptoms then excuses the child from participation in part of his or her demanding schedule.

CRPS II almost always involves injury by a high-velocity projectile. It is primarily a wartime injury, first described by Dr. Silas Weir Mitchell during the civil war. Unfortunately, with the increasing incidence of violence in civilian life, it is becoming more prevalent in community and university hospitals. The inciting injuries usually occur above the elbow or above the knee, with the brachial plexus and sciatic nerve being most commonly involved.

CLINICAL FEATURES

Pain

The pain of CRPS I and II is usually described as burning in quality, usually involving the distal portion of the extremity at minimum. However, other pain descriptors, such as deep aching, throbbing, or stabbing pain are common. Pain may follow a dermatomal or peripheral nerve distribution, but more often is seen in a stocking or glove-like pattern. Allodynia is a very common feature. Mechanical allodynia, manifested as pain on light touch, often is present in a non-dermatomal pattern. Pain on exposure to cool temperatures that are not ordinarily painful is often described. Burning distal pain and mechanical allodynia are typical of CRPS II (Box 14-1).

Hyperpathia can be a feature of either syndrome. This is the production of increasing intensity and spreading pain with repeated tactile stimulation. Tapping gently on a sensitive area typically produces this phenomenon. This is the clinical correlate to "wind-up," the production of increasing electrical responses of spinal-cord neurons to repetitive stimulation of nociceptive afferent fibers.

Autonomic Changes

CRPS I typically exhibits changes in skin color and skin temperature of the affected region. In CRPS I there may be erythema, particularly in the earliest stages of the syndrome, or, more typically, cyanosis and diminished skin temperature. The cyanosis is often patchy, as seen in patients in shock. Erythema is more typical of CRPS II. Edema is seen in most cases of both syndromes throughout their course. Both increased and decreased sweat-gland activity can be seen in CRPS I, while reduced or absent sweating is typical of CRPS II.

Motor Dysfunction

Patients with CRPS I may exhibit one or several of the following disorders of muscle: tremor, weakness, muscular incoordination, spasm, and dystonia. Dystonia in the

---

Box 14-1   CRPS I: Signs and Symptoms

These clinical findings are variable. Dystrophic changes occur later in the course of the syndrome.
Pain
    Burning in quality
    Distal extremity
Allodynia
    Mechanical
    Cold
Hyperpathia
Edema
Color changes
    Cyanosis
    Erythema
Temperature changes
    Cool
    Warm
Hyperhydrosis
Motor dysfunction
    Tremor
    Dystonia
Joint dysfunction
Dystrophic changes
    Glossy skin
    Bone demineralization
    Hair and nail growth changes

---

upper extremity is usually manifested as flexion of the fingers, or clenched fist position, while lower extremity dystonia is usually a fixed equinovarus position of the foot.

Dystrophic Changes

Several types of dystrophic changes are typical of CRPS I. These include smooth, glossy skin, changes in hair and nail growth, joint dysfunction, and osteopenia. The bone demineralization is typically most prominent in periarticular regions.

Progression and Spread of Symptoms

It has been suggested that there is a progression of symptoms, with autonomic changes presenting in the earliest stage, dystrophic changes presenting as an intermediate constellation of findings, and severe, presumably irreversible, atrophic findings seen late in the course of the illness. However, a cluster analysis has identified three subgroups of patients based on their signs and symptoms. There was no correlation between the type of symptoms seen and the duration of the condition.

Spread of symptoms to previously uninvolved areas is relatively common. Three types of spreads were identified in a retrospective study. Contiguous spread was seen in essentially all patients, with extension from distal to proximal parts of the extremity. Independent spread, the appearance of signs and symptoms in distant, non-contiguous sites was seen in about 70% of patients. Mirror-image spread, the appearance of symptoms in a similar pattern in the opposite limb, occurred in about 15% of patients.

Recurrence of CRPS I symptoms in the same or in another region occurs in about 5% to 10% of patients. These recurrences may happen months to years after the initial event and are usually preceded by another traumatic or surgical event. However, some occur without an apparent trigger.

DIAGNOSIS OF CRPS

Clinical

The diagnosis of CRPS I and II are made mainly on the basis of clinical signs and symptoms. The following are criteria for the diagnosis of CRPS I:
- The presence of an initiating noxious event or cause for immobilization.
- Continuing pain, disproportionate to the degree of injury, allodynia, or hyperalgesia.
- Evidence of edema, changes in blood flow, or abnormal sudomotor activity in the painful region.
- The absence of other condition that would otherwise account for the degree of pain and dysfunction.
- The diagnosis of CRPS II is made on similar criteria with the addition that the inciting cause involves nerve trunk injury.

Laboratory

It is important to rule out vascular conditions, particularly when vasomotor signs and symptoms are prominent. If peripheral pulses are weak or absent, flow studies are indicated. If neurological findings are prominent, electrodiagnostic testing may be indicated to determine whether there is an entrapment neuropathy or other peripheral nerve or nerve root pathology.

Plain or fine-detail radiography may reveal osteoporosis, particularly in periarticular regions, as early as 2 weeks after the onset of symptoms in CRPS I.

A three-phase bone scan may be abnormal in some cases, but is occasionally normal in patients with clearly defined clinical symptoms. In the two early phases, termed flow and gate pool (tissue uptake) phases, findings are dependent on changes in regional blood flow. There may be abnormally high uptake if regional vasodilation is prominent or low uptake if the affected area is vasoconstricted. In the third phase, there is often increased periarticular uptake in the affected limb.

Quantitative sweat testing has been used in a few centers to determine whether there is abnormally high or low sweat production in the affected areas. The quantitative sudomotor axon reflex test measures sweat output in response to iontophoresis of a cholinergic agonist. In both tests, output is measured against that of the unaffected limb.

The phentolamine test provides an indication of the role of the sympathetic nervous system in the production of pain in a given patient. Following adequate testing for a placebo response, an infusion, or multiple bolus injections of this α1-adrenergic antagonist is given intravenously. Relief of pain coincident with evidence of the onset of sympathetic blockade (decreased blood pressure, peripheral vasodilation, nasal congestion) indicates a sympathetically mediated component to the patient's pain. Unfortunately, there are no studies that indicate whether a positive response is predictive of specific therapies, such as sympathetic blocks, surgical sympathectomy, or oral adrenergic antagonists.

Diagnostic Nerve Blocks

The diagnostic role of nerve blocks is to determine whether or not pain is sympathetically mediated. Interpretation of the response to local anesthetic blockade of the sympathetic chain is not at all straightforward, and there are multiple possibilities for error.

For upper extremity CRPS, a so-called stellate ganglion block is employed. This is somewhat of a misnomer, as most techniques produce a block of the cervical sympathetic chain above the level of the stellate ganglion, and MRI studies have indicated that spread of anesthetic to the ganglion itself is unlikely. Local anesthetic is most commonly injected in front of the anterior tubercle of C-6 or the transverse process of C-7. If the drug is in the correct plane, a prompt Horner's syndrome (i.e., ptosis, meiosis, anhydrosis, and enophthalmos) is produced. However, in as many as one-third of cases, there is little or no evidence of sympathetic blockade in the affected limb. In a patient without anatomic compromise to the arterial system, the skin temperature of the palmar surface of the hand should increase to at least 34°C.

For lower extremity CRPS, the needle tip is positioned at the anterolateral surface of the L-2 vertebral body. A similar increase in temperature of the skin over the plantar surface of the foot indicates a complete block of sympathetics to the limb.

Interpretation of the response to sympathetic blocks is compounded by the fact that the incidence of placebo response may be 50% or higher in patients with acute or chronic pain. In addition, the placebo response may take as long as an hour to become manifest in some patients. It is helpful, therefore, to precede the local anesthetic block with a placebo procedure.

After injection of local anesthetic on the sympathetic chain, several assessments must be made. First, it is essential to do careful sensory testing before and after the block. Any decrease in sensory function after the block precludes the interpretation of sympathetically maintained pain. Next, the skin temperature of the blocked and contralateral limbs should be measured. An appropriate rise in skin temperature of the glabrous skin of the blocked extremity along with absent sensory blockade will help establish the diagnosis of sympathetically maintained pain. However, one can still not rule out the possibility that pain relief is associated with the systemic absorption of local anesthetics, which are sodium channel blockers.

Once the block is complete, the patient should keep a careful record of the duration of pain relief as well as the duration of the block. If the patient relates that pain relief lasted only 40 minutes but that the extremity remained warm and erythematous for 4 hours, then the role of sympathetics in the pathogenesis of that patient's pain is in doubt.

Differential Diagnosis

The most important condition to rule out in the differential diagnosis is vascular insufficiency. Peripheral pulses should be checked in all patients. If the pulse is weak or absent, Doppler flow studies are indicated. Other possible diagnoses in the differential include venous insufficiency, peripheral neuropathy, collagen-vascular diseases, and factitious disorders. Patients can voluntarily produce edema of the extremity by placing a tourniquet on the extremity prior to clinic visits. Self-induced trauma to the extremity can produce bruising that resembles the discoloration associated with CRPS. Self-induced symptoms are termed malingering if they are done with the intent of attaining financial compensation. Munchausen syndrome is a term used to describe patients who feign symptoms to gain medical attention.

PATHOPHYSIOLOGY

There is no clear consensus on the pathologic mechanisms of CRPS. An early explanation was that of a reflex increase in sympathetic tone producing vasoconstriction, increased sweating and, consequently, tissue ischemia. Clinical studies have not supported this theory. First, some of the most intense cases exhibit skin vasodilation. Second, microneurographic studies have failed to demonstrate abnormalities in sympathetic outflow in the affected limb. Third, venous catecholamine levels in the affected limb have not been shown to be different from those in the normal extremity. Lastly, some patients with CRPS fail to experience relief of pain with sympathetic blockade. There may, however, be abnormalities of autonomic regulation in some patients with CRPS. Ordinarily, sympathetic fibers to skin are under the control of hypothalamic centers, while sympathetic axons supplying muscle are controlled by medullary centers in the brain. The two types of sympathetic efferents respond differently to various stimuli, such as blood pressure changes, and have different resting discharge patterns. Following peripheral nerve injury in animals, the skin vasoconstrictor fibers appear to come under medullary control, as their discharge patterns shift such that they resemble those of the sympathetic fibers supplying muscle.

Following certain types of nerve injury in animals, there is a dramatic increase in the population and configuration of sympathetic efferents in the dorsal root ganglia (DRG). There is sprouting of sympathetic fibers and growth into the DRG producing basket-like structures surrounding certain cell bodies. While the character and purpose of these structures has not been elucidated, it seems apparent that they are associated with changes in the interactions between sympathetic nervous system and sensory functions.

Another possible consequence of nerve injury is the loss of myelin of Schwann cell sheaths that normally limit the spread of impulses from one axon to another (cross-talk). Ephaptic transmission is thus enabled, allowing sympathetic efferent traffic to activate nociceptors. Nociceptive axons thus activated transmit impulses orthodromically to the spinal cord, activating pain pathways and antidromically to the periphery, causing release of substance phosphorus (P) and other peripheral neurotransmitters that can activate or sensitize nerve endings and produce vasodilation or vasoconstriction and changes in capillary permeability.

Injured peripheral nerves have been shown to fire spontaneously, with ectopic impulses arising from either the injured nerve segment or from cell bodies in the dorsal root ganglion. This ectopic activity can be suppressed by drugs with sodium channel blocking properties or by high-frequency electrical stimulation. It is greatly enhanced by locally applied norepinephrine or by stimulation of the sympathetic chain.

Another theory proposes that nociceptive nerve endings become sensitized to the effects of norepinephrine (i.e., that norepinephrine can either activate or reduce the firing thresholds of these receptors). Despite considerable research, there is little evidence that this occurs. There is, however, evidence that increased sympathetic discharge can sensitize peripheral mechanoreceptors. Reduced firing thresholds and increased firing rates of mechanoreceptors combined with sensitization of wide dynamic range (WDR) neurons in the spinal-cord dorsal horn could explain the allodynia so prevalent in these syndromes.

There is considerable evidence that central sensitization occurs in CRPS. As mentioned previously, the symptom of hyperpathia correlates well with the phenomenon of wind-up seen in dorsal horn neurons in response to intense electrical stimulation. Repetitive activation of nociceptive afferent fibers produces sensitization of second order WDR neurons in the dorsal horn, principally through activation of N-methyl-D-aspartate (NMDA) receptors with subsequent calcium influx. Persistent sensitization gives rise to hyperalgesia (i.e., exaggerated responsiveness to painful stimuli, and allodynia–pain induced by normally nonpainful stimuli). Central sensitization may be further enhanced by the use of exogenous opioids. Persistent activation of opioid receptors is known to activate protein kinase C (PKC), which in turns enables activation of the NMDA receptor.

Sensitization of dorsal horn neurons occurs through mechanisms involving glial cells as well as neuronal cells. Activation of microglia and astrocytes by nerve injury, inflammation, nociceptor activation, and spinal immune activation (e.g., by HIV infection) causes increased production of proinflammatory cytokines, such as tumor necrosis factor (TNFα), interleukin 1 (IL-1), and IL-6. These substances in turn cause increased production and release of nitrous oxide, prostaglandins, excitatory amino acids, and substance P. These changes give rise to allodynia and hyperalgesia in animal models and to central sensitization typified by CRPS. Chronic administration of opioids to experimental animals can also cause glial activation, increased production of proinflammatory cytokines, and allodynia and hyperalgesia.

Repetitive nociceptor activation can lead to cellular injury as well. High levels of excitatory amino acids, such as glutamate and aspartate, released from central terminals of nociceptors, are capable of producing cell injury or death (excitotoxicity). Inhibitory interneurons, such as those that release the inhibitory neurotransmitter γ-aminobutyric acid (GABA) appear to be particularly susceptible to this type of injury. Loss of the tonic inhibitory effect of these cells may then produce more disinhibition of sensory systems.

TREATMENT

A multimodal approach is essential for successful treatment in most patients. A combination of physical rehabilitation, psychotherapy, patient education, medication management, and interventional pain management should be available to all patients who present with these conditions. For some patients, the clinical course is intense and rapid, with early development of severe pain, dystrophy, and disability. Those patients may require aggressive treatment with a wide range of treatment modalities. In the past, much of the emphasis of treatment was directed toward managing the autonomic dysfunction. Sympathetic nerve blocks, sympatholytic drugs, and sympathetic neu-

roablative techniques were often the principal treatment modalities. The failure of many patients to such directed therapies has led to the understanding that the sympathetic nervous system plays a variable role in the pathophysiology of these conditions; hence, the change from reflex sympathetic dystrophy to complex regional pain syndrome (Box 14-2).

Physiotherapy

Preservation and restoration of function is the primary role for physical rehabilitation therapies in CRPS. Several different approaches are needed. One goal is desensitization of the affected regions. Tactile allodynia is treated with very soft tactile stimulation that is gradually increased in intensity. Combined heat and cold stimulation, such as contrast baths, are used to desensitize cold allodynia. Another goal is restoration of function. Joint

---

Box 14-2   CRPS I

Treatment modalities
Physical therapy
   Range of motion
   Functional restoration
   Desensitization (mechanical, thermal)
   TENS
Psychotherapy
   Cognitive strategies
   Education
   Skin temperature biofeedback
   Behavior modification
Nerve blocks
   Sympathetic blocks
   Continuous regional blocks (epidural, femoral, brachial plexus)
   IV regional blocks
Medications
   Tricyclic antidepressants
   Anticonvulsants
   Sodium channel blockers
   Sympatholytics
   Bisphosphonates
   Corticosteroids
   Analgesics
      NSAIDs
      COX-2s
      Opioids
      Tramadol
   NMDA antagonists
Surgical (late, "last resort")
   Sympathectomy
   Spinal-cord stimulation
   Intrathecal drug administration

TENS, transcutaneous electrical nerve stimulation; NSAIDs, nonsteroidal anti-inflammatory drugs; COX-2, cyclooxygenase-2; NMDA; N-methyl-D-aspartate.

stiffness is treated with active and active-assisted range of motion exercises. Aggressive passive joint mobilization may result in aggravation of symptoms. Restoration of strength is accomplished using isotonic strengthening and stress-loading exercises. Edema control using exercise, position, and elastic garments is important as well. Maintenance and restoration of aerobic conditioning is critically important as well. Once it is decided that maximum benefit has been achieved, vocational and functional rehabilitation is begun.

A major concern during physiotherapy is that the activities and treatments required to achieve necessary goals will trigger increased pain, autonomic dysfunction, and dystrophic changes. It may be helpful, therefore, to initiate pain-relieving interventions prior to beginning therapy sessions. Transcutaneous electrical nerve stimulation (TENS) may be beneficial in this context. Sympathetic nerve blocks, trigger-point injections, and somatic blocks that provide temporary pain relief may be helpful as well.

Nerve Blocks

If sympathetic blocks provide temporary pain relief, they may be useful in providing a window of reduced pain that allows more effective physical therapy. In some instances, repeated blocks may produce progressive, lasting improvement in symptoms and may even bring about a complete recovery. Typically, patients will experience relief of pain for the duration of the local anesthetic. As the block wears off, pain returns, but often to a less severe level. If this is the case, blocks repeated every few days may produce gradual improvement. Blocks should be continued until no further progression in benefit is seen.

When a block is performed, the patient should be monitored for evidence of sympathetic blockade. If the sympathetic outflow to the limb is successfully interrupted, the skin temperature should rise to 34°C to 35°C. Skin temperature should be monitored on the plantar surface of the foot or toes or on the palmar surface of the hand or fingers. These areas have extensive sympathetic innervation. Horner's syndrome indicates blockade of sympathetic outflow to the face, but does not guarantee blockade of sympathetic efferent fibers to the arm and hand, many of which leave the sympathetic chain at the T1-3 level.

Cervicothoracic Sympathetic Block (Stellate Ganglion)

Blockade of sympathetics to the upper extremity is usually accomplished by blocking the sympathetic chain at the level of C-6 (Fig. 14-1). Using this technique, the term stellate ganglion block is a misnomer, as it is unlikely

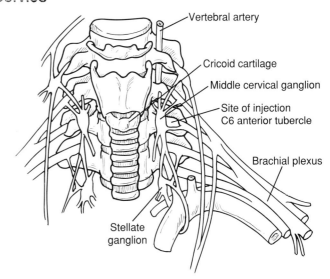

Figure 14-1   Site of injection for the C-6 paratracheal approach to the stellate ganglion block. Note the relationship of the C-6 anterior tubercle to the cricoid cartilage. The vertebral artery passes anterior to the C-7 transverse process and behind the C-6 anterior tubercle. (Redrawn from Benumof JL (ed): Clinical procedures in Anesthesia and Intensive Care. Philadelphia, JB Lippincott, 1992, p 791.)

that block of the ganglion itself, which lies caudal and posterior to the injection site, will occur. At the level of the cricoid cartilage, the sternocleidomastoid muscle and carotid artery are retracted laterally with the index and middle finger, and the tip of the anterior tubercle of C-6 is palpated. The needle is inserted straight downward onto the anterior tubercle, which usually lies 1 to 2 cm below the skin (Figs. 14-2 and 14-3). Careful aspiration is performed, and 10 ml of 1% lidocaine or its equivalent is injected using a slow, intermittent injection technique with frequent aspiration. If there is resistance to injection, the needle tip is probably within the longus colli muscle, and the needle should be withdrawn slightly. The patient may be asked to sit up briefly after the block to facilitate spread of the drug downward toward the stellate ganglion, which lies over the head of the first rib.

An alternative technique is to inject over the transverse process of C-7. This site is found by locating the sciatic notch and measuring a fingerbreadth lateral and a fingerbreadth cephalad. The needle is advanced straight downward (posteriorly) until contact is made with bone. The needle is withdrawn 1/2 cm and the local anesthetic is injected. The C-7 transverse process has a different configuration than those above, lacking an anterior and posterior tubercle, and the sympathetic chain lies superficial to its bony surface. This technique is more likely to result in needle malposition, as the target structure can not be palpated, as is the case with the C-6 anterior tubercle. Unlike the C-6 approach, the vertebral artery lies anterior to the target structure.

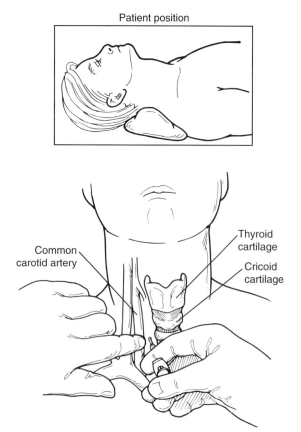

Patient position

Figure 14-2   Stellate ganglion block. (Reprinted from Rathmell JP: Sympathetic blocks. In Rathmell JP, Neal JM, Viscomicm (eds): Regional Anesthesia: The Requisites in Anesthesiology. Philadelphia, Mosby, 2004, p 132.)

Assessment of the result of the block should include the following:

1. Effect on pain level
2. Sensory exam of the extremity
   • Improvement in tactile and cold allodynia
   • Sensory function—blockade of sensory fibers
3. Evaluation of autonomic function
   • Horner's syndrome: ptosis, meiosis, anhydrosis
   • Skin temperature, color, skin moisture of the extremity
4. Functional assessment of the limb—range of motion, strength

The patient should be instructed to monitor the duration and extent of pain relief and the duration of autonomic changes. If the increased skin temperature lasts several hours but the pain returns in 30 minutes, then it is likely that the pain relief was associated with placebo effect, not sympathetic blockade.

Some patients (as many as 30% in some series) experience Horner's syndrome but do not show evidence of sympathetic denervation of the upper extremity following conventional cervical sympathetic blocks. When this occurs repeatedly, a CT-guided approach allows place-

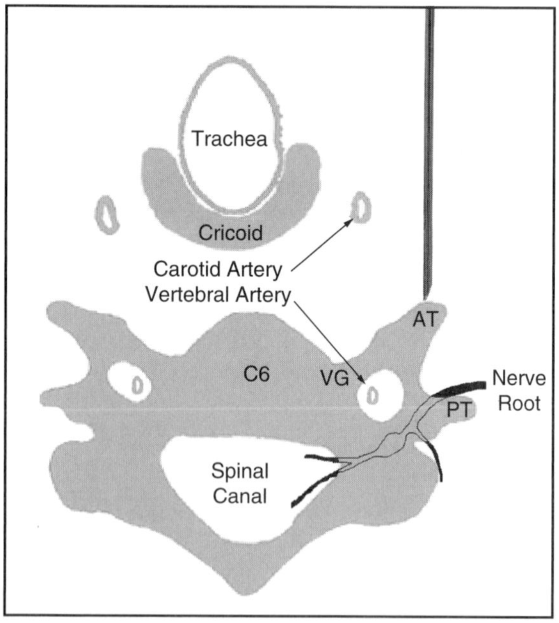

Figure 14-3   Chassaignac's tubercle and adjacent structures. Axial view of Chassaignac's tubercle (anterior tubercle, AT) and adjacent structures with needle shown in proper position. Note that angulation of the needle slightly medially will result in needle seating on the vertebral gutter (VG), an acceptable position that will lead to successful stellate ganglion block. However, more lateral angulation will result in needle placement on the posterior tubercle (PT) and will lead to somatic block of the exiting nerve root and adjacent brachial plexus. Note the close proximity of the carotid artery (shown in its usual anatomic location—the carotid artery is typically retracted laterally during stellate ganglion block). The vertebral artery lies within the transverse foramen in close proximity to the needle's final position. (Reprinted from Rathmell JP: Sympathetic blocks. In Rathmell JP, Neal JM, Viscomicm (eds): Regional Anesthesia: The Requisites in Anesthesiology. Philadelphia, Mosby, 2004, p 132.)

ment of a needle directly on the head of the first rib, the site of the stellate ganglion itself. Following initial imaging, a path for needle insertion can be delineated on the imaging screen that avoids contact with the lung and pleura. Using this technique, a profound block of sympathetics to the upper extremity can be accomplished with as little as 1 to 2 ml local anesthetic.

Side effects of the block are related to Horner's syndrome and blockade of adjacent structures, which may include recurrent laryngeal nerve block (hoarseness) and phrenic nerve block, which may cause subjective dyspnea but no serious respiratory dysfunction except in patients with severely compromised pulmonary function. To minimize risk of aspiration, patients should be warned not to eat or drink until hoarseness resolves.

Complications include intra-arterial injection of the vertebral or carotid arteries, which can produce loss of consciousness, seizures, and hypotension with as little as 2 ml of local anesthetic. If anesthetic is deposited deep to the prevertebral fascia (this will occur if the needle misses the anterior tubercle), a brachial plexus block will occur. This may also lead to intrathecal or epidural spread of drug, with resulting respiratory insufficiency, hypotension, and bradycardia. This is more likely with the C-7 approach. Pneumothorax is another possible complication and is also more likely using the C-7 technique. As with virtually any injection technique, vasovagal syncope may occur. Many physicians avoid bupivacaine and other long-acting anesthetics in order to minimize the consequences of intravascular or neuraxial injection.

Lumbar Sympathetic Block

The target for this procedure is the anterolateral surface of the L-2 vertebral body. The procedure is best done using fluoroscopy. A skin wheal is made about 8cm lateral to the midline at the level of the lower 1/3 of the L-2 vertebral body. The needle is advanced toward the lower end of the body to avoid the transverse process and the L-2 nerve root. After contact is made with the body, the needle is withdrawn and redirected at a slightly steeper angle. The best result is obtained if the needle can be felt to touch and slide past the anterolateral surface of the vertebral body. Once that sensation is felt, the needle is advanced a few millimeters. A lateral fluoroscopic view is obtained, which should show the needle tip at the anterior border of the body (Figs. 14-4 and 14-5). If radio-opaque dye is

injected, it should be seen spreading cephalad and caudad in a thin line along the front of the vertebral bodies. Injection of 5 ml of 1% lidocaine will produce prompt increase in skin temperature of the foot along with erythema and venodilation. Skin temperature of the plantar surface of the toes or heel should increase to 34°C to 35°C unless there is significant vascular compromise to the limb. Once there is documentation of sympathetic blockade and lack of somatic block, a long-acting local anesthetic, such as bupivacaine can be added. If no rise in skin temperature occurs, the needle should be repositioned and the injection repeated. There is some variation in the position of the sympathetic chain. One possible anomaly is occurrence of the chain within the psoas muscle.

Assessment of the result of the block is similar to that for the stellate ganglion block with the exception that there will be no Horner's. Evidence of sympathetic blockade and absence of somatic block confirms a successful procedure. If bupivacaine is used, the block should last 6 hours or more. This will be helpful in differentiating between sympathetically maintained pain and placebo response.

Side effects and complications are less common than with the stellate block. Orthostatic hypotension can occur because of the vasodilation of the leg, but is very uncommon unless bilateral blocks are performed. Positioning the needle into a neural foramen can produce epidural or subarachnoid spread of anesthetic. This can be avoided by observing the lateral fluoroscopic view prior to injection. Intravascular injection or the use of very large anesthetic volumes can produce systemic toxicity. Large doses may be injected if there have been multiple failed attempts.

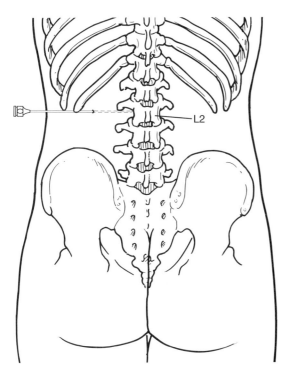

Figure 14-4   Final needle position for the lumbar sympathetic block. (Redrawn from Abram SE, Haddox JD (eds): The Pain Clinic Manual. Philadelphia, Lippincott Williams & Wilkins, 2000, p 401.)

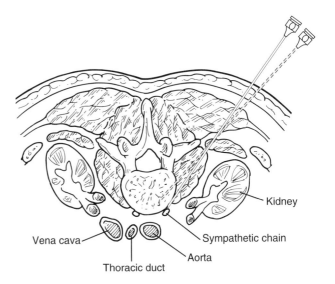

Figure 14-5   Initial and final needle position for the lumbar sympathetic block. (Redrawn from Abram SE, Haddox JD (eds): The Pain Clinic Manual. Philadelphia, Lippincott Williams & Wilkins, 2000, p 400.)

Epidural Block

For CRPS involving the lower extremity, continuous lumbar epidural analgesia may be helpful for refractory cases. Its role is mainly to provide temporary pain relief and sympathetic blockade to enable more aggressive physical rehabilitation efforts. Continuous infusions of bupivacaine or ropivacaine are generally used in an inpatient setting. For outpatients, a lumbar epidural catheter may be left in place and activated in the office or the physical therapy suite prior to therapy sessions. Treatment with epidural analgesia alone rarely produces lasting improvement. Cervical epidural anesthesia can be used in a similar manner for upper extremity CRPS, although risks are somewhat greater than for lumbar epidurals.

Peripheral Nerve Blocks

Blockade of nerve trunks to the affected area will produce both afferent and sympathetic efferent denervation. Continuous blockade of the brachial plexus is occasionally used to provide prolonged denervation. This procedure can be combined with intensive physical therapy for particularly resistant cases of upper extremity CRPS. The infraclavicular approach provides stable catheter placement with minimal risk of movement or displacement of the catheter tip. Infiltration of more distal peripheral nerves with a combination of corticosteroid and local anesthetic may be helpful if peripheral nerve injury is the trigger for the syndrome.

Intravenous Regional Block

IV regional injection of guanethidine was proposed as an alternative technique for providing temporary sympathetic block of the upper or lower limb. Glynn found that IV regional injection of 20 mg guanethidine but not saline provided pain relief and increased blood flow for up to 7 days in patients with reflex sympathetic dystrophy or Raynaud's disease. A subsequent randomized trial failed to show substantial benefit, and the injectable form of the drug is no longer available in the United States. Bretylium in doses of 1 to 3 mg/kg have been used instead, but no controlled trials have been published. IV regional bretylium is not particularly helpful in patients who have failed to respond to local anesthetic sympathetic blocks.

Psychotherapy

There has been a perception in the past that these syndromes were associated with more profound psychopathology than other chronic pain syndromes or that certain personality traits may predispose certain individuals to their development. The phrase "typical RSD personality" has been frequently used by physicians and psychologists. Several studies that compared psychological test results of patients with CRPS to those of patients with other chronic pain conditions have failed to demonstrate any differences. As with other painful conditions, the basic principles of cognitive-behavioral pain management are extremely important in managing CRPS. Stress reduction can lead to restoration of descending control mechanisms and improvement in central sensitization. Biofeedback techniques and relaxation training can produce dramatic reductions in sympathetic tone. The psychologist can play an important educational role, teaching patients the importance of their own rehabilitative efforts rather than relying on healthcare providers to provide them with a cure.

Pediatric patients who develop CRPS I may be particularly susceptible to psychopathologic mechanisms for their disease. A typical scenario is a child whose daily life is filled with stressors, such as marital discord between parents or pressures to achieve in sports or academics. Counseling and psychotherapy involving the patient and the parents coupled with an intensive rehabilitation and physical therapy program produce dramatic results for many children and adolescents.

Medications

Patients with documented sympathetically maintained pain may benefit from medications that block α-1 adrenergic receptors or that reduce overall sympathetic outflow. Phentolamine has been used intravenously as a measure of the importance of sympathetic tone on maintenance of symptoms. Patients who obtain relief from a phentolamine infusion may be more likely to benefit from pharmacologic reductions in sympathetic tone, although studies documenting the prognostic value of the technique are lacking. Oral adrenergic blockers such as phenoxybenzamine, prazosin, and terazosin have been used with variable results, and there have been no controlled trials of their efficacy. Similarly, both oral and transdermal clonidine have been reported to relieve pain and reduce associated symptoms in case reports but not in controlled studies. In the 1980s reports on the benefits of IV regional injection of guanethidine led to fairly widespread use of the technique. When injectable guanethidine was no longer available in the United States, bretylium was substituted by many practitioners. More recent controlled trials of these techniques have failed to show any lasting benefit.

Tricyclic antidepressants (TCAs) are of significant benefit for some patients. They may restore improved sleep patterns and reduce pain and allodynia. The drug is titrated up to a dose that improves sleep without causing daytime sedation. Pain relief generally begins 2 or more weeks after establishing therapeutic drug levels. Weight gain, cardiac arrhythmias, and anticholinergic side effects may limit their utility in some patients. Amitriptyline and doxepin are the most sedating drugs in this class and have considerable anticholinergic effects. Nortriptyline is less sedating, and desipramine is the least sedating.

Anticonvulsants

Gabapentin has been shown to be effective in several types of neuropathic pain, and there are several reports of benefit for patients with CRPS. Doses as high as 4800 mg/day may be needed for maximum effect. There are now many anticonvulsants that have been used successfully in neuropathic pain states. Since the mechanism of action differs considerably among drugs, it is reasonable to try several different agents if one has failed. Lamotrigine, topiramate, oxcarbazepine, zonisamide, tiagabine, and levetiracetam are drugs that have been reported to relieve pain in other neuropathic pain states. Older drugs such as carbamazepine, valproate, and phenytoin may also be of benefit, but they are more likely to produce serious side effects and require regular laboratory investigation.

Bisphosphonates, which inhibit bone resorption, have been reported to improve pain, allodynia, and autonomic dysfunction. One small randomized study of alendronate showed a tendency for reduction in pain and allodynia and improved range of motion. Calcitonin has also been reported to provide clinical benefit. Further study is needed before these drugs can be recommended for routine use.

Systemic corticosteroids have been used for refractory cases of CRPS I. A short course of high doses (e.g., 80 mg/day of oral prednisone is followed by tapering doses over 1 to 2 weeks). Some patients demonstrate persistent improvement in symptoms, while other experience on relief or improvement in symptoms for the duration of high dose therapy. IV regional corticosteroids have been used in conjunction with guanethidine or bretylium, but it is unclear how important their role has been for those patients who reported improvement in symptoms.

Systemic opioids are often used for patients resistant to blocks and nonopioid medications. While some patients experience significant and lasting improvement, others have only slight improvement with significant dose escalation. Given the current understanding of the potential for opioids to produce or worsen central sensitization, these drugs should be used with caution in both CRPS I and CRPS II. Opioid therapy should be maintained only for those patients who obtain substantial pain relief without rapid dose escalation. Patients should be informed early in the course of treatment that opioids will be discontinued if there is not dramatic improvement in pain and functional capacity. Improved ability to participate in physical rehabilitation programs should be an absolute condition to continued use. For patients on high-dose opioids who obtain only slight pain relief, one should seriously consider the possibility of opioid-induced hyperalgesia and initiate a gradual opioid withdrawal regimen.

NMDA antagonists have been shown to block or reverse the development of allodynia and hyperalgesia in mononeuropathy models in animals. They have also been shown to block the development of tolerance and hyperalgesia associated with administration of opioids in animals. It is likely that central sensitization plays a major role in the pathophysiology of CRPS I and II. It is reasonable, therefore, to administer this class of drugs to CRPS patients. Unfortunately, there are few choices among agents that are approved for human use. Ketamine provides analgesia in nearly all types of pain, but is associated with significant psychotomimetic effects and in all but very low doses produces immobilization. However, very low IV doses (10 to 30 mg) may produce significant analgesia without major central nervous system effects. The drug is effective orally, with about one-half to one-third the bioavailability of the IV route. It can be used intermittently for severe episodes of pain and may be helpful in enabling rehabilitation procedures. It may be possible that, with regular use, it will gradually reverse central sensitization. Other drugs that have NMDA antagonist effects include dextromethorphan, amantadine, methadone, and amitriptyline.

Intrathecal Drug Administration Systems

Intrathecal drug delivery systems may be considered for patients unresponsive to conventional management protocols. Unfortunately, while spinal opioids may initially provide improvement in symptoms, tolerance and treatment failure is common, as in other types of neuropathic pain syndromes. High-dose spinal morphine may produce a hyperalgesic state either through the accumulation of morphine-3-glucuronide or through central sensitization processes described above. Intrathecal clonidine may be tried in patients who have developed opioid tolerance. Bupivacaine may be added to the pump in an effort to provide a reduction in sympathetic tone as well as partial afferent block. Intrathecal baclofen has been reported to provide dramatic improvement in pain, autonomic dysfunction, and dystonia associated with CRPS I. One report described a patient with severe dystrophic symptoms for several years who achieved permanent relief after 6 months of intrathecal baclofen therapy.

Spinal-Cord Stimulation

Spinal-cord stimulation has been used successfully in patients with CRPS I that have been resistant to all other types of therapy. Successful application of this therapy is associated with improved blood flow, relief of pain, and improvement in allodynia. It has been reported to be effective in some patients who had undergone sympathectomy, indicating that the beneficial effects are not related only to changes in sympathetic tone.

Surgical Sympathectomy

Sympathectomy was shown to be highly effective in several large series of gunshot wound victims with causalgia (CRPS II). Most of these publications were published during or shortly after World War II. A more recent large series of cases published by Iranian surgeons following the Iran Iraq War again confirmed the efficacy of surgical sympathectomy. Nevertheless, aggressive treatment with sympathetic blocks, physiotherapy, anticonvulsants, and TCAs should be attempted before considering surgical intervention, as some patients will have good outcomes from these protocols.

Sympathectomy for CRPS I is more controversial. While some patients do experience good relief, many others experience temporary relief or no benefit at all. Patients with this syndrome are likely to experience new pain syndromes following any surgical procedure, and painful complications following sympathectomy, particularly if the surgery involves extensive tissue trauma, are fairly common. In a retrospective review of patients who failed sympathectomy, over half the patients experienced new pain, and more than two-thirds developed compensatory hyperhydrosis or gustatory sweating.

Prior to sympathectomy, for either syndrome, it is essential to perform careful diagnostic/prognostic blocks. Sympathetic blockade should produce expected increases in skin temperature, no somatic blockade and significant pain relief. Pain relief should outlast the duration of sympathetic blockade.

SUGGESTED READING

Abram SE, Boas RA: Sympathetic and visceral nerve blocks. In Benumof JL: Clinical Procedures in Anesthesia and Intensive Care. Philadelphia, JB Lippincott pp 787–806, 1992.

Bruehl S, Harden RN, Galer BS, et al: Complex regional pain syndrome: are there distinct subtypes and sequential stages of the syndrome? Pain 95:119–24, 2002.

Cepeda MS, Lau J, Carr DB: Defining the therapeutic role of local anesthetic sympathetic blockade in complex regional pain syndrome: a narrative and systematic review. Clin J Pain 18:216–33, 2002.

Erickson SJ, Hogan QH: CT-guided injection of the stellate ganglion: description of technique and efficacy of sympathetic blockade. Radiology 188:707–9, 1993.

Hogan QH, Abram SE: Neural Blockade for diagnosis and prognosis. Anesthesiology 86:216–241, 1997.

Hogan QH, Erickson SJ, Haddox JD, Abram SE: The spread of solutions during stellate ganglion block. Reg Anesth 17:78–83, 1992.

Kapetanos AK, Furlan AD, Mailis-Gagnon A: Characteristics and associated features of persistent post-sympathectomy pain. Clin J Pain 19:192–99, 2003.

Mayer DD, Mao J, Holt J, Price DD: Cellular mechanisms of neuropathic pain, morphine tolerance and their interactions. Proc Natl Acad Sci 96:7731–36, 1999.

Raja SN, Grabow TS: Complex regional pain syndrome I (reflex sympathetic dystrophy). Anesthesiology 96: 1254–60, 2002.

Rho RH, Brewer RP, Lamer TJ, Wilson PR: Complex regional pain syndrome. Mayo Clin Proc 77:174–80, 2002.

Stanton-Hicks M, Janig W, Hassenbusch S, et al: Reflex sympathetic dystrophy: changing concepts and taxonomy. Pain 63:127–33, 1995.

Watkins LR, Milligan ED, Maier SF: Spinal cord glia: new players in pain. Pain 93:201–5, 2001.

Myofascial Pain Syndrome

STEPHEN E. ABRAM
CARIDAD BRAVO-FERNANDEZ

INTRODUCTION

Muscle contains several types of nociceptors. Many of the A-δ and C fibers found in muscle, fascia, and tendons are not activated by normal stretching or contraction and are probably nociceptive in function. Muscle C fibers are responsive to chemical irritants, heat, and strong pressure. Some respond to strong contraction or to ischemia. Others are activated by greater than normal stretching of the muscle. Some A-δ fibers are insensitive to mechanical stimuli, but respond to certain chemicals, such as bradykinin. Others, such as those near muscle-tendon junctions, respond to local pressure, stretch, and intense contractions.

Acute muscle pain can result from direct trauma, recurrent microtrauma, such as that which occurs with repeated overloading during active contraction or over-stretching. Pain generally begins several hours following overactivity and peaks in 1 to several days.

DEFINITION AND CHARACTERISTICS

Myofascial pain syndrome is a condition characterized by localized muscle pain. Affected muscles are chronically in a shortened or contracted state and contain tender trigger points found within taut palpable bands of muscles. Pain is usually referred to distant, nondermatomal locations. Palpation of trigger points (TPs) can produce a "jump sign" or involuntary reflex movement or flinching and occasionally produces a local twitch response. The intensity can be increased by palpation and pressure on the TP, overwork, fatigue, trauma, and/or cold. The activation of a TP can sometimes cause autonomic symptoms—vasoconstriction, sweating, salivation, and dizziness. There is often restricted range of motion and subsequently weakness.

The location of TPs is fairly constant from one patient to the next. Interestingly, there is a high degree of correlation between commonly encountered myofascial TPs and acupuncture points. There are many sites of myofascial pain. Myofascial TPs are often found in patients with headaches and facial pain. TPs in the posterior cervical muscles can cause pain referred to the occipital, temporal, and frontal regions as well as to the vertex. Involvement of the trapezius, levator scapulae, infraspinatus, and rhomboids can produce multiple pain reference zones, including the occiput, the upper extremity, the anterior chest wall, and the shoulder. Multiple TPs may be found in the quadratus lumborum, producing mainly unilateral low- to mid-back pain. Involvement of the gluteus medius is extremely common, producing pain in the sacrum, posterior thigh, and calf. This syndrome is often confused with sciatica, sacroiliitis, and lumbosacral facet arthropathy. Myofascial pain of the tensor fascia lata can produce hip pain or posterolateral thigh and calf pain. Some common TPs and their pain reference zones are shown in Figure 15-1. Extensive descriptions and illustrations of most known myofascial TPs can be found in Travell and Simon's two-volume text.[1]

The syndrome can be initiated by a single or repetitive trauma, postural dysfunction, and physical deconditioning. It is often seen in conjunction with painful conditions that do not ordinarily involve muscle, such as complex regional pain syndrome, whiplash, and facet arthropathy.

All laboratory studies are usually normal, except when other medical conditions are present at the same time.

PATHOPHYSIOLOGY

A variety of theories have been proposed, none of which have been confirmed. Biopsies of TPs have usually failed to show any characteristic changes. One theory proposes an abnormally high production and release of

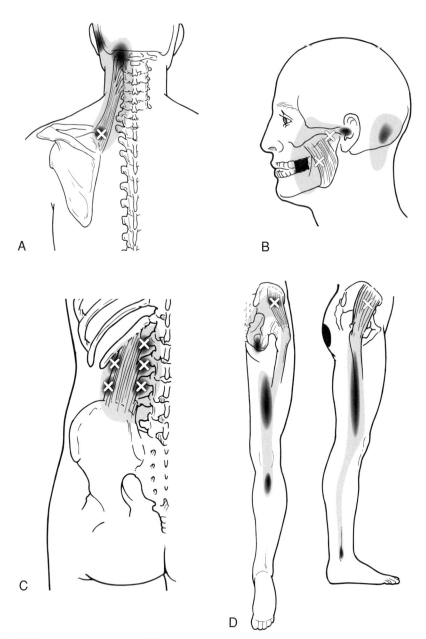

Figure 15-1   **A.** Pain pattern and TPs of the levator scapulae muscle. **B.** Masseter muscle with some of its characteristic pain reference sites. **C.** Quadratus lumborum muscle with common TPs and local pain reference pattern. **D.** Gluteus medius TPs (one of the most powerful TPs in the body, with its local pain and referral patterns to the thigh and legs), and tensor fascia lata trigger point and characteristic hip pain and lateral thigh and leg reference zones.

acetylcholine at the affected neuromuscular junctions produces intense and prolonged postjunctional depolarization with persistent shortening of sarcomeres. The sustained muscle contraction then produces inadequate arterial supply and oxygen deprivation and subsequent release of algogenic substances and inflammatory mediators.

DIAGNOSIS

The medical examination should determine whether tenderness arises from muscle contractile elements versus noncontractile structures, such as tendinous insertions, joints, or bursae. The exam will also help to determine if there is an underlying neurologic or skeletal source of pain. Posture, biomechanics, and joint function should be evaluated. A thorough physical will enable the physician to locate active TPs by palpating areas that the patient reports as symptomatic. The examiner should examine for muscle tightness, twitch with palpation, or jump sign. The patient should be questioned regarding where the pain is perceived during palpation of the TP. Range of motion of adjacent joints and spinal structures should be tested.

The differential diagnosis of myofascial pain syndrome includes a variety of muscular disorders as well as nearly every painful disorder that produces secondary muscle pain and tenderness. A list of differential diagnoses is shown in Box 15-1.

The following are findings that are characteristic of myofascial pain syndrome:
- History of trauma with an acute onset or of chronic overload with gradual onset.
- Characteristic referred pain pattern.

Box 15-1 Differential Diagnosis of Myofascial Pain Syndrome

Fibromyalgia
Muscular disorders
  Polymyositis
  Polymyalgia rheumatica
  Dermatomyositis
  Viral myositis
  Drug-induced myalgia
Arthritis with secondary muscle dysfunction
  Osteoarthritis
  Rheumatoid and other inflammatory arthritides
Neuropathic pain
  Radiculopathy
  Traumatic or entrapment neuropathies
  Systemic neuropathies
Visceral pain disorders
Neoplasm

- Restriction of range of motion and weakness in affected muscles.
- Palpable tight band.
- Focal tenderness at the TP within the tight band.
- Twitch in the muscles triggered by palpation or needling of a TP.
- Pressure on the TP reproduces the patient's pain pattern.
- Improvement or elimination of symptoms by therapies.

Factors that perpetuate the presence of myofascial TPs include:
- Structural imbalances—improper posture, scoliosis, etc.
- Pressure persisting on a muscle or nerve area.
- Nutritional imbalances—deficiencies (vitamins, amino acids, minerals), drug abuse, metabolic imbalances (e.g., diabetes), endocrine imbalances (e.g., pregnancy), drug abuse, etc.
- Psychological factors—depression, anxiety, emotional stress, etc.
- Impaired sleep.
- Chronic infection—viral, bacterial, parasitic, etc.

There is often confusion between the diagnoses of myofascial pain syndrome and fibromyalgia, and there are patients who have characteristics of both conditions. However, myofascial pain syndrome is characterized by localized muscle pain and tenderness, while fibromyalgia patients exhibit pain in muscle and nonmuscle tissue, including bony structures, ligaments, and cartilaginous structures. Myofascial pain is associated with muscle pathology while fibromyalgia is more likely associated with abnormalities in the central processing of sensory information (i.e., a diffuse hyperalgesic state). Differences between the two conditions are outlined in Box 15-2. Further discussion of fibromyalgia can be found in Chapter 19.

TREATMENT

Treatment of myofascial pain with TPs starts with the reversal of perpetuating factors. Stretching exercises are important in order to restore and maintain range of motion, in addition to the use of rest and other modalities. Many of the pain-relieving therapies are utilized to provide temporary periods of antinociception in order to enable stretching and conditioning exercises. There are specific therapies for myofascial pain, such as "spray and stretch" and "trigger point injections."

Spray and Stretch

This is used in order to restore full range of stretch to the muscle while providing temporary analgesia and reducing reflex muscle spasm. The most commonly used vapocoolant spray is chlorofluoromethane, which is non-

Box 15-2 Differences Between Myofascial Pain and Fibromyalgia	
Fibromyalgia	**Myofascial Pain**
Diffuse pain	Localized pain
Pain in muscle, ligaments, bone	Muscle pain only
Many tender points	Few TPs
Tender points locally tender	Trigger-point pressure causes referred pain
Pain is bilateral, above and below waist	Pain often unilateral, above or below waist
Onset often spontaneous	Onset usually after overuse, trauma
Frequent systemic symptoms (e.g., fatigue, insomnia, GI symptoms, headache)	Systemic symptoms uncommon
Probably a disorder of CNS sensory function	Probably a disorder primarily of muscle

GI, gastrointestinal; CNS, central nervous system; TPs, trigger points.

flammable, nonexplosive, and not irritating to skin. (There has been some controversy about the effects of vapocoolant spray on the ozone layer.) Ethyl chloride has been used, but this material is flammable and, if applied for more than a very brief exposure can freeze and injure the skin. The spray is applied to the skin over the tight muscle fibers to cover the area of referred pain. The spray is initiated over the TP then swept into the pain reference zone. Several repetitions are performed, then the patient performs active stretching exercises specific to the involved muscle. The spraying allows the muscle to gradually stretch to its full range of motion while avoiding reflex spasm.

Ice Massage

This treatment can be an effective substitute for fluoromethane spray. A small paper cup is filled with water and frozen. The top of the cup is peeled back and the TP is massaged for about 30 seconds to a minute, then stretching exercises are initiated. Another technique, which allows the patient to cool inaccessible upper back TPs without assistance, is to place a small plastic bag filled with cracked ice or a package of frozen peas over the affected TP and to compress the cold object against the back of a chair. After a few minutes of cooling, stretching exercises are initiated.

Injections

TP injections are helpful for patients who are unresponsive to spray and stretch. Injections should be done with the patient lying down to avoid any syncopal response or possible injury. Although dry needling or plain saline injection can be done, injection of local anesthetic is more common. A 25 ga (1½ in.) needle is best and causes minimal discomfort. The inactivation of TPs by needling is attributed to the mechanical disruption of contracted muscle, to release of intracellular potassium, to dilution of inflammatory substances, and/or to local vasodilatation. Some local anesthetics are thought to cause destruction of the TP by local

muscle degeneration and to interrupt the sensory-motor interaction between a TP and the CNS. Bupivacaine has the greatest capacity for producing muscle degeneration, but there is no evidence that it is more effective than other less myotoxic agents, such as procaine or lidocaine. Long-acting steroids should not be injected repeatedly, as muscle destruction and cushinoid reactions can occur. While some practitioners advocate the use of steroid-local anesthetic mixtures, there is no evidence that corticosteroids provide any added efficacy. Most studies have indicated that simple needling of the TP or injection of saline are as effective as local anesthetic injections. An advantage to the use of local anesthetics is more immediate relief. There is also a diagnostic benefit, as prompt relief indicates that the affected muscle is likely to be a pain generator.

Injection Procedure

Communication with the patient is important throughout the procedure. Both hands are used with one hand maintaining contact with the skin to palpate the TP and to feel any reaction to needling. The skin is antiseptically prepared and each TP is injected with 1 to 2 ml of local anesthetic, moving the needle back and forth through the TP several times during the injection. This should be followed with gentle active stretching exercises. A description of the technique for local anesthetic injection is shown in Box 15-3.

A series of several injections carried out at intervals of 1 to several weeks may be required to produce lasting benefit. Some patients experience temporary relief lasting a few days to several weeks, but no progressive improvement over time. Prolonged repeated use of injections appears to be of limited benefit in such patients.

Transcutaneous Electrical Nerve Stimulation

Transcutaneous electrical nerve stimulation (TENS) can be an effective means of providing temporary antinoci-

Box 15-3   Trigger-Point Injections

Locate and mark TPs
Note current location(s) and intensity of pain
Note any restriction of motion
Prepare skin antiseptically
Immobilize muscle with thumb or between thumb and forefinger
Using a fine (25 to 27 ga) needle, advance into trigger point until patient reports reproduction of pain
Inject 1 to 2 ml local anesthetic (e.g., 1% lidocaine) while moving needle several millimeters back and forth at the painful site
Reassess location and intensity of pain, range of motion
Have patient perform appropriate stretching exercises
Instruct patient to record pain intensity, ability to do physical activity over the next few days
Instruct patient to continue stretching exercises at prescribed intervals at home

ception that enables the initiation of stretching exercises. The electrodes are most often placed over or adjacent to active TPs. High-frequency TENS, using conventional stimulation or modulated modes, utilizes pulse frequencies in the 30 to 100 Hz range and current amplitudes adjusted to levels perceived by the patient to be strong but not painful. Intensities that produce muscle contraction are generally too high. Stimulation is typically carried out for at least 30 minutes prior to starting exercises and may be continued throughout the stretching exercise regimen. If high-frequency TENS is not effective at reducing pain intensity, low-frequency or acupuncture-like TENS can be utilized. Individual pulses or short bursts of high frequency are repeated at 2 to 4 Hz, and the current is adjusted to fairly high intensities that may cause discomfort and/or muscle contraction. Stimulation is only continued for short periods (e.g., 5 to 10 minutes and is discontinued just prior to the exercise session).

For persistent pain, TENS can be continued for longer periods of time to provide antinociception to enable increased general activity. The amount of use is determined by the period of relief that occurs when stimulation is discontinued.

Botulinum Toxin

Botulinum Toxin A (Botox) injection produces temporary interruption of function at the neuromuscular junction lasting 3 to 4 months. It is Food and Drug Administration approved for dystonias. There are anecdotal results of beneficial effects, but this treatment is by no means universally effective. The dose ranges from 10 units for small muscles such as the temporalis to 50 units for large muscles such as gluteus medius. It should be

reserved for patients who experience very temporary relief from local anesthetic injections. Combining Botox with other drugs such as local anesthetics is not recommended, as it may become denatured and inactivated. Use around the eye can result in prolonged ptosis, and use in the anterior neck muscles can produce difficulty swallowing, both of which can last for several months. Electromyogram (EMG) localization of the muscle is usually used for dystonias, but it is not clear whether this is advantageous for myofascial pain syndromes.

Physical Therapy and Other Modalities

Muscle-stretching exercises are the mainstay of therapy for myofascial pain. Assessment and correction of postural abnormalities is an important aspect of therapy. Modification of the workplace environment and scheduling of frequent short breaks for keyboard operators can provide significant help. A regimen of daily home stretching exercises combined with reconditioning and aerobic exercise can be initiated for most patients unless other illnesses or underlying disabilities prevent their initiation. Ultrasound can be helpful for providing temporary relief during sessions in the clinic but rarely provides lasting relief. Acupuncture can also be an effective means of providing the relief needed to facilitate the initiation of a supervised exercise program.

Psychotherapy

Patients with myofascial pain benefit from those treatment strategies that are effective for all chronic pain conditions. Patient education can be extremely helpful for these patients. It is useful for them to understand that their condition is treatable and that it is not a progressive degenerative condition. They need to understand that the increased pain they experience with activity is not causing further injury and that it will improve as a result of improving their physical condition and range of motion. They also need to learn that opioid use is generally not a first-line treatment for their condition and that their use may be associated with hyperalgesia, cognitive and sexual dysfunction, constipation, and depression. Cognitive-behavioral therapy is helpful for most patients whose pain has become chronic. EMG biofeedback can be particularly effective for patients whose stress response involves increased muscle tone.

MEDICATIONS

Nonsteroidal anti-inflammatory drugs (NSAIDs) are variably effective. Most patients who present to a pain clinic have failed to obtain significant relief from NSAIDs. Cyclooxygenase-2 antagonists are generally not more effective than NSAIDs but are better tolerated by patients who experienced gastrointestinal side effects.

Opioids should be considered only when other therapies have failed to provide progressive benefit. It should be made clear to the patient that their purpose is to facilitate a therapeutic exercise program and that it is the resultant increase in strength and flexibility that will produce lasting improvement without the opioids. Patients who obtain only slight reduction in pain or who require frequent dose escalation should not continue opioid use. Occasional patients will experience significant relief over long periods of time with little or no tolerance development. Patients who respond in this way and who have failed more conventional therapies may be candidates for prolonged use. Tramadol is an analgesic that has mild opiate receptor agonist effects and inhibits reuptake of norepinephrine and serotonin. Its mode of analgesic action is not well understood. It is effective in some patients with mild to moderate pain and is beneficial in some patients who are poorly responsive to pure µ-opiate antagonists. It is of limited use in patients with myofascial pain. There is a risk of seizures, which is increased in patients on opioids, tricyclic antidepressants (TCAs), and serotonin specific reuptake inhibitor antidepressants (SSRIs). Combining tramadol with monoamine oxidase inhibitors is particularly risky.

TCAs can be helpful in restoring normal sleep patterns in patients whose sleep is interrupted by pain. In addition, these drugs are capable of providing reduction in pain levels, particularly in patients with a neuropathic component to their pain. The dose is initially titrated to a level that restores better sleep patterns without causing daytime drowsiness. Analgesic effects generally do not occur for 1 to several weeks. If no benefit is seen at doses of 50 to 100mg in the first few weeks, blood levels should be checked, as some patients metabolize these drugs rapidly.

Amitriptyline is the most commonly prescribed TCA. It is one of the most sedating with significant anticholinergic effects. Doxepin has a similar pharmacologic profile. Nortriptyline is slightly less sedating and has less anticholinergic effect. Desipramine is still less sedating. Daytime sedation, cardiac arrhythmias, orthostatic hypotension, dry mouth, constipation, and increased intraocular pressure are relatively common side effects of TCAs. These drugs can also produce significant weight gain.

SSRIs have not proved to be useful for pain control in most chronic pain studies. There is little data on their efficacy in myofascial pain syndrome. They may be helpful when depression is a significant associated symptom.

There is little information about the efficacy of anticonvulsants in myofascial pain syndrome. Gabapentin is a reasonable drug to try in patients with combined neuropathic and myofascial pain.

In general, muscle relaxants are of limited benefit in myofascial pain. Baclofen and tizanidine are occasionally of some benefit and are less sedating and less likely to lead to abuse than benzodiazepines. Carisoprodol and diazepam may provide some pain relief but are generally very sedating and can produce habituation and dependence with prolonged use.

REFERENCE

1. Travell JG, Simons DG: Myofascial Pain and Dysfunction: The Trigger Point Manual, vol 1. Baltimore, Lippincott Williams & Wilkins, 1983.

SUGGESTED READING

Bennett RM: Emerging concepts in the neurobiology of chronic pain: evidence of abnormal sensory processing in fibromyalgia. Mayo Clin Proc 74(4):385-398, 1999.

Cummings TM, White AR: Needling therapies in the management of myofascial trigger point pain: a systematic review. Arch Phys Med Rehabil 82:986-992, 2001.

Davidoff RA: TPs and myofascial pain: toward understanding how they affect headaches. Cephalgia 18:436-448, 1998.

Harden RN, Bruehl SP, Gass S, et al: Signs and symptoms of the myofascial pain syndrome: a national survey of pain management providers. Clin J Pain 16:64-72, 2000.

Myofascial pain syndrome and fibromyalgia: a critical assessment and alternate view. Clin J Pain 14:74-78, 1998.

Porta M: A comparative trial of botulinum toxin type A and methylprednisolone for the treatment of myofascial pain syndrome and pain from chronic muscle spasm. Pain 85:101-105, 2000.

Sola AE, Bonica JJ: Myofascial pain syndromes. In Loeser JD (ed): Bonica's Management of Pain, 3rd ed. Philadelphia, Lippincott Williams & Wilkins, 2001, pp 530-542.

Travell JG, Simons DG: Myofascial Pain and Dysfunction: The Trigger Point Manual, vol 2. Lippincott Williams & Wilkins, 1992.

Wheeler AH: Myofascial Pain Disorders: Theory to Therapy. Drugs 64:45-62, 2004.

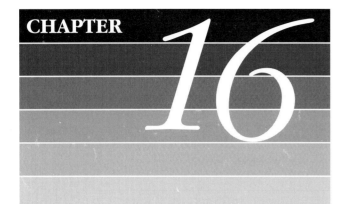

CHAPTER 16

Headache

STEPHEN E. ABRAM

INTRODUCTION

The most common headaches are those that are primary painful disorders. These include migraine, tension-type, cluster, and chronic daily headaches. A substantial number of patients with chronic, persistent headache have ongoing pain either caused by or exacerbated by medication overuse. Cervical spine pathology, including whiplash injury, upper cervical radiculopathy, and cervical facet arthropathy, is another common source of persistent headaches. Direct head trauma can result in a syndrome that includes chronic headache. Environmental factors, such as cigarette smoke, fluorescent lighting, and a variety of foods or food additives can evoke or worsen headache symptoms. Finally, there are a number of medical illnesses, many of which are potentially life-threatening, that produce headache symptoms. While they are by no means the most common causes, they must be ruled out before beginning definitive therapy.

HEADACHES CAUSED BY UNDERLYING MEDICAL CONDITIONS

Sudden Onset Severe Headache

While patients with sudden onset headache rarely present to a pain management center for their initial management, patients with chronic headaches or other chronic pain conditions may consult their pain clinic physician for new or worsening headache symptoms. It is essential, therefore, that the pain management physician be familiar with the conditions that can produce rapid increases in headache severity. A severe, rapid-onset migraine may have symptoms that are difficult to distinguish from more serious conditions. Symptoms that suggest a serious neurologic event include:

- Abrupt onset with rapid progression of headache over seconds to a few minutes.
- Associated symptoms such as nausea, fever, stiff neck, sensory or motor changes, or changes in mental status.
- Persistence of symptoms beyond a few hours.

Serious Conditions Causing Headache

Intracranial Hemorrhage

Rupture of an intracranial aneurysm produces severe, usually bilateral headache, often accompanied by nausea, vomiting, and photophobia. A change in mental status is an ominous sign. The so-called sentinel headache is a sudden severe headache that improves temporarily and may signal a subsequent catastrophic bleed. Bleeding from an atrioventricular (A-V) malformation is also associated with severe headache, although the onset may be somewhat slower. Spontaneous parenchymal hemorrhage can also produce sudden severe headache and is usually associated with neurologic changes. Hypertension is a predisposing factor, and hemorrhage into the substance of the brain may be more likely in migraine patients.

Careful neurologic evaluation, CT scan, and lumbar puncture are the classical means of working up a suspected intracranial bleed. MR angiography is becoming more accepted as a diagnostic tool and may be approaching conventional angiography in its diagnostic accuracy.

Internal Carotid Artery Dissection

This is an uncommon cause of sudden onset headache. It is unilateral and may present with pain in the orbit, frontal region, or neck. It is usually accompanied by neurologic changes and often produces pupillary changes and/or Horner's syndrome. Cervical MRI or ultrasound will provide the diagnosis.

Acute Hypertension

Sudden increases in blood pressure can be accompanied by severe headache. Hypertensive encephalopathy can produce associated neurologic signs. If hypertension is associated with pheochromocytoma, symptoms associated with elevation of catecholamines (e.g., palpitations, diaphoresis, anxiety) may be present.

Acute Glaucoma

Rapid onset of increased intraocular pressure can cause eye pain, headache, and pupillary changes.

PRIMARY HEADACHES

A variety of medical conditions can produce headaches with slow or subacute onset. While many of these conditions are not immediately life-threatening, most of them require treatment in a timely fashion. Conditions that produce a fairly rapid onset of headache include A-V malformation, cerebral vein thrombosis, obstructive hydrocephalus, stroke, and viral meningitis. Chronic subdural hematoma, pseudotumor cerebri, brain tumor, brain abscess, temporal arteritis, AIDS, Lyme Disease, and chronic sinusitis can produce more chronic headache symptoms with subacute to slow, insidious onset. The differential diagnosis of medical conditions causing headache is listed in Box 16-1.

Headache Induced by Foods

A variety of common foods can produce or exacerbate headache. It may be useful for patients to begin a very simplified diet with a very few items, such as rice and one or two meats, vegetables, and fruits. They should diligently avoid simple sugars, caffeine, artificial sweeteners, nitrites, sulfites, and monosodium L-glutamate. If the headache improves, they can add additional foods or additives one by one, noting whether the headache recurs. A list of foods that are likely to induce headaches in susceptible individuals is found in Box 16-2.

Migraine Headache

Migraine is an extremely common, complex neurophysiologic condition characterized by episodic or, in many cases, daily headaches. It is somewhat more common in women. It is divided into two major categories:

Box 16-1 Medical Conditions Associated with Severe Headache

Subarachnoid hemorrhage
Intracerebral hemorrhage
Severe acute hypertension
Acute glaucoma
Carotid artery dissection
Acute obstructive hydrocephalus
Encephalitis
Viral or bacterial meningitis
Brain abscess
Cerebral vein thrombosis
Stroke
Sinusitis
Optic neuritis
A-V malformation
Intracranial tumor
Temporal arteritis
Pseudotumor cerebri
AIDS
Lyme Disease

Box 16-2 Foods that Induce Headaches

Aged cheese
Chocolate, especially dark
Sugar
Milk, ice cream, yogurt
Pickled foods
Nitrites in packaged meats
Monosodium glutamate
Artificial sweeteners
Caffeine
Alcohol
Sulfites
Yeast
Some fruits and vegetables

migraine with aura and migraine without aura. About one-third of attacks are accompanied by aura, and some patients experience both types. It is now believed that many patients who were previously diagnosed with persistent tension or chronic daily headaches have a variant form of migraine that has progressed to a daily or persistent form. These patients may have nearly constant headache with superimposed severe, typical migraine attacks.

Migraine is often preceded by prodromal symptoms, such as mood changes, chills, stiff neck, diarrhea or constipation, anorexia, fatigue, and fluid retention. These symptoms can occur hours to days preceding an attack. The aura consists of focal neurologic signs that begin in the minutes to hours preceding the headache or begin coincidentally with the headache. The most common aura symptoms are visual. The familiar scintillating scotoma, or fortification spectra, is commonly a bright zigzag image across the visual field.

The headaches can be unilateral or bilateral and can occur anywhere in the head and neck. They may be throbbing in quality, although this characteristic is not always present. They are often accompanied by nausea and vomiting, photophobia and phonophobia. Attacks usually last at least 4 hours, and may persist for days to weeks. Severe, prolonged attacks are referred to as status migrainosis.

Migraine is fairly common in children. Attacks are often less severe than in adults. Abdominal pain and other gastrointestinal complaints are common. Biofeedback and other types of psychotherapy may be very effective, eliminating the need for pharmacotherapy.

Concepts of the pathophysiology of migraine have evolved through the years. Once thought to be a primary vascular disorder, it is now considered to arise from neuronal structures in the upper brainstem. Trigeminal sensory neurons release several peptide neurotransmitters, triggering neurogenic inflammation, dilation of meningeal vessels, and extravasation of plasma proteins. Serotonin released from nerve endings adjacent to meningeal vessels appears to play an important role in mediating some of the pathologic processes. Aura is associated with a spreading wave of reduced blood flow.

There is some evidence of comorbidities between migraine and other conditions. The most important comorbid conditions are stroke and epilepsy. Some cases of stroke occur coincidentally with a migraine attack, while others are temporally unrelated. The highest incidence of comorbidity between migraine and stroke occurs in younger women who smoke and/or use high estrogen oral contraceptives. The prevalence of migraine among epileptic patients is in the range of 10% to 20% while the incidence of migraine in the general population is about 6%. Drugs that have both antimigraine and anticonvulsant effects are reasonable therapeutic options in such patients, while drugs that lower seizure thresholds [e.g., tricyclic antidepressants (TCAs) and meperidine] should be avoided.

Acute Treatment

Treatment of an acute attack may be with nonspecific drugs such as opioids, nonsteroidal anti-inflammatory drugs (NSAIDs), and antiemetics. Specific drug treatment includes ergot derivatives and $5\text{-HT}_{1B/1D}$ agonists (triptans).

NSAIDs may be very effective first-line therapy for some patients. While opioids have traditionally been a common emergency room treatment for severe attacks, recent studies suggest that the majority of migraine patients experience incomplete relief of acute episodes and do not benefit appreciably from long-term opioid therapy. Recent evidence that migraine is related to neuroimmune activation and that opioids can independently produce glial cell activation helps to explain the poor response to these drugs for many patients with this disorder.

Phenothiazines such as promethazine and prochlorperazine, butyrophenones such as droperidol and haloperidol, and metoclopramide can be useful in treating the associated nausea. An uncommon but potentially life-threatening prolongation of the Q-T interval can occur with droperidol.

Before the introduction of the triptans, ergotamine derivatives were the mainstay of specific acute migraine therapy. Dihydroergotamine (DHE) can be given intranasally or IM. Repeated intravenous DHE can be useful for episodes refractory to more conventional therapy.

The triptans were introduced into clinical practice in the early 1990s. They produce vasoconstriction of meningeal vessels and inhibit both primary afferent trigeminal fibers and second-order neurons in the trigeminal nucleus caudalis. Sumatriptan was the first of these drugs introduced and is available as a subcutaneous injectable, a nasal spray, and an oral preparation.

The other preparations are available as oral or oral transmucosal preparations. The advantages of some of the newer drugs include more rapid onset with oral administration and longer duration of action, with less need for repeated dosing (Table 16-1). The triptans can produce coronary vasoconstriction in susceptible patients and are contraindicated in patients with severe ischemic heart disease as well as those with basilar and hemiplegic migraine.

Preventive Treatment

Preventive therapy is indicated for patients who do not obtain satisfactory control of their headaches with acute intermittent therapy. Patients with very frequent headaches or those who have intolerable side effects from acute therapy drugs are candidates. Patients with hemiplegic migraine and those who experience persistent neurologic dysfunction after migraines should also be considered.

The usual first-line drugs for preventive treatment are β-adrenergic blockers and TCAs. Divalproex is a reasonable choice for patients who also have bipolar disorder or seizures. Other less toxic anticonvulsants, such as gabapentin and topiramate, have been undergoing trials as well, but their efficacy has not yet been established. Calcium channel blockers, selective serotonin reuptake inhibitor and monoamine oxidase inhibitor antidepressants, and NSAIDs have been used as well. The ergot preparations methysergide and methylergonovine are effective for some patients, but can cause retroperitoneal fibrosis. The medication selected should be started at a low dose and increased slowly while monitoring efficacy and adverse effects. A list of commonly used preventive medications is shown in Table 16-2. Previously ineffective acute therapies can be retried once a maintenance dose of preventive drug has been established if attacks are not completely controlled.

Table 16-1 Triptan Preparations		
Drug	**Route**	**Dose**
Sumatriptan	Oral	50–100 mg
	Nasal spray	5–20 mg
	Subcutaneous	6 mg
Zolmitriptan	Oral	2.5–5 mg
	Oral transmucosal	2.5–5 mg
Naratriptan*	Oral	1–2.5 mg
Frovatriptan**	Oral	2.5 mg
Rizatriptan	Oral	5–10 mg
	Oral transmucosal	5–10 mg
Eletriptan	Oral	20–40 mg
Almotriptan	Oral	6.25–12.5 mg

*Long half-life (6 hours)
**Longest half-life (25 hours)

Table 16-2 Preventive Therapies for Migraine		
Drug Type	**Drug**	**Daily Dose**
β-Adrenergic blockers	Metoprolol	100–200 mg
	Atenolol	100–200 mg
	Propranolol	80–240 mg
Tricyclic Antidepressants	Amitriptyline	10–100 mg
	Doxepin	10–100 mg
	Nortriptyline	10–100 mg
	Desipramine	10–100 mg
Calcium Channel Blockers	Verapamil	160–480 mg
	Nimodipine	90–180 mg
	Diltiazem	90–180 mg
	Flunarizine	5–15 mg
Ergotamine Derivatives	Methysergide	3–10 mg
	Methylergonovine	0.6–1.2 mg
Anticonvulsants	Divalproex sodium	800–2000 mg
	Topiramate	100–400 mg
	Carbamazepine	300–1200 mg
	Gabapentin	1800–3600 mg

Other Forms of Migraine

Basilar Migraine

This is a subgroup of migraine with aura. Vasoconstriction involving the basilar artery was initially thought to be the underlying pathology but it is likely that, as with other types of migraine, the initial event is neuronal dysfunction. The aura is not typical of classical migraine and may include diplopia, visual field loss, vertigo, tinnitus, changes in consciousness, ataxia, and dysarthria.

Ophthalmoplegic Migraine

This form is characterized by headache, diplopia, and pupillary dilation.

Hemiplegic Migraine

This condition is characterized by an aura that involves hemiplegia that can last an hour or longer. There is a familial form that is associated with a specific genetic finding. Hemiplegic migraine often begins in childhood and often resolves in later life.

Retinal Migraine

Visual impairment involving one eye characterizes the aura associated with this condition.

Cluster Headache

Cluster headache is a condition typified by severe, episodic unilateral headaches that are accompanied by signs of autonomic dysfunction. It is more common in men, and often begins in early adulthood.

Episodes occur in clusters separated by periods of remission lasting weeks to years. During periods of frequent headaches, attacks occur up to 6 times per day. Attacks can be precipitated by alcohol, and many cluster headache patients are heavy users of alcohol and tobacco. Attacks are much shorter than those of migraine headaches, lasting less than an hour in many cases. During attacks, the patient experiences ipsilateral lacrimation, nasal congestion, ptosis, pupillary changes, and conjunctival injection. In some patients, the episodic attacks evolve to a more constant, chronic form.

Treatment

Acute symptomatic treatment options include oxygen inhalation, dihydroergotamine (intranasal or IV), triptans, intranasal lidocaine, indomethacin, and opioids. Oxygen should be given at high flows, approaching 100%, for 15 minutes. Subcutaneous sumatriptan is usually rapidly effective.

Preventive therapy is the principal of treatment, since episodes are severe and relatively short. Verapamil is the first-line therapy, and is administered in fairly high doses (120 to 160 mg tid to qid). Since the onset of the verapamil effect may be delayed, transitional therapy with corticosteroids (60 mg/day prednisone for 3 days) can be initiated at the beginning of an active headache period. Oral ergotamine can be effective as well. Other options include lithium, methysergide, divalproex sodium, oral or transdermal clonidine, and topiramate.

Tension-Type Headache

This is the most common type of headache. It is characterized as episodic if it occurs fewer than 15 days per month and chronic if it occurs 15 or more days per month. The headache is bilateral, tight, or pressing in quality and may be accompanied by photophobia or phonophobia. Nausea is not a prominent feature. There is no aura and no neurologic symptoms.

Tension-type headache (TTH) is probably the result of both central and peripheral mechanisms. Alterations of sensory processing may play a role. Generally, decreased pain threshold is a common finding. In addition, there is often increased tone and tenderness of pericranial muscles.

TTH often occurs in patients with a history of migraines and may represent mild migraine episodes in some of those patients.

Treatment

Acetaminophen, aspirin, and NSAIDs are effective for many patients. Caffeine may be a helpful adjunct for some patients. TCAs are affective in preventing episodes for some patients. Relaxation training and electromyo-gram biofeedback can be extremely effective and should be tried in most patients.

Chronic Daily Headache

This is a term that is controversial and somewhat confusing. It probably includes several distinct pathophysiologic mechanisms. The majority of patients are likely to have transformed migraines or chronic tension-type headaches. Treatment with medications recommended for migraine has usually been tried and has often failed. If not previously initiated, TCAs, β blockers, calcium channel agonists, ergot derivatives, divalproex, and other anticonvulsants may be tried. Patients treated with chronic opioid medications are likely to benefit from discontinuing these drugs, particularly if they have developed substantial tolerance. Patients whose pain levels remain high (≥ 7/10) despite relatively high opioid doses should be encouraged to discontinue opioids for at least 3 months. Lifestyle changes, such as smoking cessation, interventions for substance and alcohol overuse, exercise programs, stress management, and family counseling should be encouraged. Biofeedback and relaxation training should be tried. Acupuncture and other alternative therapies can be beneficial.

Another diagnosis associated with chronic daily headaches is medication overuse headache. Frequent use of nonopioid analgesics, triptans, ergot preparations, and opioids can produce these headaches. The diagnosis is confirmed when headaches improve following medication withdrawal.

Triptan-induced overuse headaches often take the form of increased frequency of migraine attacks or transformation to migraine-like daily headaches. In about one-third of patients the headaches are tension-type daily headaches. Withdrawal symptoms are rarely problematic, and patients note a reduction in migraine attacks within a few days to weeks. Caffeine can produce withdrawal type headaches. Combination drugs containing barbiturates, such as butalbital will produce medication overuse headache at a substantially higher rate than NSAIDs or opioid/analgesic combinations without barbiturate.

LESS COMMON PRIMARY HEADACHES

Hemicrania Continua

The diagnosis of hemicrania continua should be entertained in cases of chronic unilateral headaches. This condition produces stabbing, ice-pick–like pain and is brought on or exacerbated by physical exertion. It almost always responds dramatically to indomethacin.

Chronic Paroxysmal Hemicrania

This condition occurs mainly in women. It produces daily short-lived attacks that are often provoked by certain neck movements. It can produce ipsilateral autonomic symptoms similar to those seen in cluster headache, including ptosis, meiosis, lacrimation, and regional perspiration. Indomethacin is the most reliable form of treatment.

SUNCT Syndrome

The syndrome of short lasting, unilateral, neuralgiform headache with conjunctival injection and tearing is more common in men and produces very brief attacks of neuralgia-like pain lasting a minute or less. It occurs episodically, with periods of reduced or absent attacks. No reliably effective treatment has been identified.

Hypnic Headache

This is a nocturnal condition that usually affects elderly patients. There is no gender specificity. Patients are awakened by the headaches, which can last a few minutes to several hours. Headaches are usually unilateral and throbbing. Lithium carbonate 300 to 600 mg at bedtime is usually helpful. Indomethacin may also provide relief.

CERVICOGENIC HEADACHE

Structures in the cervical spine and surrounding tissues can produce symptoms of headache. This is not surprising, since afferent nerve fibers from the upper three cervical nerve roots as well as trigeminal afferents synapse in the trigeminal cervical nucleus. Pain of cervical origin is often perceived in the orbital or frontal regions. Structures that can produce pain perceived as headache include the atlanto-occipital joint, the atlantoaxial joint, the C2-3 zygapophyseal joint, posterior cervical muscles, the vertebral artery, and the C2-3 disc. Upper cervical radiculopathy usually produces pain in the occipital region, but may be referred to the frontal area as well.

C2 neuralgia is a syndrome that produces occipital, temporal, and frontal pain, often accompanied by lacrimation and conjunctival injection. It is easily confused with cluster headache. It is thought to be related to entrapment of the C2 spinal nerve. In some cases there is a dense venous network around the nerve root. Entrapment can also occur as the nerve traverses the posterior aspect of the atlantoaxial joint. Degenerative or inflammatory changes in the joint capsule can

produce irritation or entrapment of the nerve. Radiofrequency ablation of the nerve can provide relief in some cases.

Entrapment or irritation of the C3 nerve by inflammation or osteophytes of the C2-3 zygapophyseal joint is a fairly common cause of occipital headache. The facet joint as well as the C3 nerve can be anesthetized by injecting over the lateral aspect of the joint. The addition of corticosteroid may produce prolonged relief for some patients. Pathologic changes in this joint and the overlying nerve root may account for occipital pain in some cases of whiplash. Entrapment of the occipital nerve as it perforates the suboccipital muscles can produce pain that is indistinguishable from C2 or C3 radiculopathy. Injection of the occipital nerve provides temporary relief. Steroid injection of the nerve or repeated injection of suboccipital trigger points may provide lasting benefit. Radiofrequency lesioning or implantation of a peripheral nerve stimulator has been utilized for resistant cases.

POSTDURAL PUNCTURE HEADACHE

Pain management clinics are often called upon to treat dural puncture headaches. Many of the referrals come from Radiology, Internal Medicine, and Neurology departments. Many of these headaches can be managed conservatively as the large majority caused by small gauge needles (22 ga or less) will resolve within 2 to 3 days. Those caused by accidental dural puncture with epidural needles or by cerebrospinal fluid (CSF) drains employed during neurosurgical procedures are more likely to persist longer and are likely to require epidural blood patch.

Postdural puncture headache is thought to be caused by a reduction in intracranial CSF pressure with sagging of the brain, especially in the upright position, and traction on blood vessels, meninges, and other pain sensitive structures. Traction on the acoustic nerve produces varying degrees of hearing loss, while traction on cranial nerves supplying the extraocular muscles, particularly the abducens nerve, can produce diplopia. Dural puncture headaches are much more common in teenagers and young adults, and the incidence is directly related to the size of the needle used. Pencil-point needles are less likely to produce headaches than cutting point needles of the same gauge, and approaching the dura tangentially, as with a paramedian approach, reduces the incidence. Following accidental dural puncture with a large gauge needle there is a 30% to 80% incidence of postdural puncture headache. While prophylactic blood patch has not been shown to be consistently effective, intrathecal injection of 10 ml preservative free saline prior to withdrawal of the needle was shown to significantly reduce the incidence of headache.

Headaches are usually bitemporal or bifrontal. Almost invariably, they are aggravated by sitting or standing and at least partially relieved by lying down. Nausea and mild neck stiffness are common. Photophobia may be present, but is not often seen, and it may signal other causes of headache. Fever, mental status changes, and neurologic dysfunction, other than diplopia and hearing loss, indicate other, potentially serious diagnoses. Most headaches begin 12 to 48 hours after dural puncture.

Treatment

Conservative treatment consists of bedrest and mild analgesics. Forced hydration does not increase CSF production and has not been shown to help. Abdominal binders, caffeine, and sumatriptan have all been recommended, but have not been proven effective in controlled trials. Epidural saline provides temporary relief, but recurrence is common.

Epidural blood patch is the treatment of choice for resistant cases. Many physicians will choose this treatment early if the dural puncture was done with a large gauge needle. The procedure must be done with strict aseptic technique. The epidural level should be at or below the site of dural puncture, as there is preferential spread of the injectate in a cephalad direction. The optimal dose is 15 to 20 ml. The injection should be stopped if the patient begins to experience significant back pain, neck pain, or radicular symptoms. Complications of the technique are rare and include epidural abscess and transient cranial nerve palsies. Back and leg pain lasting 1 to several days are fairly common. Patients who experience recurrence of postural headaches after initial relief will most likely benefit from a repeat blood patch.

SUGGESTED READING

Ashkenazi A, Silberstein SD: Headache management for the pain specialist. Reg Anesth Pain Med 29:462-475, 2004.

Charsley MM, Abram SE: The injection of intrathecal normal saline reduces the severity of postdural puncture headache. Reg Anesth Pain Med 26:301-305, 2001.

Goadsby PH: The pharmacology of headache. Prog in Neurobiol 62:509-525, 2000.

Lake AE, Saper JR: Chronic headache. Neurology 59(suppl 2):S8-S13, 2002.

Olesen J, Lipton RB: Headache classification update 2004. Curr Opin Neurol 17:275-282, 2004.

Safa-Tisseront V, Thormann F, Malassine P, et al: Effectiveness of epidural blood patch in the management of post-dural puncture headache. Anesthesiology 95:334-339, 2001.

Saper JR, Silberstein SD, Gordon CD, et al: Swidan S: Handbook of Headache Management, 2nd ed. Philadelphia, Lippincott Williams and & Wilkins, 1999.

Toth C: Medications and substances as a cause of headache: a systematic review of the literature. Clin Neuropharmacol 26:122-136, 2003.

CHAPTER 17

Facial Pain

CONSTANTINE SARANTOPOULOS

INTRODUCTION AND BASIC CONCEPTS

Pain in the face is associated with a very broad and heterogeneous etiology, and may originate from diseases or pathologic conditions involving extracranial, intracranial, musculoskeletal, vascular, or neural tissues. Pathologic lesions in any of the organs in the orofacial area, such as the eyes, ears, nose, throat, sinuses, nerves, tongue, or teeth can result in painful sensations, which are being perceived on the face and the oral cavity, or may project beyond these areas. Intracranial pathologic processes, such as neoplasms, hematomas, vascular malformations, infectious processes, among others, may also manifest with facial pain that needs to be distinguished from the original conditions.

Facial pain of musculoskeletal origin may be of myofascial etiology (commonly accompanying other disorders), may originate from temporomandibular joint problems, systemic collagen diseases, or manifest as a referred pain pattern from pathologic conditions affecting the cervical spine. Pain of vascular etiology includes temporal arteritis as well as migraines or cluster headaches, which, although are typically classified as "headaches," may need to be included in the differential diagnosis of facial pain as well. Pain in the face may be of neuropathic etiology, and includes various neuralgias, such as trigeminal or glossopharyngeal neuralgia. These may be idiopathic or secondary to other disorders, including benign tumors or malignancy. Not infrequently, facial pain does not fit in any of the above classifications and is characterized as "atypic facial pain," or constitutes a part or the primary manifestation of psychological dysfunction.

Overall, the vast majority of all orofacial pain, in terms of frequency, is of dental origin, produced by lesions of the teeth, including the pulp and periodontal tissues. Most of these conditions are being identified and treated by dental or oral surgeons and are rarely being referred to a pain clinic. Pain originating from the sinuses is also very common, not necessarily accompanied by fever or discharge in the chronic phase. Likewise, most of these conditions are being treated etiologically by ear, nose, and throat (ENT) specialists and are not being very commonly encountered amongst the population of patients who receive treatment through a pain clinic. In contrast, conditions such as trigeminal or glossopharyngeal neuralgia, other neuropathies, pain from temporomandibular joint (TMJ) disorders, myofascial pain, and atypic facial pain are more prevalent amongst the latter population of patients.

NEUROANATOMY RELEVANT TO OROFACIAL PAIN

Neural pathways that contain nociceptive primary afferent fibers conveying pain from the orofacial structures include mainly cranial nerves V (trigeminal) and IX (glossopharyngeal) as well as lesser contributions from the superficial cervical plexus and afferent fibers contained in cranial nerve VII (facial) (Table 17-1).

The trigeminal nerve divides into three major branches: (1) ophthalmic, (2) maxillary, and (3) mandibular, which convey sensory information (including nociception) from the upper, middle, and inferior face, respectively. The neuronal somata of the primary afferent fibers conveying nociception from sensory distribution of the trigeminal nerve are contained within the trigeminal or gasserian ganglion, while they proximally project on to second-order neurons located within the spinal nucleus of the trigeminal nerve, in the medulla (Table 17-2).

The ophthalmic branch exits through the superior orbital fissure and passes through the orbit to provide innervation to the skin of the forehead and top of the head. The maxillary nerve passes through the foramen rotundum into the pterygopalatine fossa. It provides sensory branches via the inferior orbital fissure to the middle face, cheek, and upper teeth, and via the pterygopalatine canal to the soft and hard palate, nasal cavity, and pharynx. There are also meningeal sensory branches that enter the trigeminal ganglion within the cranium. The mandibular nerve contains sensory fibers conveying general sensory information from the mucosa of the mouth and cheek, the anterior two-thirds of the tongue, lower teeth, skin of the lower jaw, side of the head and scalp, and meninges of the anterior and middle cranial fossae. A branch of the mandibular nerve, the auriculotemporal nerve, provides innervation to the TMJ.

The glossopharyngeal nerve, as the name implies, innervates the tongue and the pharynx. It exits the skull through the jugular foramen. The nerve contains sensory as well as motor and parasympathetic fibers, mainly to the parotid gland. The motor fibers supply the stylopharyngeus muscle, which elevates the pharynx during swallowing and talking. Sensory neuronal somata are located within two sensory ganglia in the jugular foramen: the superior and inferior glossopharyngeal ganglia. General sensory signals—including nociceptive ones—from the external ear, inner surface of the tympanic membrane, posterior third of the tongue, and the upper pharynx are conveyed through fibers of the superior or inferior glossopharyngeal ganglia. The ganglia project centrally into the caudal part of the spinal trigeminal nucleus in the medulla. The nerve also contains visceral sensory fibers innervating the carotid body (responding to oxygen tension changes) and carotid sinus (responding to blood pressure changes) as well as conveying taste from the tongue (Table 17-3).

Sensory fibers conveying nociceptive information from the posterior tongue, tonsils, oropharynx, soft palate and ear, via the glossopharyngeal nerve (IX), also project to second-order neurons within the same nucleus. This

Table 17-1	Neural Pathways Conveying Nociceptive Information from the Orofacial Structures
Major contribution	Cranial nerves V (trigeminal)
	Cranial nerve IX (glossopharyngeal)
Minor contribution	Superficial cervical plexus
	Afferent fibers in cranial nerve VII (facial)

Table 17-2	Branches of the Trigeminal Nerve
Ophthalmic	Skin of the forehead and top of the head
Maxillary	Middle face, cheek, and upper teeth
	Soft and hard palate, nasal cavity, and part of nasopharynx
Mandibular	Mucosa of the mouth and cheek
	Anterior two-thirds of the tongue, lower teeth, skin of the lower jaw
	Side of the head and scalp and meninges of the anterior and middle cranial fossae
	TMJ
	Motor fibers to the muscles of mastication

Table 17-3	Glossopharyngeal Nerve: Innervation
Sensory fibers	External ear, inner surface of the tympanic membrane, posterior third of the tongue, tonsils, and the upper pharynx
	Visceral sensory fibers from carotid baroreceptors and chemoreceptors
Motor fibers	To stylopharyngeus muscle (elevates pharynx during swallowing and talking)
Parasympathetic fibers	To parotid gland

converge constitutes the neuroanatomic basis for various referred pain patterns relevant to the perception of nociceptive signaling from the facial structures.

A lot of times headache and facial pain are difficult or impossible to distinguish clinically, or they may coexist. The brain tissue itself is not sensitive to noxious stimuli resulting in pain; however, pain may originate from the meninges and supporting structures, which are densely innervated. Inflammatory changes involving these structures, traction, or distortion may result in pain, which may be perceived as headache or facial pain.

Considering the convergence of neural nociceptive pathways, pathologic processes inside the cranial cavity may produce pain patterns referred to areas of the face, including the mandible, even the neck. The possibility of referred pain patterns needs to be taken into consideration at the diagnostic evaluation of pain of the face, and pertinent pathologic conditions need to be ruled out. Pathologic conditions within the anterior or middle cranial fossae may elicit pain that is referred to the scalp or face anterior to the coronal suture, while lesions in the posterior fossa may result in pain projecting in the more posterior portions of the head and upper neck. Pain arising from processes in the sphenoid or sella may present with patterns referred to the vertex. Generalized intracranial disease, such as meningitis or subarachnoid hemorrhage as well as lesions of the incisura may also present with simultaneous facial pain and posterior headache. In addition to intracranial pathology, other conditions may present with pain referred to the face, and these also need to be ruled out during diagnostic evaluation of these patients. Lesions involving the sinuses and the structures of the nasal cavity are a frequent source of acute and/or chronic facial pain. The mucosa of the nose and paranasal sinuses receive sensory innervation from the ophthalmic and maxillary branches of the trigeminal nerve, with some minor contributions from the greater superficial petrosal branch of the facial (VII) nerve. So, pain originating from processes within the sinuses is frequently referred to the corresponding cutaneous dermatome innervated by the trigeminal nerve, or sometimes to the auricular or periauricular region due to the contributions of the facial nerve.

The innervation of the frontal sinus is derived from the ophthalmic branch of the trigeminal nerve. Inflammation of the mucosa of the frontal sinus from sinus infection or a malignant process may therefore result in pain referred to the forehead or anterior cranial fossa, explained by the convergence of the primary afferents that innervate the sinus and the dura, with those arising from the cutaneous distribution of the nerve.

The anterior ethmoidal nerve, a branch of the nasociliary division of the ophthalmic division of the trigeminal nerve also innervates the anterior ethmoid structures. The anterior ethmoid nerve has a relatively large receptive field, which includes innervation within the nasal cavity as well the anterior septum and lateral nasal wall, including the superior, middle, and inferior turbinates and middle meatus. In addition, the anterior ethmoids may also receive some innervation from the small supraorbital branch that supplies the frontal sinus. All these patterns imply that pain over the distribution of the ophthalmic division of the trigeminal nerve may originate from sources of nociception anywhere in the above mentioned areas of innervation. The maxillary division of the trigeminal nerve provides nerve branches, which include the posterior superior alveolar, infraorbital, and anterior superior alveolar nerves, and these provide innervation to the maxillary sinuses. Pain arising from the latter may thus refer to the cutaneous area of distribution of the maxillary division of the trigeminal nerve. The maxillary division also innervates the posterior nasal septum and a significant area of the superior and middle turbinates. However, some portions of the posterior ethmoid and sphenoid sinuses receive innervation from branches of the greater superficial petrosal branch of the VII cranial nerve, and the ophthalmic branch of the trigeminal nerve.

Patients suffering from facial pain, frequently also complain of pain in the ear (otalgia). Ear pain may be secondary to pathologic conditions within the ear; however, otalgia frequently constitutes a referred pain pattern from a distant process, such as lesions within the oropharynx. The sensory innervation of the ear and the nearby area is complex and obtained from four cranial nerves (V, VII, IX, and X) as well as from the cervical plexus. So, nociception originating anywhere within the receptive field of any of these nerves may produce referred pain projecting to the ear. Thus, pathologic lesions of the anterior tongue or oral cavity as well as problems of the temporomandibular joint may cause referred otalgia via the third division (mandibular nerve) and auriculotemporal branch of the trigeminal nerve. Lesions of the base of the tongue, tonsils, and tonsillar fossae may result in referred otalgia through the petrosal ganglion and Jacobson's branch of the glossopharyngeal nerve. Likewise, lesions of the hypopharynx and supraglottic area of the larynx may also cause ear pain by nociceptive signals transmitted via fibers of the jugular ganglion and Arnold's branch of the vagus nerve.

EVALUATION OF PATIENTS SUFFERING FROM FACIAL PAIN

A detailed and thorough medical history followed by a meticulous physical and neurologic exam are highly important in the evaluation of facial pain, even if a patient referred to the pain clinic has been already evaluated by other specialties. Considering the nature of most chronic facial pain entities, the most valuable information leading in an accurate diagnosis would emanate mainly from the patient's history. This requires very detailed and targeted questioning with regard to all aspects and descriptors of pain, including precipitating events, exact location and radiations, intensity, quality, temporal characteristics, and aggravating and alleviating factors. Treatments, which have been tried, with all specific details (such as medications and doses) and response to them should be recorded.

Special attention should be attributed to the exact location, frequency, and timing of attacks, associated symptoms as well as the subjective description of the quality of the pain since all these provide helpful differential diagnostic features. Pressure-like or aching pain commonly originates in inflamed cavities, while sharp, lancinating, and shooting pains are more suggestive of neuropathic or neuralgic pain. Throbbing pain is typical in vascular headaches. Burning and aching pain, worse with movement or chewing, suggests muscular pain. Associated symptoms, such as nausea and vomiting, fever, diplopia, lacrimation, nasal congestion, photophobia, and phonophobia, should be also noted. The presence of preceding symptoms, such as aura prior to the attacks may be suggestive of migraines. Precipitating, aggravating, and alleviating factors should be recorded also, since they not only guide diagnosis, but may be indicative of treatments as well.

Pertinent issues from the past medical history include information about prior head trauma, infections, tumors, or past surgeries. Any past or current coexistent medical conditions should also be documented as well as detailed information relevant to all previous and current medications, including the type, dose, and timing of use of over-the-counter analgesics, oral contraceptives, herbal medicines, and topical agents used on the head and face.

A complete family and social history with information about the use of tobacco, alcohol, and other drug use should follow. Psychological conditions, work-related information, and possible life stressors should be investigated next, and finally a complete review of systems should be obtained.

A physical examination should follow, within the context of which a complete head and neck exam and a neurologic examination are mandatory. With regard to the latter, the evaluation of all the cranial nerves needs special focus.

Furthermore, limited or asymmetric jaw opening as well as any crepitus in the temporomandibular joint with opening and closing of the mouth may be suggestive of TMJ disorders. Normal TMJ motion is nonpainful. With regards to the mobility of the TMJ, opening of the mandible allows normally an interincisal distance ranging between 3.5 and 5 cm, while closure is normally smooth with no lateral deviation of the midline of the mandible and no midline shift when the teeth move to maximal closure.

Inspection and percussion of the teeth may indicate pain originating from these organs, while inspection and palpation of the oral cavity, the cheeks, and the floor of the mouth may reveal ulcerations, tumors, or lymphadenopathy. Meticulous palpation over the face, with special attention to the muscles of mastication may reveal diffuse tenderness or specific tender or trigger points. The latter may provide targets for future injections as therapeutic interventions. Trigger points within the trapezius or posterior cervical triangle should be sought. The temporal arteries should be palpated for tenderness or nodules.

Findings from the medical history and examination should further guide the ordering of further laboratory tests and imaging studies as well as the possibility of referral to other health specialists, such as ENT surgeons, dentists, ophthalmologists, or neurologists. Imaging studies, depending on the indication, may include CT and MRI scans, and the latter may be helpful in ruling out intracranial pathology in patients with facial or head pain. Tenderness of the TMJ may be further evaluated by radiographic imaging of the joint. Pain in the face with atypic characters, abnormal cervical postures, and trigger points may be also evaluated with cervical spine imaging.

Psychological evaluation definitely also has an important role in the evaluation and treatment of selected patients with headache and facial pain, so referral to a specialist might be indicated in certain cases.

SPECIFIC CLINICAL ENTITIES RELATED TO FACIAL PAIN

Trigeminal Neuralgia

Trigeminal neuralgia was first reported by Aretaeus, a Greek physician from Capadocia, in the second century AD. Later, Dr. John Fothergill gave the first full and accurate description of trigeminal neuralgia in a report to the Medical Society in London in 1773. The 18th century French surgeon, Nicolaus Andre reported the condition as "tic douloureux," which means "painful spasm."

Trigeminal neuralgia is a rare condition, occurring in approximately 150 million people per year, and usually affects those over 50 years of age, although it may be seen also in younger individuals.

Clinical Characteristics

Trigeminal neuralgia is characterized by sudden, paroxysmal attacks of severe pain in the face lasting from a few seconds to a few minutes. The pain is unilaterally localized over one or more of the branches of the trigeminal nerve and is of severe intensity, and of a sharp, lancinating, stabbing, or burning quality. Between attacks the patient is completely asymptomatic, and with no neurologic manifestations of any kind, but several attacks can follow each other, in bursts, within minutes. The pain is completely absent during periods of remission, which can last days, weeks, months, even years. These pain-free periods are unpredictable, and without medical treatment, the pain usually returns. Most patients can identify factors (such as chewing food or eating, talking, washing the face, shaving, or brushing the teeth), which may precipitate the attacks by acting on specific trigger areas in the face or oral cavity. Also, even simple touch of these trigger points on the face may trigger attacks (Table 17-4).

Etiology of Trigeminal Neuralgia

Any traumatic condition affecting any branches of the trigeminal nerve may result in painful neuropathy with or without dysesthesia and/or anesthesia dolorosa. In several cases of trigeminal neuralgia, no underlying etiologic associations could be identified. In 2% to 4% of the cases, trigeminal neuralgia is a manifestation of multiple sclerosis, of which rarely it can be the first symptom, and is a sequela of neural demyelinization at the trigeminal nerve entry zone in the pons. Patients much younger than 50 years of age, or those with bilateral pain should be further evaluated with higher degree of suspicion for multiple sclerosis.

Other factors that have been implicated in the pathogenesis of trigeminal neuralgia include compression of the trigeminal ganglion or dorsal root entry zone by aberrant or ectatic blood vessels or tumors (usually posterior fossa meningiomas or neuromas) or traumatic injury to the trigeminal nerve fibers as a result of trauma or surgery. It has been suggested that pain secondary to vascular compression is usually of a more constant pattern and accompanied by allodynia and loss of sensation.

The International Association for the Study of Pain (IASP) distinguishes between primary trigeminal neuralgia (in which neuralgia from multiple sclerosis is also included) and secondary neuralgias caused by tumors or other lesions, except multiple sclerosis.

Diagnosis

The diagnosis of trigeminal neuralgia is mainly clinical, and most times made on the history alone. The diagnosis is clear in cases that manifest with the classical symptoms (sudden paroxysms of shooting or stabbing pain interrupted by pain-free intervals). In any case, a meticulous medical history is the most useful tool in establishing the diagnosis, but manifestations may cover a very wide spectrum ranging from the classical to other, atypic presentations. As a result, sometimes diagnosis is missed and made only after several years have gone by, and after patients have been seen by several health practitioners. In contrast, other times the condition is over-diagnosed as a result of misinterpretation of symptoms. Favorable response to carbamazepine has been used also as a criterion indicating the diagnosis of trigeminal neuralgia.

A thorough medical history as well as a meticulous physical and neurologic exam are essential. The exam is usually negative or noncontributory. There is no facial numbness or weakness. The presence of sensory deficits or cranial nerve dysfunction may be suggestive of secondary trigeminal neuropathies from traumatic, demyelinating, or other lesions, such as tumors. Not infrequently, observation of the nonverbal behavior of the patient reveals patterns, such as various "tics" or speech interruption, while some patients show aversion to touch on the face. Differential diagnosis includes painful conditions of the face (from the teeth, sinuses, nose, TMJ, etc.) as well as headaches of neuralgic nature or other cranial neuralgias, such as glossopharyngeal or occipital.

Initially, testing is required to rule out any serious conditions, and this may include an MRI scan with contrast, and/or a special MRI technique called high-definition MRI angiography (MRTA). The latter may identify whether the nerve is compressed by a blood vessel. Positive findings in MRTA usually correlate well with identification of neurovascular compression after posterior fossa surgical exploration.

Treatment

The initial treatment for trigeminal neuralgia is based on anticonvulsant medications, while most practitioners still consider carbamazepine as the drug of first choice, based on several studies. This is administered at

Table 17-4	Trigeminal Neuralgia
Clinical features	Sudden, paroxysmal attacks of severe pain in the face (unilaterally)
	Sharp, lancinating, stabbing, or burning quality
	Duration from a few seconds to a few minutes
	Between attacks asymptomatic
	Identifiable precipitating factors
Diagnosis	Medical history (most important)
	Physical and neurologic exam
	MRI scan
	MRI angiography
Treatment options	Anticonvulsants (carbamazepine, gabapentin, lamotrigine)
	Microvascular decompression
	Neurolytic injections or radiofrequency ablation
	Stereotactic neurosurgery ("Gamma knife")

daily doses of 400 to 1200 mg, after careful escalation, starting from doses 100 mg qd or bid. Patients should be monitored closely with repeated complete blood counts, since carbamazepine may produce hematologic toxicity (bone-marrow suppression). Nevertheless, considering the good safety profile of gabapentin as well as some existing evidence from the biomedical literature, the latter is also used first in selected patients, titrated to total daily doses of 900 to 3600 mg, starting from 300 mg daily. However, much lower doses and careful titration are needed in patients with renal impairment, considering the renal elimination of the drug.

Either medication should be initiated in escalating doses, titrated carefully, and patients should be warned about potential side effects. In case of treatment failure or intractable side effects it is reasonable to switch to the other. Baclofen and lamotrigine, also in escalating doses, are considered to be drugs of next choice.

Today, microvascular decompression has been established as an acceptable surgical method for treating this condition. This is performed after a suboccipital craniotomy, posterior fossa exposure, and mobilization and separation of the aberrant blood vessel compressing the nerve. Mortality of the procedure is less than 1%, while the incidence of cerebellar injury or VIII nerve injury is 0.5% to 0.8%. Most patients (87% to 98%) experience immediate pain relief, while at 1 or 2 years the incidence of complete pain relief is 75% to 80%. However, after 8 years, this proportion drops to about 60%. Some neurosurgeons attempt re-exploration and neuroablative procedures in the failed cases. Neuroablative procedures include injection of alcohol, glycerol, or phenol into the Meckel's cave, wherein the trigeminal ganglion resides. Radiofrequency gangliolysis, which involves a selective partial lesioning of the affected ganglion or retrogasserian root, is considered to be more precise and safer than the former techniques. The ganglion is approached with a radiofrequency needle through the foramen ovale under fluoroscopy, and after confirmation with electrical stimulation, a thermal lesioning is performed. Persisting dysesthesias, in approximately 8% of the patients, is the main complication of the technique, while anesthesia dolorosa or keratitis from corneal anesthesia occur less frequently (1% to 2%).

With regard to chemical neurolysis, the use of glycerol seems to be the most popular, but some studies indicate poor long-term results or more significant adverse effects (dysesthesias or keratitis).

Stereotactic radiosurgery (using the "gamma knife") has also been utilized to produce well-localized lesions in the trigeminal nerve, using 201 focused intercepting beams of gamma radiation. Other methods that have been tried include peripheral neurectomies or various nerve blocks with tetracaine, lidocaine, and streptomycin.

GLOSSOPHARYNGEAL NEURALGIA

Glossopharyngeal neuralgia resembles trigeminal neuralgia. It is characterized by pain attacks similar to those in trigeminal neuralgia, but located unilaterally in the distribution of the glossopharyngeal nerve. It is also much less common than trigeminal neuralgia. Pain of sharp, electric, or stabbing nature is most common in the posterior pharynx, soft palate, base of tongue, ear, mastoid, or side of the head. Swallowing, yawning, coughing, or phonation may trigger the pain. There is usually no abnormality on the physical exam, but oropharyngeal tumors may manifest with similar pain patterns. In 2% of the cases, glossopharyngeal neuralgia is bilateral. In this case, like in the trigeminal neuralgia, multiple sclerosis needs to be ruled out.

Etiology

Pain conveyed by the glossopharyngeal nerve may be secondary to conditions associated with nociception over its receptive field area, from tumors or inflammation, or may be a manifestation of a true neuralgia. The latter category includes various causes of neuropathic pain, including vascular compression of the nerve on its course from the medulla towards the jugular foramen. Glossopharyngeal neuralgia can also be seen, rarely, in patients with multiple sclerosis.

Diagnosis

Symptoms include pain with various neuropathic characteristics, such as "electrical shock"-like pain in the region of the tonsillar fossa, pharynx, or base of the tongue. It can radiate to the ear or the angle of the jaw or into the upper lateral neck. The trigger zone is often in the same area, and patients frequently report that swallowing, yawning, clearing the throat, or talking is the precipitating stimulus. The pain often appears to be spontaneous. Chewing or touching the face does not precipitate an attack.

Treatment

The pharmacologic management is the same as that for trigeminal neuralgia, based mainly on anticonvulsant medications (e.g., carbamazepine, gabapentin, lamotrigine). In refractory cases, suboccipital craniectomy with exploration of the glossopharyngeal nerve for microvascular decompression has been tried.

TEMPORAL ARTERITIS

Temporal arteritis, also known as "giant cell arteritis" is an inflammatory condition that affects the medium-sized arteries that supply the head, eye, and optic nerve. The exact cause is unclear. The disease usually affects the elderly and is associated with inflammatory changes in arteries of the face and head. The pathophysiology leading to clinical manifestations includes decreased blood flow leading to jaw or tongue claudication, scalp tenderness, and visual changes with anterior ischemic optic neuropathy, amaurosis, or optic atrophy leading to blindness in as many as 60% of patients.

Histologically, it is characterized by a granulomatous inflammatory process that is most pronounced along the internal elastic lamina of the arterial wall. Temporal artery biopsy demonstrates a predominance of mononuclear cells or multinucleated giant cells with fragmentation of the intima. Inflammation may be followed by intimal proliferation and eventual stenosis or occlusion of the involved arterial segment.

Diagnosis

The clinical manifestations of temporal arteritis include pain in the head, face, periorbital area, or jaw, which occurs daily and is of moderate to severe intensity. This may be accompanied by jaw or tongue claudication, various visual disturbances, scalp sensitivity, fatigue, and various nonspecific complaints with a general sense of illness. The pain is usually unilateral, but less frequently can be bilateral or occipital in location. The quality is of a continuous aching nature, with occasional sharp, shooting paroxysms. Because the pain may be similar to that encountered in cluster headaches, the latter should be included in the differential diagnosis, although it tends to occur in much younger patients (Table 17-5).

Erythrocyte sedimentation rate (ESR), angiography, and biopsy may be helpful in the diagnosis. Diagnostic criteria, established by the American College of Rheumatology, may facilitate the diagnosis. Identification of 3 out of 5 of the following criteria may establish the diagnosis with a sensitivity and specificity higher than 90%:
1. Age older than 50 years
2. New onset of localized headache
3. Tenderness over the temporal artery or decreased temporal arterial pulse
4. Increased erythrocyte sedimentation rate (>50 mm/h)
5. Arterial biopsy showing necrotizing arteritis characterized by a predominance of mononuclear cell infiltrates or a granulomatous process

Treatment

The treatment is based chiefly on steroid administration. Glucocorticoids, administered in relatively high doses, usually reduce significantly the manifestations of temporal arteritis, including the pain. Failure to respond to steroid therapy with a negative biopsy should place the diagnosis into question. It has also been suggested that if the diagnosis seems likely based on history and physical examination, steroids should be started immediately to avoid vision loss, which may occur in 30% of untreated cases. Steroids are then tapered to a maintenance dosing after pain resolves and ESR normalizes. The disease is usually active for 1 to 2 years, during which time steroids should be continued to prevent vision loss. Angioplasty and stent placement have been also used in patients with symptoms of ischemia who have not responded well to steroids.

ATYPIC FACIAL PAIN

Atypic facial pain is nothing but "facial pain of unknown origin." This diagnosis is based not on positive identification, but is reached by elimination, after other recognizable entities causing pain in the face have been ruled out by a reasonable differential diagnostic process.

Atypic facial pain is often described as burning, aching, or cramping, usually occurs on one side of the face, often in the region of the trigeminal nerve, and can extend into the upper neck or the scalp. The term is applied by some physicians to pain that has features, or an area of distribution, that are not suggestive of other identifiable disorders. Any apparently nerve-related pain that crosses the midline of the face may fall into this category. In this condition usually no specific cause can be identified.

Differential Diagnosis

Differential diagnosis describes patients diagnosed as suffering from atypic facial pain who perceive pain in the territory of innervation of the trigeminal nerve, but the symptoms and signs are not typical of trigeminal neuralgia. The location of pain is within the area of the trigeminal innervation. The intensity of the pain may be as severe as in the trigeminal neuralgia, but the temporal pattern and quality of pain are different—the duration of

Table 17-5 Temporal Arteritis

Diagnostic criteria (3 out of 5 required for diagnosis):
1. Age older than 50 years.
2. New onset of localized headache.
3. Tenderness over the temporal artery or decreased temporal arterial pulse.
4. Increased erythrocyte sedimentation rate (>50 mm/h).
5. Arterial biopsy showing necrotizing arteritis with mononuclear cell infiltrates or a granulomatous process.

the individual painful episodes facilitates the distinction. Whereas trigeminal neuralgia is characterized by quick episodes of shooting, stabbing, or lancinating pain, atypic facial pain is usually more constant, and of burning, dull, or aching quality. Furthermore, the attacks or episodes of the atypic facial pain usually last longer than a few seconds, commonly minutes or hours, and occasionally are continuous. It is important to distinguish atypic facial pain from trigeminal neuralgia because of different treatment choices between the two conditions.

Another variation of atypic facial pain includes painful sensations with qualities similar to those of trigeminal neuralgia (shooting, stabbing, lancinating) but in locations other than the area of innervation by the trigeminal nerve. Many of these painful conditions may represent neuralgias of other nerves.

Atypic facial pain should also be distinguished from TMJ syndrome, migraine, and cluster headaches, in addition to trigeminal neuralgia. The incidence and prevalence of atypic facial pain is much lower than that of the trigeminal neuralgia, although there is no consensus on that due to lack of agreement on criteria for classification. Males and females are affected with equal frequency.

With regard to the distinction from TMJ syndrome, the location and quality of pain may be quite similar between the two conditions; nevertheless, pain from TMJ syndrome is usually aggravated by activity, such as chewing, talking, and lateral movements of the mandible, while this is not the case in the atypic facial pain. The former condition also may be associated with focal tenderness on one or both temporomandibular joints.

Migraine can be differentiated from atypic facial pain, on the basis of recurrent, severe unilateral pain on one side of the head, with normal neurologic examination, most commonly prevalent in females. Aura usually precedes the onset of migraines, some scalp tenderness may be present, and in most cases nausea, photophobia, and phonophobia are common characteristic-associated symptoms, usually not present in atypic facial pain. Finally, pharmacologic therapy effective for migraine, including serotonin receptor agonists, is ineffective in atypic facial pain.

Cluster headache is another condition, which in terms of pain location and quality sometimes may be confused with atypic facial pain. Characteristics of cluster headaches, helpful in differential diagnosis, include a higher prevalence in males (6:1), intense, crushing, or burning quality, frequent recurrence up to several times a day in clusters of several days to weeks, and accompanying conjunctival injection and nasal congestion.

In patients suffering from atypic facial pain physical and neurologic examinations are usually normal or noncontributory. Trigger points are rare. Significant tenderness at one or both temporomandibular joints is indicative of TMJ syndrome. Imaging studies, such as MRI scans or CT scans, can be helpful in ruling out tumors or other lesions. Most times, patients also need proper psychological or psychiatric evaluation.

Treatment

Medical management of atypic facial pain is not as successful as that of trigeminal neuralgia, reflecting the unclear pathophysiology and etiologic associations of the former disorder. Both pharmacologic and psychotherapeutic approaches should be considered, reflecting the nature of this condition.

Opioids or other drugs with addictive properties should be avoided or patients should be gradually weaned-off. In case patients exhibit any signs of addiction, referral to an addiction specialist is necessary.

Tricyclic antidepressants may be a reasonable choice in most patients as well as trial of an anticonvulsant, such as gabapentin, in case of the presence of suggestive qualitative characteristics of the pain. For example, in case of lancinating or electrical-shooting quality of pain in an atypic location, gabapentin, lamotrigine, or carbamazepine may be reasonable choices for a trial. Traditionally, it has been considered that painful sensations of a continuous, burning nature are more likely to respond to tricyclic antidepressants. The majority of patients (75%) usually respond to the latter. For pain of a more aching or dull nature, nonsteroidal anti-inflammatory drugs or acetaminophen may be tried. Depending on the circumstances pertaining in each particular patient, psychotherapy, physical therapy, or biofeedback may also be beneficial.

Trigger points, indicative of a facial myofascial condition, should be sought in a meticulous physical exam and treated with local anesthetic injections. Opioid medications should be avoided.

HEADACHE SYNDROMES WITH FACIAL PAIN

Tension-Type Headache

Tension-type headache is the most common type of headache and sometimes needs to be distinguished from conditions presenting with pain in the face. Within a lifetime period, this type of headache affects approximately 70% of men and 90% of women. This disorder can be episodic or chronic and is distinguished from other headaches or conditions that manifest with pain in the face by its quality (pressing or tightening), intensity (mild to moderate), location (bilateral, over the temples), and duration (30 minutes to 7 days) of the pain. Usually there is no nausea, vomiting, photophobia, or phonophobia.

Migraine

Migraines are prevalent in 17% of the female and 6% of male population, usually starting in the second or third decade. Headaches are of moderate to severe intensity, unilateral, and of a pulsating quality. Attacks last from 4 to 72 hours, accompanied by nausea, vomiting, photophobia, or phonophobia and may be preceded by aura (most commonly with visual disturbances). Various triggering factors, such as stress, certain foods (e.g., red wine, cheese), hormonal factors (e.g., menstruation, pregnancy, oral contraceptive pills), infections, trauma, and various environmental factors have been implicated in precipitating the attacks. Changes in the serotoninergic transmission in the central nervous system have been implicated in the pathogenesis of the condition, and serotoninergic agents (sumatriptan) are helpful in the therapy.

Cluster Headache

Cluster headache, another condition that needs to be considered in the differential diagnosis of pain in the face, is characterized by attacks of severe pain, of burning quality, usually unilateral, in the orbit, supraorbital, or temporal area. It is more common in males. Attacks last from 15 to 180 minutes and may follow an episodic or chronic pattern. Symptoms of autonomic hyperactivity (e.g., lacrimation, nasal congestion, rhinorrhea, conjunctival injection, forehead and facial sweating, miosis, ptosis, or eyelid edema) usually accompany the attacks. Frequency of the attacks ranges between 1 every 2 days to several per day. Nausea and vomiting is uncommon and there is no aura. Attacks may be precipitated by alcohol. Treatments aim at preventing or aborting attacks, and include trials of calcium channel blockers, low-dose daily ergotamine, lithium carbonate, anticonvulsants, antihistamines, and glucocorticoids. Oxygen inhalation, serotonin receptor agonists, intranasal lidocaine instillation, and sphenopalatine ganglion blocks have also been used with success in the management of cluster headaches.

Chronic Daily Headache

Chronic daily headache is described as occurring at least 6 days a week for a period of at least 6 months, as bilateral, frontal, or occipital, nonthrobbing, and of moderate intensity pain. The pain is associated with the overuse or abuse of many common prescription or over-the-counter analgesics (e.g., aspirin, acetaminophen, ibuprofen), barbiturates, and opioid analgesics. A meticulous history usually reveals the problems and indicates a transformation of the original head or facial pain to a new, qualitatively different headache.

The treatment is based on the weaning off of the causative medication. Psychotherapy, physical therapy, biofeedback, and tricyclic antidepressants may be helpful.

SUGGESTED READING

Burchiel KJ: A new classification for facial pain. Neurosurgery 53:1164-1166, 2003.

Filipchuk D: Classic trigeminal neuralgia: a surgical perspective. J Neurosci Nurs 35:82-86, 2003.

Haddox JD, Biondi DM: Facial pain. In Abram SE, Haddox JD (eds): The Pain Clinic Manual, 2nd ed. Philadelphia, Lippincott Williams & Wilkins, 2000, pp 20-212.

Horowitz M, Horowitz M, Ochs M, et al: Trigeminal neuralgia and glossopharyngeal neuralgia: two orofacial pain syndromes encountered by dentists. J Am Dent Assoc 135:1427-1433, 2004.

Jaaskelainen SK: Clinical neurophysiology and quantitative sensory testing in the investigation of orofacial pain and sensory function. J Orofacial Pain 18:85-107, 2004.

Liu JK, Apfelbaum RI: Treatment of trigeminal neuralgia. Neurosurgical Clinics N America 15:319-334, 2004.

Loeser JD: Cranial neuralgias. In Bonica JJ (ed): The Management of Pain, 2nd ed. Philadelphia, Lea and Febiger, 1990.

Madland G, Feinmann C: Chronic facial pain: a multidisciplinary problem. J Neurol Neurosurg Psychiatry 71:716-719, 2001.

Pollock BE: Percutaneous retrogasserian glycerol rhizotomy for patients with idiopathic trigeminal neuralgia: a prospective analysis of factors related to pain relief. J Neurosurg 102:223-228, 2005.

Rozen TD: Trigeminal neuralgia and glossopharyngeal neuralgia. Neurol Clinics 22:185-206, 2004.

Spiera R, Spiera H: Inflammatory disease in older adults. Cranial arteritis. Geriatrics 59:25-29, 2004.

Turp JC, Kowalski CJ, Stohler CS: Pain descriptors characteristic of persistent facial pain. J Orofacial Pain 11:285-290, 1997.

Wahlund K, List T, Dworkin SF: Temporomandibular disorders in children and adolescents: reliability of a questionnaire, clinical examination, and diagnosis. J Orofacial Pain 12:42-51, 1998.

CHAPTER 18

Central Pain

STEPHEN E. ABRAM
RANDA NOSEIR

CENTRAL POSTSTROKE PAIN

Central poststroke pain (CPSP), for many years known as thalamic pain, was eloquently described by Dejerine[1] and his students in the early 20th century. It is fairly common and is characterized by severe unilateral pain and sensory disturbance that is frequently refractory to treatment. Loss of temperature perception and spontaneous and evoked dysesthesias are very common among CPSP patients.

Incidence and Epidemiology

Poststroke pain occurs in about 8% of stroke patients and 18% of patients following strokes that are accompanied by somatosensory disturbances. Pain is moderate to severe in only 5% of cases. Nevertheless, with a stroke prevalence of 5 per 1000 in the general population, it represents an important public health concern. In one study, patients who developed CPSP were found to be younger (median age 57) than the average stroke patient (median age 75). However, another study failed to show such a difference. The onset of pain is usually delayed, usually for 1 to several months following the stroke. Less than half of cases involve thalamic strokes. Brainstem lesions and injury to extrathalamic supratentorial structures are fairly common antecedents to poststroke pain.

Pathophysiology

Several theories have been proposed to explain poststroke pain, none of which can be proven conclusively. Bursting activity in thalamic relay cells that project to the cortex are thought to occur in response to changes in inputs to these neurons. This can occur if there is loss of input to the reticular nucleus, a shell-shaped group of γ-aminobutyric acid (GABA)-ergic cells surrounding the dorsal and lateral aspects of the thalamus, that ordinarily inhibit activity of relay neurons. Changes in activity of the reticular nucleus can result from injury to corticospinal fibers or from injury to spinothalamocortical projections. Thus, lesions in the spinal cord, thalamus, or cortex can lead to similar pain syndromes.

Treatment

Antidepressants

Tricyclic antidepressants (TCAs) are considered by many physicians to be the first line treatment for CPSP. Amitriptyline was the first drug shown to be effective in CPSP in a placebo-controlled trial. Significant improvement compared to placebo was documented after 2 weeks of treatment. Selective serotonin reuptake inhibitor (SSRI) antidepressants have not been studied for this condition, but in light of their relative lack of efficacy for other types of neuropathic pain, they are not likely to be of benefit for CPSP. However, venlafaxine and duloxetine, which have substantial norepinephrine reuptake inhibitory effects, may be more likely to be effective. Data regarding these drugs in CPSP is lacking.

Anticonvulsants

There is anecdotal evidence for the benefit of gabapentin in CPSP. Lamotrigine was effective in a single, small placebo-controlled trial. Carbamazepine was shown to be of limited benefit in a placebo-controlled trial. Several newer anticonvulsants, including topiramate, zonisamide, oxcarbazepine, tiagabine, pregabalin, and levetiracetam have been useful in some patients with neuropathic pain states and are reasonable options for patients who are resistant to amitriptyline or gabapentin.

Antiarrhythmics

Intravenous lidocaine has been shown to be transiently effective in several studies. One study showed efficacy for both spontaneous and evoked pain, while another only reduced the severity of tactile allodynia and mechanical hyperalgesia. Mexiletine was beneficial in only one study.

Opioids

Most discussions of opioid use for CPSP indicate that the condition is poorly responsive. One study of 15 patients demonstrated initial improvement in seven cases, but only three experienced any relief for a year or more. As with other central pain states, the general consensus is that most patients respond poorly, but a small minority may experience significant and lasting relief. There is considerable evidence from animal models that opioids may produce a hyperalgesic state with prolonged use, particularly when administered to nerve-injured animals.

NMDA Antagonists

Low-dose ketamine produced temporary relief in about half of a group of CPSP patients. One case report documented improvement in pain in a patient treated with long-term oral ketamine at a dose of 50 mg three times a day. There is no information regarding other drugs with NMDA-antagonist effects, such as dextromethorphan, amantadine, memantine, or methadone.

Motor Cortex Stimulation

Motor cortex stimulation has been reported to be efficacious in over 50% of CPSP patients in several small case series.

PAIN AFTER SPINAL-CORD INJURY

Classification of Spinal-Cord Injury Pain

While there is no widely accepted classification scheme for pain following spinal-cord injury (SCI), the International Association for the Study of Pain has proposed categorizing it into neuropathic and non-neuropathic. Neuropathic pain is subdivided into three categories: at the level of injury, below the level of injury, and above the level of injury. Nociceptive pain is further divided into somatic or musculoskeletal pain and visceral pain. In cases of complete spinal-cord transsection, all nociceptive pain is located above the level of injury, and, with few exceptions, treated no differently than nociceptive pain in non-SCI patients. Similarly, neuropathic pain whose source is above the level of the cord injury is likely to be treated like neuropathic pain in non-SCI patients. Pain that arises at or below the level of the cord injury is more likely to fit the definition of central pain, is refractory to most therapies, and will be the focus of this discussion.

Pathophysiology

A wide variety of anatomic and functional changes occur after injury to the spinal cord. Transsection of tracts leads to Wallerian degeneration. Less complete injury leads to loss of myelin and Schwann cells, permitting cross talk between adjacent axons. Denervation of afferent fibers supplying higher centers in the spinal cord or brain leads to deafferentation hyperexcitability. Neuronal plasticity is stimulated, leading to sprouting of axons, a high proportion of which contain neurotransmitters that are typical of nociceptors.

Following injury to the central nervous system (CNS), exceedingly high concentrations of excitatory amino acids are released. These compounds initiate a cascade of neuronal events leading to sensitization of remaining neurons and to long-term potentiation. Some of these changes are mediated by NMDA-receptor activation, and early administration of NMDA antagonists have been shown to block the development of allodynia and hyperalgesia in animal SCI models. Inhibitory neurons in the CNS, such as GABA-ergic cells, are particularly susceptible to injury from high levels of glutamate. Other substances that are found in high concentrations after SCI include calcium, reactive oxygen species (ROS), nitric oxide (NO), protein kinase C, substance P, and dynorphin, all of which are capable of either neuronal sensitization or inhibition of or injury to inhibitory interneurons.

Any injury to the CNS initiates intense activation of glial cells. Microglia are initially activated, producing proinflammatory cytokines, NO, chemokines, ROS, and prostaglandins. Glutamate transport systems are inactivated, leading to increased concentrations of excitatory amino acids in the vicinity, contributing to the enhanced excitotoxicity. Changes in the blood brain barrier permit the influx of inflammatory cells and antibodies from the blood stream, further contributing to the inflammatory process and to the subsequent degree of injury. Astrocytes are subsequently activated, thus prolonging the processes that can lead to prolonged hypersensitivity of neurons in the spinal cord.

Spontaneous and evoked pain associated with SCI is poorly responsive to opioids. Chronic administration of opioids has been shown to initiate both neuronal and glial mediated hyperalgesia. Similarly, hyperalgesia initiated by either NMDA-receptor activation or glial-cell activation is affected minimally by opioid administration. Even spinally-administered opioids have little effect on the hypersensitivity induced by ischemic injury to the spinal cord.

Some of the most widely accepted pain mechanisms involved in SCI pain are shown in Box 18-1.

Box 18-1   Pathophysiologic Mechanisms of Chronic Pain in Spinal-Cord Injury

Denervation hypersensitivity and spontaneous activity of higher CNS neurons

Regeneration and sprouting involving nociceptors disproportionately

Excitotoxicity (glutamate) causing loss of non-nociceptive neurons and inhibitory cells

Ephaptic transmission (cross-talk) between injured axons

NMDA-mediated sensitization of spinal-cord pain projection cells

Glial activation with production of proinflammatory cytokines, other mediators

Loss of descending inhibitory pathways leading to sensory disinhibition, autonomic dysfunction and muscle spasm

---

At-Level Pain

Neurons in the dorsal horn of the spinal cord just above the level of experimental spinal-cord transsection show hyper-responsiveness to afferent activation, prolongation of after-discharge responses, and marked increases in spontaneous activity. Those neurons that exhibit abnormal spontaneous activity can not be activated by stimulation of peripheral nerves, suggesting that their abnormal activity is the result of deafferentation, possibly by injury to the adjacent dorsal roots or dorsal root ganglia (DRG). Abnormal spontaneous activity has also been recorded from human dorsal horn neurons just rostral to the level of cord injury. This abnormal hypersensitivity and background activity is the basis for the use of dorsal root entry zone lesions as a therapy for at-level pain.

Below-Level Pain

It has been theorized that interruption of spinothalamic tracts leads to hypersensitivity of deafferented centers in the thalamus. Spinothalamic tractotomy has been shown to produce exaggerated spontaneous and evoked firing in the ventrobasal thalamus. Allodynia and hyperalgesia often occur after cordotomy in humans. There is also evidence that interruption of the dorsal columns contributes to below-level pain. Various stimuli, particularly visceral stimulation, such as bladder distension, can induce or exacerbate pain. Stimulation of a few remaining ascending fibers appears to drive deafferented neurons to high firing rates.

There appears to be considerable correlation between at-level and below-level pain. At-level pain often appears first, followed by below-level pain or a combination of both. At-level pain generators may be important in the initiation and maintenance of pain perceived below the cord lesion. Evidence for a pain generator in the region just rostral to the cord transsection comes from the observation that spinal anesthesia that extends above the level of injury relieves below-level pain in some SCI patients while anesthesia that affects only levels below the transsection has no effect.

Treatment

Pain associated with SCI is one of the most difficult painful disorders to treat. Recommended therapies at best provide modest reduction in pain. For many patients there is little or no relief.

Pharmacologic Treatment
Antidepressants

TCAs are uniformly recommended for pain following SCI, and there is anecdotal evidence that they can be effective. However, in the only controlled trials comparing antidepressants to placebo, neither amitriptyline nor trazodone was effective. Nevertheless, it is reasonable to initiate therapy with a TCA, particularly if sleep disruption is a significant problem. In addition to the usual side effects of drowsiness and xerostomia, SCI patients may have problems with increased spasticity and urinary retention.

Anticonvulsants

The only controlled trials of antidepressants failed to show significant improvement with valproate or lamotrigine. There are case reports of benefit from carbamazepine. Gabapentin has been tried fairly extensively, but its effects have been disappointing. Since it is effective for a variety of peripheral neuropathic conditions, one might expect better results in patients with incomplete cord injuries or with at-level pain.

NMDA Antagonists

Ketamine has been shown to transiently reduce SCI pain. Patients who experience relief from intravenous trials of subdissociative doses (10 to 40 mg) may benefit from chronic oral administration. The oral dose is titrated to an amount that provides pain relief without significant psychotomimetic effects. This is generally in the 30 to 60 mg range. Since there is no oral preparation available, the injectable form can be measured and diluted in water or juice. Several opioids, including methadone and propoxyphene, have NMDA-antagonist effects, and may have some beneficial effects independent of their opioid-agonist properties. Dextromethorphan, amantadine, and memantine all have NMDA-antagonist effects, but none have been shown to be particularly helpful in SCI pain.

Sodium Channel Blockers

Intravenous lidocaine has been shown to reduce spontaneous pain in SCI patients. It is less effective in blocking mechanical allodynia. There is little data regarding the effects of mexiletine on SCI pain.

Opioids

Systemic opioids are clearly less effective for SCI pain than for nociceptive pain. One study reported that intravenous morphine had no effect on spontaneous pain but provided some reduction in mechanical allodynia. A randomized controlled trial showed that intravenous alfentanil provided better analgesia in neuropathic SCI pain than placebo. However, no studies have evaluated the use of chronic opioid administration in SCI patients. Typically, they experience slight to modest benefit at the initiation of therapy, but become rapidly tolerant. It is likely that chronic opioid administration produces hyperalgesia in some patients with SCI and neuropathic pain.

Intrathecal Drug Administration

An early study of spinal morphine administration in SCI patients reported reduction in pain and spasticity in 8 of 12 patients. Six patients had good long-term results with minimal development of tolerance. A more recent study reported minimal benefit from intrathecal morphine or clonidine alone, but significant benefit when the two drugs were administered together. Intrathecal baclofen has been shown to be effective for spasticity and for muscle spasm-induced pain in SCI patients. In addition, central pain that is unrelated to muscle spasm is significantly reduced in some patients. Baclofen may provide still better analgesia when combined with morphine or clonidine. When there is some preservation of function below the level of cord injury the addition of low concentrations of bupivacaine to the intrathecal infusion may be of some benefit. The initial human trials of intrathecal ziconotide, an ω-conopeptide that selectively blocks N-type calcium channels, showed significant pain reduction in patients who were resistant to spinal opioids. Patients with SCI pain were among those who showed a beneficial response.

Surgical Intervention

Cordectomy

Resection of the spinal cord at or just above the injured segment is sometimes successful for treating pain perceived at the level of the injury. Occasionally, it is helpful for pain below the injured segment, but this is less likely. It is postulated that cordectomy is effective when there is an ectopic generator of abnormal neuronal activity in cord segments adjacent to the cord injury.

Dorsal Root Entry Zone Lesions

Dorsal root entry zone (DREZ) lesions have been used mainly for patients with brachial plexus avulsion injuries. It is thought to provide relief by destroying cells responsible for initiating spontaneous activity. The procedure consists of creating multiple small radiofrequency lesions in the dorsal horn at the site where the nerve rootlets enter the cord. In SCI, this procedure works best in patients with at-level pain and in patients with unilateral pain. It is less effective in patients with below-level pain.

Spinal-Cord Stimulation

Implanted spinal-cord stimulators have provided some benefit for patients with at-level pain and in patients with incomplete cord lesions. Pain perceived below the level of transsection in patients with complete lesions is poorly responsive.

PHANTOM LIMB PAIN

Amputation of a limb is associated with a high incidence of persistent postoperative pain. Phantom limb pain, or pain perceived to originate in the absent limb, is generally considered to be a form of central pain, while stump pain is usually thought of as a peripheral somatic or neuropathic type of pain. It is likely, however, that both central and peripheral mechanisms contribute to both types of pain.

Following amputation, phantom sensations are nearly always present. They are well-defined and, at least early in the postoperative course, quite vivid. Fortunately, most phantom sensations are not painful. When phantom limb pain occurs, it is often severe, very distressing, and difficult to treat.

Epidemiology and Pain Characteristics

Phantom limb pain has been reported to be as low as 2% and as high as 97%. Most series report an incidence of 60% to 80%. Some patients fail to report phantom limb pain for fear that they will be thought of as mentally disturbed by physicians or family members. This is particularly true of patients who experience somewhat strange painful sensations, such as a tightly clenched fist with fingernails digging into the palm or tight bands around the fingers or toes. It is helpful, therefore, to discuss this condition with the patient preoperatively. There is no difference in incidence associated with age or gender. Some studies have demonstrated higher likelihood of phantom pain with more proximal surgery, especially following hemipelvectomy or hip disarticulation.

Several series have indicated that the incidence of phantom limb pain is higher among patients who had severe or prolonged pain before amputation. For this reason, some researchers have attempted to determine whether preemptive regional analgesia might reduce the incidence. One study compared patients undergoing epidural analgesia 3 days preoperatively and continued through the operation to patients treated with epidural anesthesia begun immediately preoperatively. The incidence and duration of phantom pain was higher in the group that did not receive prolonged block, but the numbers were insufficient to show a significant difference. While some patients report phantom pain that is similar in quality and location to their pre-existing pain, this is certainly not true of all patients.

In the large majority of patients, phantom pain begins within a few days of amputation. Some patients, however, can experience the onset months or even years later. The pain is constant in some patients, but is usually intermittent. Pain is most often experienced at least several times a day but is occasionally felt only every few days or even weeks. The quality of the pain is quite variable and occasionally very unusual, sometimes taking the form of painful distortions of the limb. Pain is usually felt in the distal part of the limb, most often involving the hand or foot, occasionally the ankle or wrist.

The duration of phantom limb pain is variable, but often very prolonged. While pain subsides spontaneously in weeks or a few months in some patients, it is not uncommon for pain to persist for 10 years or more. Typically, the frequency and duration of attacks diminishes with time, but the intensity often remains constant. With time, the phantom limb is often perceived to "telescope" proximally, with shortening of the limb but preservation of perception of the hand or foot.

The epidemiology and characteristics of phantom limb pain are reviewed in Box 18-2.

Pathophysiology

While phantom limb pain is thought to be primarily a central type of pain, peripheral contributions are evident. In some patients, cessation of the phantom pain coincides with healing of pathologic processes in the stump. Neuroma formation in the stump is nearly inevitable. Neuromas formed after nerve transsection in animals have been shown to be foci of spontaneous nerve activity. In addition, changes in excitability of cells in the DRG, including persistent spontaneous activity originating from DRG cells, occur following nerve transsection. It is likely that such neural activity contributes to phantom pain sensations. Palpation or percussion of stump neuromas often reproduces phantom pain, and local anesthetic block of the neuroma or associated nerve relieves phantom pain in some patients.

Sympathetic nervous system activation is associated with increased firing of neurons originating in a neuroma. Similarly, local infiltration of norepinephrine around a neuroma activates some axons to very high firing rates. In addition, following nerve injury in animals, sympathetic nerve sprouts appear in the DRG, most in close proximity to neuronal cell somata. While it is not known how these changes affect sensory processing, it is likely that such neuronal plasticity changes are related to certain types of persistent pain. Indeed, some patients

---

Box 18-2   Epidemiology and Characteristics of Phantom Limb Pain

Incidence: 60% to 80%.
Usually felt in distal limb.
Quality: Shooting, throbbing, stabbing, squeezing, burning.
Painful distortions of the limb may be felt.
Onset: 1 to 2 weeks postoperatively. May be delayed after months or years.
Sometimes subsides in a few weeks. Often persists many years.
More common when preoperative pain present; often resembles preoperative pain.

with phantom limb pain experience reduction or relief of pain following sympathetic blockade.

Sensitization of neurons in the dorsal horn probably plays an important role in the pathophysiology of phantom limb pain. Intense nociceptive inputs from tissue injury or nerve damage can lead to activation of neuronal and glial mechanisms of hyperalgesia. Deafferentation of projection neurons in the spinal cord and brain predispose to spontaneous firing.

Reorganization of centers in the thalamus and cortex that are responsive to nociceptive inputs undergo reorganization following amputation. In animal models, there is expansion of regions that are responsive to painful stimuli, and these regions become hyper-responsive to peripheral inputs. Cortical reorganization has been observed in humans following amputation using magnetoencephalography.

Treatment

Medical Therapy

TCAs are mentioned in nearly all discussions of medication therapy for phantom limb pain. An uncontrolled trial of doxepin was reported to be helpful, but no controlled trials have been done. A variety of anticonvulsants have been used, and case reports of benefit from carbamazepine in individual patients have been reported, but no controlled trials are available. Drugs that are commonly used for peripheral neuropathic pain, including gabapentin, lamotrigine, and topiramate are often tried. Substantial benefit is uncommon with either the anticonvulsants or TCAs. SSRIs are generally ineffective for neuropathic pain and are unlikely to benefit patients with phantom limb pain. The sodium channel blocker mexiletine was shown to provide some relief in a single open label study.

NMDA antagonists are of theoretic benefit since they can block or reverse central sensitization associated with nerve injury. Ketamine can be administered orally or intravenously at subdissociative doses. Memantine was shown to be more effective than placebo for postamputation pain. Dextromethorphan has been used with limited success in neuropathic pain, but there is no data regarding its use for phantom pain.

Opioids are considerably less effective for phantom limb pain than for nociceptive pain, and there is substantial concern about opioid induced hyperalgesia in neuropathic and central-pain states. However, there are patients who obtain some benefit from them. They should be reserved for patients who obtain substantial relief with relatively low doses and who do not require substantial dose escalation over time. Methadone, which has some NMDA-antagonist effect, might be a reasonable opioid choice.

Calcitonin was reported to provide pain relief when administered soon after the onset of phantom limb pain. Nonsteroidal anti-inflammatory drugs have been uniformly ineffective.

Other Therapies

Transcutaneous electrical nerve stimulation (TENS) is occasionally helpful, although it is more likely to provide benefit for stump pain than for phantom limb pain. Spinal-cord stimulation is beneficial for some patients, although the success rate is low compared to other conditions, such as radiculopathy and complex regional pain syndrome. There is anecdotal evidence for benefit from acupuncture and from surface electrical stimulation of acupuncture points.

Local anesthetic blocks rarely provide more than temporary benefit. Deafferentation can be associated with pain aggravation. It is not uncommon for phantom pain to appear or to be aggravated during spinal anesthesia. There is limited evidence that sympathetic blocks performed soon after the onset of phantom pain can be effective.

Cognitive strategies, including hypnosis and distraction techniques, as well as biofeedback and relaxation training can be useful therapies. Since the chances of treatment success with medical or surgical interventions is low, it is important that patients receive supportive psychotherapy to help them cope with pain and to avoid becoming inactive and isolated.

Neuroablative techniques are rarely beneficial and are associated with a high incidence of adverse effects. Neuroma resection is occasionally beneficial for stump pain, rarely for phantom pain. Rhizotomy, DREZ lesions, cordotomy, and sympathectomy have all been used with very limited success.

REFERENCE

1. Dejerine J, Roussy G: Le syndrome thalamique. Rev Neurol 14:521–532, 1906.

SUGGESTED READING

Anderson G, Vestergaard K, Ingeman-Nielsen M, Jensen TS: Incidence of central post-stroke pain. Pain 61:187–193, 1995.

Boivie J, Leijon G, Johansson I: Central post-stroke pain—a study of mechanisms through analyses of the sensory abnormalities. Pain 37:173–185, 1989.

Bowsher D: Central pain: clinical and physiological characteristics. J Neurol Neurosurg Psychiat 61:62–69, 1996.

Burchiel KJ, Hsu PK: Pain and spasticity after spinal-cord injury. Spine 26:S146–S160, 2001.

Finnerup NB, Jensen TS: Spinal-cord injury pain—mechanisms and treatment. Eur J Neurol 11:73–82, 2004.

Hansson P: Post-stroke pain case study: clinical characteristics, therapeutic options and long-term follow-up. Eur J Neurol 11(Suppl 1):22–30, 2004.

Hord AH, Shannon C: Phantom Pain. In Raj PP (ed): Practical Management of Pain. St. Louis, Mosby, 2000, pp 212–222.

Nikolajsen L, Jensen TS: Phantom limb pain. Br J Anaesth 87:107–116, 2001.

CHAPTER 19

Painful Medical Diseases

THOMAS J. WHALEN

INTRODUCTION

The medical illnesses considered in this chapter are in general chronic and associated with long-term nociceptive stimulation and/or neuropathic mechanisms that may be either continuous or intermittent. Prolonged nociceptive stimulation causes the peripheral and central changes that are routinely associated with the emergence of peripheral and central sensitization. Therefore, these diseases may each have components of somatic, visceral, neuropathic, and central pain. Long-term treatment often results in tolerance to medications used for treatment. Acute exacerbations of pain may be difficult to control with medications, especially if the underlying disease is poorly controlled. Behavioral and/or psychological problems (including substance abuse) may have preceded the onset of the medical illness or may develop as a result of the illness. It is in the patient's best interest to approach treatment from a multidisciplinary approach, including in the treatment model, the treating physician, psychiatry and psychology, rehabilitation techniques, and other tools, such as stress reduction, acupuncture, neuromodulation, and massage.

PANCREATITIS

Acute Pancreatitis

Acute pancreatitis has a prevalence of 4.8 to 24.2 cases per 100,000 people. Pancreatitis can present in childhood, but is more often a disease of adults. The predominant causes are listed in Box 19-1.

Acute pancreatitis presents as poorly localized epigastric pain, often continuous and boring, with interspersed spasms, in association with nausea, vomiting, abdominal distension, and tachypnea. Physical findings include fever, tachycardia, hypotension (all associated with intraperi-

---

Box 19-1 Causes of Acute Pancreatitis

1. Gallstones (35%)
2. Alcohol (10%)
3. Hypertriglyceridemia (3%)
4. Hypercalcemia from any cause
5. Drugs (low incidence)
   Didanosine, pentamidine, Flagyl, tetracycline, sulfonamides, furosemide, thiazides, sulfasalazine, L-asparagine, azathioprine, tamoxifen, estrogen, valproic acid, sulindac
6. Infections
7. Trauma
8. Genetic
   Pancreas divisum
9. Vascular insufficiency
10. Pregnancy
11. Post-ERCP
12. Idiopathic

---

toneal fluid sequestration and/or sepsis), arrhythmias (may be due to sepsis, hypocalcemia, hypomagnesemia), decreased bowel sounds, peritoneal signs, crackles on pulmonary auscultation (pneumonia, chronic heart failure, atelectasis, acute respiratory distress syndrome), and petechiae [diffuse intravascular coagulation (DIC)]. Laboratory changes may include increased white blood cell count, increased or decreased hematocrit (hemoconcentration, DIC, hemorrhagic pancreatitis), hypocalcemia, hypomagnesemia, hyperglycemia, hypertriglyceridemia, increased blood urea nitrogen (BUN) and creatinine, hypoxemia, and increased serum lipase. Plain films may show only a nonspecific ileus. All of the above mentioned findings are consistent with numerous intra-abdominal pathologic processes (see Box 19-2 for a partial list of differential diagnoses).

The histopathologic changes seen in acute pancreatitis are the result of proteolytic enzymes (primarily trypsin) and autodigesting pancreatic and peripancreatic tissues. There is damage to pancreatic endocrine and exocrine cells; pancreatic ductal tissue; vascular tissue leading to hemorrhage; peritoneum; and retroperitoneal tissues including connective tissue (retroperitoneal fibrosis) and the celiac plexus. Serum amylase levels above 200 Somogyi units per 100 ml should be present; the duration of elevation of amylase correlates better with the severity of disease than does the absolute level. CT scan shows evidence of edema, hemorrhage, and may show calcium deposition. Pancreatic pseudocysts develop in 10% of acute pancreatitis. Pancreatic pseudoaneurysms develop in 10% of pseudocysts.

The treatment of acute pancreatitis includes decreasing pancreatic secretory drive by making NPO and instituting nasogastric suction, prompt fluid resuscitation, correction of electrolyte abnormalities, antibiotic therapy, treatment of cardiac and pulmonary abnormalities, institution of diuretic therapy in the face of prerenal acute renal failure, blood products as necessary, and identification and elimination of inciting factors (including prescribed medications). Pain control should begin with parenteral narcotics [patient-controlled analgesia (PCA) if possible, avoiding meperidine] and ketamine (5 to 20 mg IV q6h). Continuous thoracic epidural analgesia or celiac plexus blockade can be utilized in selected patients.

Chronic Pancreatitis

The emergence of chronic pancreatitis from acute pancreatitis is poorly understood. Chronic pancreatitis is characterized by abdominal pain and/or pancreatic endocrine/exocrine dysfunction. Up to 20% of patients are pain free. Two distinct pain patterns are described: episodic pain lasting less than 2 weeks with pain-free intervals lasting months to years and prolonged periods of daily pain associated with clusters of severe pain. Pancreatic endocrine/exocrine insufficiency is a late finding, usually only occurring after greater than 90% of function is lost.

The differential diagnosis includes pancreatic cancer, peptic ulcer disease, chronic cholelithiasis, biliary carcinoma, and pancreatic pseudocyst (Box 19-3).

The pathophysiologic basis of chronic pancreatitis has not been elucidated. Therefore, there is no consensus as to diagnostic criteria. Serum amylase and lipase may be slightly elevated, but are usually normal. Plain films show calcifications in 30% of cases. CT scan (sensitivity 75% to 90%, specificity 85%) and abdominal ultrasonography (sensitivity 60% to 70%, specificity 85%) may show calcium deposits, stones, ductal dilatation (>4 mm), pancreatic enlargement, or cysts. If calcium deposition or stones are not present, endoscopic retrograde cholangiopancreatography (ERCP) is the test of choice, and typically shows "beading" of the ducts. Pancreatic function testing should be used if the diagnosis is suspected but other studies are not diagnostic; function testing has sensitivity 85%, specificity 90%. IV secretin administration shows decreased $NaHCO_3$ secretion measured in the duodenum. Oral bentiromide administration shows decreased para-aminobenzoic acid measured in urine.

Box 19-2 Differential Diagnosis in Acute Pancreatitis

1. Bowel obstruction
2. Perforated viscus
3. Acute cholecystitis
4. Abdominal aortic aneurysm
5. Mesenteric artery occlusion; renal artery/vein occlusion
6. Nephrolithiasis
7. Inflammatory bowel disease
8. Diverticulitis
9. Myocardial infarction
10. Diabetic ketoacidosis
11. Pneumonia
12. Sepsis

Box 19-3 Differential Diagnosis in Chronic Pancreatitis

1. Pancreatic cancer
2. Peptic ulcer disease
3. Chronic cholelithiasis
4. Irritable bowel syndrome
5. Inflammatory bowel disease

Histologic studies have shed light on some of the possible causes of pain in chronic pancreatitis. A low-level inflammatory infiltrate may be present causing focal fibrosis. Intrinsic ductal obstruction secondary to stones may be present. There is often evidence of edema and increased pancreatic tissue pressure secondary to obstruction from stones and/or fibrosis. Fibrosis of sensory nerves can occur, but is not a common finding. Compared to controls, there is an increase in the number and diameter of sensory nerves in the pancreas and inflammation of the perineural sheath. In addition, there is increased staining for both calcitonin gene-related peptide and substance P.

The pain of chronic pancreatitis is characterized by midepigastric/thoraco-lumbar pain that is often constant, aching, burning, or gnawing. The pain has both visceral and neuropathic qualities. There may be acute exacerbations not associated with laboratory changes. Nausea and vomiting are inconsistent findings. Peritoneal signs are rarely present. Bone pain may be present due to intramedullary fat necrosis; subcutaneous tender nodules may be present due to fat necrosis.

The first caveat of treatment of chronic pancreatitis is "Be sure of the diagnosis" (Box 19-4). Chronic pancreatitis is then best treated with a multidisciplinary approach. Psychological comorbidities occur in greater than 80% of patients.

Box 19-4   Treatment of Chronic Pancreatitis

1. General
   a. Rule out coexisting disease
      Peptic ulcer disease, pancreatic cancer, biliary obstruction, pancreatic pseudocyst, pancreatic duct obstruction
   b. No ethyl alcohol
   c. Small meals low in fat
2. Pancreatic enzyme supplementation
3. Medium chain triglyceride supplementation
4. Analgesics
   Opiates, TCAs, COX-2s
5. Antioxidant therapy
   Vitamin C, vitamin E, allopurinol, methionine, selenium
6. Specialized treatments
   a. Celiac plexus blockade
   b. Endoscopic stenting and/or stone removal
   c. Extracorporeal shockwave lithotripsy
   d. Surgery
      Decompression
      Resection
      Denervation
      Intrathecal drug delivery system

Patients should cease all alcohol consumption and should eat small meals that are low in fat. Women should avoid pregnancy. Pancreatic enzyme supplementation combined with H_2 blocker or proton pump inhibitor can be beneficial, although less likely to be successful in the presence of very large ducts or disease secondary to alcohol. Medium chain triglycerides can be beneficial.

Medication management should begin with adjuvants, including cyclooxygenase-2 (COX-2) inhibitors, tramadol, tricyclic antidepressants, anticonvulsants, and ketamine. Opiate medications can be used, including methadone and sustained release formulations, to achieve analgesia with a stable, nonescalating dose. Short-acting opiates should be avoided. Opioid abuse is a significant concern, especially among patients with a history of alcohol or other substance abuse. Strong consideration should be given to the inclusion of an addictionologist in the multidisciplinary treatment team.

Specialized treatments may be used in patients who are not responsive to these more conservative treatments. Specialized treatments include celiac plexus blockade, endoscopic therapies including stenting, extracorporeal shockwave lithotripsy, and surgery. It must be noted that none of these specialized procedures has been evaluated in controlled trials. In selected studies, each of these procedures have been shown to provide 70% to 90% significant response rate for 6 months, but less than 50% response at 2 years.

Celiac plexus blockade has long been considered a treatment option for patients whose pain is poorly controlled with other measures. Either percutaneous (transaortic or retrocrural) or endoscopic ultrasound guided transgastric approaches may be employed. Non-neurolytic blockade with local anesthetic with or without steroid may provide months of pain relief. Neurolytic blockade can be considered in patients who have had an excellent response to local anesthetic blockade. However, response to local anesthetic blockade does not guarantee a similar response to neurolytic blockade. Patients with a history of alcohol abuse, substance abuse, physical/sexual abuse, or chronic opioid use are less likely to have a successful response. Their pain complaints are likely to continue and a reduction in opioid use is unlikely. Other potential complications of neurolytic blockade include: short-term hypotension; deafferentation pain; change in intestinal motility, which may alter the absorption of po medications; further disruption of local anatomy, perhaps complicating future surgery; and visceral deafferentation, which can mask intra-abdominal pain of other etiology (e.g., perforating ulcer; cardiac arrhythmias).

Other treatment options include 4-day, low-dose phentolamine infusion; case reports of 6 months of pain relief are reported. No controlled studies are reported. In selected patients, intrathecal drug delivery may be the best pharmacologic treatment option.

SICKLE CELL DISEASE

Sickle cell disease (SCD) is a hemoglobinopathy. Hemoglobin (Hb) S has a valine substitution for glutamic acid at position 6 of B globin chain. SCD is present in individuals with homozygous Hb SS. Sickle trait, heterozygous Hb S, occurs in asymptomatic carriers. The incidence of SCD per 10,000 live births is: 29.9 for African-Americans; 2.5 for Mediterranean, Saudi Arabian and Indian heritage; 0.3 for Hispanics; and 0.1 for Whites. There is some overlap of clinical features and treatment with Hb SCD, Sickle-β(o)Thalassemia disease, and Sickle-β(+)Thalassemia disease. The diagnoses are made with hemoglobin electrophoresis.

The diagnosis is often suspected after the occurrence of dactylitis (hand-foot syndrome), which is the result of vaso-occlusive events in the marrow-containing digits of children. Other clinical features include vaso-occlusive crises, cerebral vascular accident (CVA), renal failure, splenic sequestration syndrome, septicemia secondary to splenic failure, acute chest syndrome, osteomyelitis, septic arthritis, chronic hemolytic anemia, avascular necrosis of humerus/hip, vertebral compression fractures, and liver dysfunction secondary to iron overload (Box 19-5).

Vaso-occlusive crises are the most common manifestation accounting for 90% of ER visits and 70% of hospitalizations of SCD patients. In infants, it occurs most often in the digits (dactylitis). In children and adults, it occurs most often in the humerus, then tibia, and then femur. Vaso-occlusive crises must be distinguished from osteomyelitis (Salmonella > E coli > S aureus) and septic arthritis (S aureus > Salmonella).

Water content in erythrocytes red blood cells (RBC) is governed by several passive gradient systems. A K-Cl cotransport (KCC 1,3,4) system in which K and Cl are transported out of the cell with concurrent passive water efflux. In normal RBC, this cotransport is inhibited by decreased hydrostatic pressure, pH below 6.7, increased magnesium level, and decreased PO_2. In normal RBCs, it is activated by increased hydrostatic pressure, increased urea concentration, oxidation, and positively charged hemoglobin. In Hb SS RBC, K-Cl cotransport is independent of PO_2 and is activated by decreased pH and increased urea concentration. The end result is loss of K, Cl, and water from Hb SS RBC. The K-Cl cotransport is likely the site of action of hydroxyurea.

A second mechanism is the calcium-activated K channel, also known as the Gardos channel (after the discoverer), the IK channel, or the KCNN4 channel. Calcium influx causes K efflux, with passive efflux of water. The channel is activated by calcium 0.3 to 2.0 umol/L. As Hb SS RBC deoxygenates, there is an increase in calcium permeability, activating the Gardos channel. Clotrimazole specifically inhibits the Gardos channel. Arginine and nitric oxide also inhibit the Gardos channel.

Dehydration of the RBC leads to increased concentration of Hb SS. Above a critical concentration, the Hb SS polymerizes, changing the structure of the cytosolic skeleton and sickling occurs. Sickled RBCs interact with adhesion proteins of the vascular endothelium initiating the inflammatory cascade. Vascular occlusion by sickled cells and the edema of the inflammatory reaction lead to decreased PO_2, decreased pH, and increased intracellular calcium, all of which lead to further propagation of the cycle.

Preventive treatments should be initiated in infancy (Box 19-6). Immunization with conjugate strep pneumoniae vaccine, H. influenza type B vaccine, hepatitis B vaccine, and influenza virus vaccine should be completed. Prophylactic penicillin should be given until age 5 and folic acid 1 mg/day. Chronic transfusion therapy to keep hemoglobin concentration at 10.0 mg/dL and/or Hb SS concentration <30% of total hemoglobin is indicated if transcranial doppler indicates increased risk of CVA. In the face of recurrent events, hydroxyurea at a starting

---

Box 19-5 Clinical Features of Sickle Cell Disease

1. Vaso-occlusive events in marrow containing bones
   Infants: dactylitis
   Children and adults: humerus, tibia, and femur
2. Septicemia
   Salmonella, E. coli, Staph aureus
3. Cerebral vascular accident
4. Renal failure
5. Splenic sequestration
6. Acute chest syndrome
7. Peripheral thromboembolic events
8. Chronic hemolytic anemia
9. Hepatic dysfunction secondary to chronic iron overload
10. Avascular necrosis of hip, humerus
11. Vertebral compression fracture

Box 19-6 Preventive Treatment in Sickle Cell Disease

1. Immunizations
   Conjugate strep pneumoniae vaccine, H. influenza type B vaccine, hepatitis B vaccine, influenza virus vaccine
2. Prophylactic penicillin until age 5
3. Folic acid 1 mg/d
4. Chronic transfusion therapy if high risk for CVA
5. Hydroxyurea if recurrent events
   15 mg/kg/d
6. Clotrimazole (experimental)

dose of 15 mg/kg/d is approved above age 12 and is safe to age 2. Clotrimazole is currently being evaluated.

The pain of acute events is often undertreated. One study found that 53% of ER physicians and 23% of hematologists felt that more than 20% of sickle cell patients were addicts. Patients often know from their frequent episodes of pain what works and what doesn't work. Listen to the patient and the family. Requests for particular medications are more likely to be "pain-relieving behavior" rather than "drug-seeking behavior." Acute management (Box 19-7) includes: IV hydration; supplemental O_2, only if SaO_2 is low; warm packs (avoid cold ambient temperatures); antibiotics if clinically indicated; medication management; and transfusion therapy, including possible blood substitutes.

Medication management can include:
- Parenteral opiates (PCA if possible);
- Tramadol; magnesium supplementation;
- Ketorolac (maximum 5 days) or COX-2 inhibitors;
- Ketamine; anticoagulation with heparin 5000 to 7500 units bid (warfarin not shown to be effective);
- Parenteral corticosteroids effectively decrease acute pain but have a high incidence of rebound pain;
- Epidural analgesia, if not anticoagulated;
- Hydroxyurea starting at 15 mg/kg/d;
- Poloaxemer 188 (ReothRx; a surfactant to decrease endothelial adhesion) 100 mg/kg over 1 hour, then 30 mg/kg continuous infusion over 47 hours; and
- Inhaled nitric oxide.

Box 19-7 Acute Pain Management in Sickle Cell Disease

1. IV hydration
2. Supplemental O_2 if SaO_2 low
3. Magnesium supplementation
4. Parenteral opiates
5. Ketamine
6. Ketorolac (maximum 5 days); COX-2s
7. Tramadol
8. Warm packs; avoid cold ambient temperature
9. Anticoagulation with heparin 5000 to 7500 U bid
10. Parenteral corticosteroids (high incidence rebound pain)
11. Poloxamer 188
    100 mg/kg × 1hr, then 30 mg/kg/hr × 47 hrs
12. Hydroxyurea 15 mg/kg/d
13. Inhaled nitric oxide
14. Transfusion therapy
    Maintain hemoglobin 10.0 mg/dL
    Exchange transfusion to keep Hb SS <30% total hemoglobin
    Artificial blood substitutes
15. Clotrimazole (experimental)

Chronic pain is best managed by a multidisciplinary approach. In addition to the pain of chronic complications from vaso-occlusive disease (e.g., avascular necrosis, vertebral compression fractures) and possible visceral and neuropathic pain, there is invariably the pain of depression and social isolation. Medication management can include acetaminophen, nonsteroidal anti-inflammatory drugs (NSAIDs), COX-2s, tramadol, ketamine, and long-half-life or sustained release opiates. Neuropathic and visceral pain can be treated with tricyclics, antiepileptics, and ketamine. Bone pain may be responsive to IV pamidronate.

HIV DISEASE

HIV disease covers the range from asymptomatic HIV infection to full-blown AIDS. A small percentage of the clinical manifestations are due to direct effects of the HIV virus; as the success of antiretroviral treatment has improved, maintaining CD4 counts and minimizing viral load, manifestations of direct viral effect have decreased. Many of the clinical manifestations are due to the myriad opportunistic infections and/or malignancies that develop and must be treated. Other manifestations are due to treatment side effects and drug toxicities. Depression or anxiety occurs in nearly 100% of patients. Substance abuse is a frequent comorbidity. Therefore, a multidisciplinary approach to treatment is ideal.

The prevalence of chronic pain in HIV is estimated from 40% to 70% and increases as life-expectancy increases. The chronicity and severity of pain parallels the progression of the underlying disease(s). More than one pain syndrome can occur sequentially or simultaneously (opportunistic infection and/or malignancy and/or drug toxicity).

It is estimated that up to 85% of HIV patients receive inadequate treatment of their pain. Risk factors for inadequate treatment are female gender, lower socioeconomic class, low level of education, and history of IV drug abuse.

Pain can be due to direct HIV effects (e.g., headache due to HIV encephalitis), although as noted above, direct effects are in the minority. The pain of malignancies and opportunistic infections can be: somatic due to invasion/compression of other structures; neuropathic due to wind-up from chronic somatic stimulation, direct nerve infiltration, or paraneoplastic syndromes; visceral due to bowel infiltration or obstruction; and central. The pain of drug toxicities is primarily neuropathic. Pain can be secondary to invasive procedures.

Common sites of pain are listed in Box 19-8.

Central Pain and Headache in HIV

An accurate diagnosis must be made. Diagnostic studies must include lumbar puncture and MRI. If no diagno-

Box 19-8 Common Sites of Pain in HIV

1. Pulmonary
   a. Infection, malignancy, postprocedural
2. Gastrointestinal
   a. Oral, esophageal, gastric ulcers
      Medications, candida, CMV, herpes simplex, etc.
   b. Hepato-biliary tract
      Hepatitis B and C, drug induce hepatitis, CMV, cryptosporidium cholecystitis, acalculous cholecystitis, cholangitis, hepatic carcinoma, metastatic carcinoma
   c. Pancreatitis
      Drug induced: pentamidine, didanosine
   d. Bowel
      Obstruction secondary to non-Hodgkin's lymphoma, Kaposi's.
      CMV
      Idiopathic abdominal pain associated with diarrhea and malabsorption
   e. Genito-urinary
      Renal cell carcinoma, bladder infection, bladder carcinoma, prostatitis, epididymitis
   f. Central pain and headache
      HIV encephalitis, HIV dementia, primary CNS lymphoma, cryptococcal meningitis, CMV, herpes simplex, herpes zoster, papovavirus, tuberculosis, syphilis, toxoplasmosis, drug toxicity
   g. Peripheral neuropathy
      DSP
      Mononeuritis multiplex
      Acute demyelinating polyneuropathy (Landry-Guillain-Barre)
      Chronic inflammatory demyelinating polyneuropathy
      Lumbosacral polyradiculopathy (cauda equina)
      Diffuse infiltrative lymphocytosis syndrome
      Autonomic neuropathy
      Mononeuropathy
      Herpes zoster

The most common cause of headache due to opportunistic infection in HIV is cryptococcal meningitis. Other opportunistic infection causes are CMV, herpes simplex, herpes zoster, Papova virus, Epstein-Barr virus (EBV), tuberculosis, syphilis, and toxoplasmosis. Primary central nervous system (CNS) lymphoma, another cause of headache and central pain, is associated with EBV. Headache can be due to drug toxicity (e.g., azathioprine). HIV can cause headache directly via HIV encephalitis or HIV dementia; these can be treated with antiretrovirals and human recombinant neurotrophic factor.

Peripheral Neuropathy in HIV

The prevalence of peripheral neuropathy is increasing. Distal sensory polyneuropathy is now present in one-third of HIV patients.

The diagnosis should be confirmed with electrophysiologic studies (EPS), nerve conduction velocities (NCV), and electromyography (EMG). Blood tests should then be done to rule out other reversible causes of peripheral neuropathy (Box 19-9). If the peripheral neuropathy is associated with encephalopathy, myelopathy, Cauda Equina syndrome, rapid progression of symptoms, fever, weight loss, prior history of lymphoma, or a prior history of CMV infection, a lumbar puncture must be performed (see above for interpretation of lumbar puncture results). Ultimately, a nerve

Box 19-9 Diagnostic Studies in the Evaluation of HIV Peripheral Neuropathy

1. Blood tests to rule out other reversible causes
   Liver function tests, B12, folate, TSH, hemoglobin A1C, ESR, BUN, Cr, SPEP, serum immunoelectrophoresis, RPR, cryoglobulins
2. EPS
   NCV
   EMG
3. Lumbar puncture
   Obtain in any peripheral neuropathy that is associated with encephalopathy, myelopathy, cauda equina syndrome, rapid progression of symptoms, fever, weight loss, prior history of CMV or lymphoma
4. Nerve biopsy
   May be necessary to rule out CMV and necrotizing vasculitis

TSH, thyroid-stimulating hormone; ESR, erythrocyte sedimentation rate; BUN, blood urea nitrogen; Cr, calcification rate; SPEP, serum protein electrophoresis; RPR, rapid plasmin reagin; EPS, electrophysiologic studies; NCV, nerve conduction velocity; EMG, electromyography; CMV, cytomegalovirus.

sis is made by these studies, biopsy may be necessary. Lumbar puncture testing should include: complete blood cell count (CBC); glucose; protein; IgG and oligoclonal bands; gram stain; acid fast stain; culture for bacteria, tuberculosis, fungi, and viral organisms; antigen specific reactions for virus [e.g., cytomegalovirus (CMV) polymerase chain reaction]. Sixty-three percent of asymptomatic HIV-positive patients have at least one abnormality on lumbar puncture. However, it is agreed that protein >1.2 g/L and cell count >50/mm^3 indicates the presence of a disease process.

biopsy may be necessary, especially to rule out CMV and/or necrotizing vasculitis.

Distal symmetric polyneuropathy (DSP) is now present in one-third of HIV-positive patients. EPS shows symmetric sensorimotor polyneuropathy, predominately axonal. DSP can be due to direct effects of HIV and/or antiretroviral drug toxicity (dideoxynucleosides).

The incidence of DSP due to direct HIV effect increases as CD4 counts decrease and viral loads increase. There is no clear evidence that highly active antiretroviral therapy (HAART) to prevent the development of DSP. (The picture is complicated by the fact that drug toxicity from HAART can cause DSP.) No spontaneous remissions have been documented. However, it may change from a painful to a painless syndrome, with persistence of the EPS changes. Recombinant human nerve growth factor has been shown to decrease pain, without changes in EPS. Propentofylline and pentoxifylline may decrease pain by increasing levels of endogenous neurotrophic growth factor.

DSP caused by drug toxicity is reversible with decrease in dosage or discontinuation of the drug. Symptoms often worsen during the first 1 to 6 weeks after dosage decrease or discontinuation. Recovery then occurs over the ensuing 3 to 20 weeks.

Mononeuropathy multiplex is characterized on EPS shows an asymmetric, axonal sensorimotor polyneuropathy. Severe cases may be so widespread as to closely mimic DSP. Therefore, the electrophysiologist must be sensitive to *any* asymmetry on the EPS. Causes of mononeuropathy multiplex include CMV, necrotizing vasculitis, diabetes mellitus, hereditary neuropathy, and rarely to polyclonal cryoglobulinemia. Patients with CD4 counts <200 cells/uL must be evaluated for CMV infection (lumbar puncture with CMV culture and CMV polymerase chain reaction and serum CMV antigen and examination of other organs for possible CMV infection). If the neuropathy is widespread or rapidly progressive and CMV is not diagnosed by these methods, a nerve biopsy should be done to rule CMV inclusions or necrotizing vasculitis. Specific causes should be specifically treated. CMV can be treated with ganciclovir 5 mg/kg q12 h × 14 d, then 5 mg/kg/d. Necrotizing vasculitis can be treated with IV immunoglobulin 400 mg/kg/d × 5 d and or prednisone 1.5 mg/kg/d and/or plasma exchange. Cryoglobulinemia can be treated with plasma exchange.

Lumbosacral polyradiculopathy is characterized by preservation of sensory action potentials, with abnormalities on the EMG, which vary according to the stage of presentation. CMV must be looked for with LP, serum antigen, and evidence of HIV. An MRI with and without gadolinium should be performed to rule out Cauda Equina due to disc herniation, vertebral compression fracture, hematoma, and other intrinsic or extrinsic mass lesion. CMV therapy is lifelong ganciclovir and/or foscar-

net, although life expectancy is on average 3 months. Mass lesions may require surgical decompression or chemotherapy aimed at reducing the bulk of malignancies. If a definitive diagnosis can not be made, the current treatment recommendation is ganciclovir plus foscarnet plus first-line antituberculous drugs.

Landry-Guillain-Barre syndrome, or inflammatory demyelinating polyradiculoneuropathy (IDP), is characterized on EPS by decreased conduction velocity, reduced sensory and motor amplitudes, prolonged distal latencies, conduction block, decreased motor unit recruitment, and muscle denervation potentials. Lumbar puncture shows elevated protein (>100 mg/dL) and lymphocytosis (usually 10 to 50 cells/mm^3). Acute IDP is treated with IV immunoglobulin 400 mg/kg/d × 5d; plasma exchange is second-line treatment and carries increased risks in immunocompromised patients. Chronic IDP is treated with IV immunoglobulin 400 mg/kg/d × 5d then 500 to 1000 mg every 3 weeks as maintenance therapy; prednisone 1.5 mg/kg/d may also be added to the regimen.

Diffuse infiltrative lymphocytosis syndrome presents with EPS showing a predominantly axonal polyneuropathy, either symmetric or asymmetric. Laboratory testing is key, showing a CD8 count >1200/uL. Biopsy shows perineural, endoneural, and endovascular infiltration with CD8 lymphocytes. Treatment is with zidovudine and corticosteroids.

Compressive mononeuropathies occur in HIV patients. The EPS findings of conduction delay at the site of compression are identical in HIV-infected and noninfected individuals. However, vasculitis is a much more common cause of mononeuropathy in HIV-infected patients and should be investigated.

Treatment of Pain in HIV

Underlying disease processes may alter the pharmacologic treatment options. Oral, esophageal, or gastric ulcers may limit the ability to use oral medications. Diarrhea and malabsorption may affect bioavailability. Hepatic dysfunction, renal dysfunction, and competition with other treatment drugs may alter pharmacokinetics. Encephalitis and dementia can alter central pharmacodynamics, leading to unacceptable sedation or confusion.

See Box 19-10 for medications used in treatment of HIV pain. It should be remembered that no drug or class of drug has been shown to be superior to other individual drugs or classes of drugs.

Acetaminophen has risks of hepatic and renal toxicity. NSAIDs and COX-2s can increase the risk of gastrointestinal (GI) ulceration. Tramadol can cause seizures in patients with CNS lesions; blood levels and seizure risks are increased with concurrent use of opiates, tricyclic antidepressants (TCAs), and selective serotonin reuptake

---

Box 19-10   Pharmacologic Treatment of Pain in HIV

1. Acetaminophen
    Risk of hepatic toxicity
2. NSAIDs and COX-2s
    Risks of GI ulcer, impaired coagulation, renal and hepatic toxicity
3. Tramadol
    Increased risk of seizures in patients with CNS lesions
    Blood levels increase with opioids, TCAs, SSRIs
4. TCAs
5. SSRIs, SNRIs
6. Anticonvulsants
7. Sodium channel blockers
8. NMDA antagonists
9. α-2 agonists
10. GABA agonists
11. Opiates
12. Corticosteroids
13. Propentofylline, pentoxifylline

Remember: oral, esophageal, and gastric ulceration may limit the effectiveness of the oral route; diarrhea and malabsorption may decrease bioavailability; hepatic dysfunction, renal dysfunction, and competition with other treatment drugs may alter pharmacokinetics.

Box 19-11   Differential Diagnosis in Fibromyalgia

1. Regional myofascial pain syndrome
2. Tendonitis/tendonosis and bursitis
3. Chronic fatigue syndrome
4. Neuropathic pain syndromes; CRPS
5. Temperomandibular joint syndrome
6. Hyermobile joint syndrome
7. Musculoskeletal asymmetry
8. Endocrine abnormalities
    Hypothyroid, hypoparathyroid, hyperparathyroid, menopause, adrenal insufficiency, diabetes
9. Infection
    Lyme disease, hepatitis B and C, parvovirus, HIV, Epstein-Barr virus
10. Musculoskeletal/autoimmune
    Rheumatoid arthritis, systemic Lupus, polymyalgia rheumatica, polymyositis, seronegative spondyloarthropathies
11. Neurologic disease
    Multiple sclerosis, Parkinson's, Myasthenia gravis
12. Malignancy, paraneoplastic syndromes
13. Primary sleep disorders
14. Somatiform disorders

---

inhibitors (SSRIs). TCA levels are increased with concurrent use of SSRIs. HIV-infected patients have significant autonomic dysfunction as compared to controls and are therefore at greater risk for arrhythmias. *N*-methyl-D-aspartate (NMDA) antagonists can cause psychosis when used in patients with underlying encephalitis or dementia. Opiates carry the risk of opiate induced hyperalgesia.

In selected patients, implanted intrathecal or epidural drug delivery systems, neuroaxial blockade, or spinal-cord stimulators may be beneficial.

Nonpharmacologic treatments include acupuncture, physical therapy, occupational therapy, psychological therapy, cognitive-behavioral therapy, mindfulness-based stress reduction, and electroceutical therapy (transcutaneous electrical nerve stimulation, neuromuscular re-education).

FIBROMYALGIA

Fibromyalgia affects 2% of the U.S. population (7 to 11 million people). The incidence increases with increasing age. It is 10 times more common in women than men. Women from mid-thirties to late-fifties account for 75% of cases. However, it must also be noted that 25% of new patient visits to *pediatric* rheumatologists are diagnosed with fibromyalgia.

The differential diagnosis is broad (Box 19-11). It is therefore important to have a systematic approach to the patient who presents with polymyalgias and polyarthralgia (Box 19-12).

No specific cause for fibromyalgia has been found. There are common antecedent events: infections with hepatitis B, hepatitis C, Lyme disease, parvovirus, viral flu syndromes; trauma including whiplash and surgery; and persistently elevated life stressors.

Measurable pathophysiologic changes occur in fibromyalgia. Muscle histology shows ragged red fibers. Muscle cytochemistry shows decreased high energy phosphates. There is an altered hypothalamic-pituitary axis with decreased growth hormone, decreased thyroid hormone, decreased cortisol levels post exercise, and increased prolactin. There are altered cerebrospinal fluid neurotransmitters including increased substance P, decreased homocysteine, decreased serotonin, decreased dopamine, and decreased tryptophan. Dolorimetry testing shows that fibromyalgics report the same level of pain as controls at half the applied pressure. Functional MRI combined with dolorimetry shows that fibromyalgics have decreased blood flow in the thalamus and anterior cingulate gyrus and increased blood flow in the primary somatosensory cortex as compared to controls. Sleep studies document α wave intrusion into non-REM sleep.

Box 19-12   Approach to the Patient with Polymyalgia/Polyarthralgia

History and Physical			
No Synovitis		**Synovitis**	
Symptoms >6 weeks	Tender Points **Symptoms <6 weeks**	Tender Points	No Tender Points
Fibromyalgia or multiple sites of bursitis or tendonitis	Viral arthralgia Osteoarthritis Hypothyroidism Neuropathic pain Metabolic bone disease Depression	Systemic rheumatic disease	Viral arthritis; early rheumatic disease Careful follow-up
Lyme disease testing	Liver function tests, hepatitis B and C, TSH, radiographs, calcium, albumin, alkaline phosphatase	CBC, ESR, RF, ANA, Creatinine, urinalysis, joint aspiration, Lyme disease testing	CBC, liver function tests, hepatitis B and C, parvovirus serology, Lyme disease testing

(Adapted from American College of Rheumatology Ad Hoc Committee on Clinical Guidelines. Arthritis Rheum 39:1, 1996.)
CBC, complete blood cell count; ESR, erythrocyte sedimentation rate; RF, rheumatoid factor; ANA, antinuclear antibody; TSH, thyroid-stimulating hormone.

Signs and symptoms that may be present include: widespread pain and tender points; generalized weakness and aching joints *without* synovitis; nonrestorative sleep; fatigue; stiffness; headache; irritable bowel symptoms; urinary urgency; dysuria; increased perimenstrual and menstrual pain; paresthesias; restless legs or cramps; cognitive dysfunction; psychological comorbidities including depression, anxiety, post-traumatic stress disorder (PTSD), personality disorders, and eating disorders (Box 19-13).

The accepted diagnostic criteria include at least 11 of 18 standard tender points (Box 19-14) with at least one tender point in three quadrants, nonrestorative sleep, fatigue, cognitive dysfunction, and mood disturbance (Box 19-15).

Successful treatment of fibromyalgia requires attention to the multiple facets of the syndrome. The pain of

Box 19-13   Common Clinical Features of Fibromyalgia

1. Widespread pain and tender points
2. Generalized weakness and aching joints *without* synovitis
3. Nonrestorative sleep
4. Fatigue
5. Stiffness
6. Headache
7. Irritable bowel symptoms
8. Urinary urgency
9. Increased menstrual pain
10. Paresthesias
11. Restless legs, cramps
12. Cognitive dysfunction
13. Psychological changes
    a. Depression
    b. Anxiety
    c. Post-traumatic stress disorder
    d. Personality disorder
    e. Eating disorder

Box 19-14   Diagnostic Tender Points in Fibromyalgia

The following tender points are present bilaterally in most cases:
1. Occiput: suboccipital muscle insertion
2. Low cervical: scalene muscles
3. Upper trapezius
4. Levator scapulae insertion: upper medial scapular border
5. Upper costochondral junction: medial to second rib insertion
6. Lateral epicondyle
7. Gluteus medius: upper outer portion of buttocks
8. Greater trochanter: at or posterior to trochanteric bursa
9. Knee: medial joint line

Box 19-15   Diagnostic Criteria for Fibromyalgia

1. Widespread musculoskeletal pain
   a. 11 of 18 tender points
   b. Tender points present in at least three quadrants
2. Nonrestorative sleep
3. Fatigue
4. Cognitive dysfunction
5. Mood disturbance

---

fibromyalgia is often undertreated. At the same time, it is critical to recognize that attempts to treat *just* the pain of fibromyalgia are doomed to failure. Misunderstanding about the disease process must be addressed through patient and family education. Deconditioning should be addressed through a prescribed program of graded exer-

---

Box 19-16   Pharmacologic Treatment of Pain and Depression in Fibromyalgia

(Each of these medications alone has a low success rate for controlling pain. Combinations may improve mood, sleep and sometimes pain in selected cases.)
1. Acetaminophen
2. NSAIDs, COX-2s, methylsulfonylmethane (metabolite of DMSO)
3. Tramadol
4. Topical agents
   a. Lidoderm, capsaicin
5. TCAs; low-dose for pain
6. Anticonvulsants
   Carbamazepine, oxcarbamazepine, lamotrigine, gabapentin, zonisamide, toperamate, phenytoin, valproic acid
7. GABA agonists
   Tiagabine, baclofen
8. NMDA antagonists
   Ketamine, amantadine, propoxyphene, dextromethorphan
9. α-2 agonists
   Tizanidine, clonidine
10. Opiates (low doses; avoid if at all possible: may exacerbate hyperalgesia)
11. Muscle relaxants
   Cyclobenzaprine, chlrozoxazone, metaxalone, methocarbamol, orphenadrine
12. SSRIs
13. SNRIs
14. Benzodiazepines
15. Neuroleptics/antipsychotics

---

cise, but only after pain has been adequately treated. Psychological distress must be treated with pharmacologic and nonpharmacologic modalities. Nonrestorative sleep must be treated, including primary sleep disorders. Comorbidities must be identified and treated, as they may serve to exacerbate the underlying fibromyalgia pain. Comorbidities include: spinal degenerative joint disease (DJD) and degenerative disk disease and peripheral DJD; traumatic injuries, including repetitive strain injuries; headache; temporomandibular jaw syndrome; chronic pelvic pain, including interstitial cystitis and endometriosis; irritable bowel syndrome; and other rheumatologic diseases.

Pharmacologic treatment (Box 19-16) can include: acetaminophen; NSAIDs; COX-2s; methylsulfonylmethane (MSM), a metabolite of dimethyl sulfoxide (DMSO); tramadol: topical agents, such as Lidoderm, capsaicin, Traumeel (a homeopathic preparation); TCAs, that provide analgesia as well as improving sleep; anticonvulsants; γ-aminobutyric acid (GABA) agonists; α-2 agonists; skeletal muscle relaxants other than GABA agonists; NMDA antagonists; opiates, with sustained-release preparations or methadone preferred; vitamins and minerals, including magnesium, vitamin B complex, vitamin C, vitamin E; and supplements, such as Coenzyme Q 10, L-carnitine, Gingko biloba, and α lipoic acid, all of which support mitochondrial respiration.

Pharmacologic treatment of depression and anxiety includes: TCAs (can be selected on basis of anticholinergic profile); SSRIs (onset of action 3 to 4 weeks, except for Lexapro with onset in 7 to 10 days); serotonin norepinephrine reuptake inhibition (Effexor has analgesic properties above 200 mg/d; Paxil has hyperalgesic properties); benzodiazepines; neuroleptics and antipsychotics, including Risperdal, Zyprexa, Seroquel, and Geodon.

Nonrestorative sleep must be addressed. Consideration should be given to evaluation for a primary sleep disorder, such as obstructive sleep apnea. Basic sleep hygiene needs to be observed. This includes avoiding evening stimulants, such as caffeine and perhaps television, use of a proper mattress and pillow, creating an environment conducive to sleep (appropriate light and temperature, lack of intrusive noise), and actually going to bed at a reasonable time. Esophageal reflux can worsen when lying supine and with certain evening foods. Nocturnal reflux can cause esophageal pain or lead to aspiration, either one interrupting sleep. Efforts should be made to minimize fibromyalgia pain and psychological distress at night. This may require adjustment of evening medications. Medications that can be used as sleep-aids include short-acting sedative-hypnotics, TCAs, muscle relaxants, α-2 agonists, tiagabine, zonisamide, and opiates.

Treatment of deconditioning should wait until an effective analgesic regimen has been stabilized. The patient should begin with a prescribed program of low impact aerobic exercise (e.g., pool therapy, stationary bicycle, Nordic skiing devices). Any exercises that create eccentric muscle contractions should be avoided (weights, isometric exercises, etc.).

Many nonpharmacologic therapies can be used to improve pain and quality of life for the fibromyalgia patient. Postural corrections include correction of the typical head-forward-shoulder forward slouch, correction of scoliosis, attention to leg length discrepancy often with orthotics, and correction of abnormal foot mechanics with corrective shoes or orthotics. Nutritional changes to encourage weight loss and avoidance of alcohol, caffeine, and refined sugars. Smoking cessation is *always* helpful. Psychological therapy can include supportive counseling, simple education, cognitive-behavioral therapy, desensitization training, and mindfulness based stress reduction. Acupuncture, physical therapy, and occupational therapy are often beneficial. Electroceutical treatment with neuromuscular re-education has been shown in controlled studies to be beneficial. Help with vocational rehabilitation may be vital.

PELVIC PAIN

Chronic Pelvic Pain

Chronic pelvic pain (CPP) is a disease predominantly of women. On formal questionnaires, 15% of all women age 18 to 50 report symptoms of CPP within the last 3 months. The prevalence of CPP in women between ages 12 to 70 presenting to their primary care physician is estimated is estimated to be 38 per 1000. The prevalence is similar to migraine, back pain, and asthma. Two percent of all gynecologic visits are for CPP. Ten percent of all laparoscopies (2 million per year) are performed for CPP, either diagnosis or treatment. Ten percent of all hysterectomies (600,000 per year) are performed to treat CPP.

The pain of CPP is often poorly localized, described as being abdominal in 80%, urethral in 74%, low back in 66%, and vaginal and/or vulvar in 52%. It is described as cramping, aching, throbbing, sharp, burning, and pressure. Menstruation and intercourse often aggravate the pain. Associated symptoms include urinary urgency and frequency in up to 75% of patients, and dyspareunia in up to 50% of patients. Autonomic symptoms, such as sweating, abnormal temperature regulation, and intestinal bloating are often noted.

The differential diagnosis is listed in Box 19-17.

The gynecologic literature estimates that in women with a low risk for sexually transmitted disease, endometriosis accounts for 70% of chronic pelvic pain (see section on endometriosis). The urologic literature notes that 75% of women at gynecologic evaluation for CPP complain of urinary urgency, frequency, or irritative voiding symptoms. The urologic literature suggests that many cases of CPP are misdiagnosed as due to endometriosis and should be accurately diagnosed as due to interstitial cystitis. Estimates have been made that 1 in 5 women have interstitial cystitis and that 33% to 70% of CPP is due to interstitial cystitis (see section on interstitial cystitis).

The gastroenterology literature estimates that 10% of the general population has symptoms of irritable bowel disease with a ratio of 2.5 women to 1 man. Mental health disease can also present as the primary pathology in CPP or as a comorbidity. Physical and/or sexual abuse is noted to be present in 25% of cases in the gynecologic literature and in 80% of cases in mental health-literature. Depression can be the primary pathology or secondary to CPP. Substance abuse is present in 8% to 10% of the general population and can be intimately associated with CPP. Somatization disorder can present with pelvic pain. The diagnostic criteria for somatization disorder are: at least 4 sites of pain; two GI symptoms other than pain; one neurologic symptom other than pain; and one sexual or reproductive problem other than pain. Pelvic inflammatory disease, myofascial pain, fibromyalgia, prostatitis, diverticulosis, adenomyosis, GI malignancies, genitourinary malignancies, pelvic vein thrombosis, postoperative adhesions, and postradiation therapy inflammation are also potential causes.

Box 19-17   Differential Diagnosis of Chronic Pelvic Pain

1. Interstitial cystitis
2. Endometriosis
3. Infectious
   a. Pelvic inflammatory disease
   b. Prostatitis
4. Irritable bowel syndrome
5. Mental health disease
   a. Physical and/or sexual abuse
   b. Depression
   c. Substance abuse
   d. Somatization disorder
6. Pelvic myofascial pain
7. Fibromyalgia
8. Diverticulosis
9. Adenomyosis
10. Gastrointestinal and genitourinary malignancy
11. Lymphoma
12. Pelvic venous thrombosis
13. Postop adhesions
14. Postradiation inflammation

CPP should be considered as a form of complex regional pain syndrome (CRPS), with the disease entities listed in the differential diagnosis acting as triggers to the development of CPP. The pelvic and abdominal viscera have a shared efferent innervation. Thirty to 80% of visceral C-fiber afferents are normally "silent," activated only by prolonged stimulation or by particularly intense stimulation. The source of the stimulus can be bladder urothelium, visceral or parietal endothelium, intestinal endothelium, vaginal epithelium, vulva epithelium, or prostatic stroma. C-fiber firing causes dorsal horn "wind-up." Dorsal horn wind-up causes antidromic firing of nociceptive afferents that results in the peripheral release of substance P and neurotrophic growth factor, mast cell stimulation, and the release of proinflammatory mediators. The release of these substances results in peripheral sensitization and orthodromic firing of the nociceptive afferents and perpetuation of a pain cycle. Viscera-visceral hyperalgesia develops through shared innervation. Viscera-muscular reflexes are activated and present in 85% of patients with CPP. The viscera-muscular reflex results in a hypertonic and contracted pelvic floor, voiding dysfunction, perineal trigger points, and dyspareunia. The viscera-muscular component can be treated with myofascial release.

Evidence from laparoscopic pain mapping under conscious sedation lends support to the categorization of CPP as a form CRPS. Three patterns of pain are identified from gentle stimulation of the superficial peritoneum at multiple sites in women being evaluated for CPP. The first pattern is of localized pain at the site of stimulation that reproduces the patient's symptoms; this is usually associated with endometriosis, adhesions, and hernias. The second pattern is one in which bilateral stimulation in multiple compartments causes unilateral pain in one or several compartments; this pattern is not associated with definable local lesions and is usually seen in patients with unilateral pain. The third pattern is one in which bilateral stimulation in multiple compartments causes more generalized pain that can be ipsilateral, contralateral, or bilateral to the stimulation; this pattern is not associated with definable lesions and is usually seen in patients with diffuse pain. The overwhelming numbers of patients fall into categories two and three.

The treatment of CPP is clearly most successful with a multidisciplinary approach (Box 19-18). Specific treatment for the underlying pathogenetic trigger(s) should be instituted as well as general multidisciplinary treatments used to treat chronic pain of any etiology. One study showed that oral medications alone gave >75% pain relief in 80% of patients if the diagnosis was made and treatment begun within 2.5 years of the onset of symptoms. Unfortunately, symptoms are often present for 4 to 7 years before diagnosis.

Box 19-18   Treatment of Chronic Pelvic Pain

1. Multidisciplinary approach ideal
2. Specific treatments aimed at underlying pathogenetic triggers
   As example, endometriosis or interstitial cystitis
3. Pharmacologic treatment of pain
   a. NSAIDs, COX-2s
   b. Tramadol
   c. NMDA antagonists
   d. Adjuvants
       TCAs, anticonvulsants, α-2 agonists, GABA agonists, sodium channel blockers, etc.
   e. Opiates
4. Pharmacologic treatment of depression, anxiety, PTSD
   a. TCAs
   b. SSRIs, SNRIs
   c. Benzodiazepines
   d. Antipsychotics
5. Psychological treatment of depression, PTSD, pain
   a. Supportive counseling
   b. Cognitive-behavioral therapy
   c. Desensitization therapy
   d. Mindfulness based stress reduction
6. Acupuncture
7. Physical therapy, massage therapy
8. Interventional procedures
   a. Sympathetic blockade superior hypogastric plexus
   b. Spinal-cord stimulator
   c. Sacral nerve root stimulator
   d. Intrathecal drug delivery system

INTERSTITIAL CYSTITIS

Interstitial cystitis (IC) is thought to be secondary to a glycosaminoglycan deficiency covering the bladder urothelium. Urinary components, such as potassium and urea, are able to penetrate the urothelium and initiate an inflammatory reaction. Common symptoms include urinary urgency, frequency, pelvic pain, pelvic pressure, bladder spasms, dyspareunia, dysuria, nocturnal pain, pain exacerbated by menses, and pain that persists for several days after intercourse. Fifty to 60% of patients report an increase in pain with acidic foods, carbonated drinks, alcohol, and caffeine. The pain is located in the lower abdomen in 80%, the urethra in 74%, the lower back in 66%, and the vagina in 52%. The pain often presents episodically (often misdiagnosed as recurrent UTI) before progressing to continuous pain with flares. Symptoms are typically present for 4 to 7 years before diagnosis.

The differential diagnosis includes chronic bladder infections, bladder carcinoma, and radiation or medication induced cystitis (see Box 19-17).

The diagnosis can be suggested by administering the O'Leary-Sant questionnaire or the pelvic pain, urgency, frequency (PUF) questionnaire. A score of >10 on the PUF is 75% to 94% predictive of a positive intravesical potassium sensitivity test (PST). The intravesical PST is positive in 80% of patients who meet all diagnostic criteria for IC as established by the National Institute for Diabetes and Digestive and Kidney Disease. The intravesical PST is positive in 82% of patients with CPP, 86% of patients with endometriosis, 79% of patients with vulvodynia, and 91% of patients with dyspareunia. A urinalysis and urine culture and sensitivity should be done for all patients that present with pelvic pain. Cystoscopy should be performed on any patient with gross hematuria, microscopic hematuria on repeat testing, or patients with onset of symptoms after age 50. There are both ulcerative and nonulcerative forms of IC. Therefore, visual findings on cystoscopy do not correlate with either presence or absence of disease.

A multidisciplinary approach to treatment is ideal (see Box 19-18). This can include psychological supportive treatment, cognitive-behavioral treatment, desensitization treatment, mindfulness-based stress reduction, specific treatment of PTSD associated with physical or sexual abuse, dietary changes to avoid food triggers, acupuncture, and massage/physical therapy to relieve pelvic floor trigger points.

Specific treatments for IC are outlined in Box 19-19. TCAs provide 50% to 64% total relief of symptoms. Anticholinergic properties decrease urinary frequency. Sedation minimizes nocturnal pain effects that interfere with sleep. Catecholamine reuptake inhibition decreases neuropathic pain. Pentosan polysulfate sodium (PPS) 100 mg tid has a response rate of 42% when used alone and 80% when used in conjunction with TCAs. PPS stimulates reemergence of glycosaminoglycans on the urothelium and can take 2 to 12 months to show its effect. Gabapentin has a response rate of 50% in patients refractory to TCAs. Hydroxyzine has a 40% response rate, with the effect taking 2 to 3 months to appear. Calciumglycerophophate (Prelief) provides a 70% decrease in food related symptoms in both IC and irritable bowel syndrome.

Intravesical DMSO has a 50% to 90% efficacy rate, but a 35% to 40% relapse rate. Retreatment with DMSO shows only a maximum 50% response rate.

Intravesical heparin can be used alone or in combination with intravesical DMSO. Intravesical heparin has a 50% to 95% response rate. The relapse rate is less than 35%. Retreatment is equally effective as initial treatment.

Posterior tibial nerve stimulation can be applied percutaneously with either needle probes or cutaneous gel electrodes. Stimulation at 2Hz, voltage just below pain threshold, 30-minute sessions weekly, for 8 to 10 weeks have been shown to significantly reduce symptoms of urgency, frequency, and bladder pain and pressure. Stimulation is carried out just proximal to the medial malleolus.

Botulinum toxin is effective injected intravesical, intrasphincteric, and as well in levator antitrigger points. Botulinum toxin acts both by direct muscle relaxation and by direct effects on nociceptive neurons inhibiting the release of glutamate.

Sacral nerve root stimulation is reserved for patients refractory to other forms of treatment. Seventy-three to 92% of patients achieve a greater than 50% improvement in their symptoms.

Box 19-19   Specific Treatment of Interstitial Cystitis

1. Pharmacologic
   a. TCAs
   b. Gabapentin
   c. Pentosan polysulfate sodium 100 to 300 mg tid
   d. Hydroxyzine
   e. Calciumglycerophosphate (Prelief)
2. Intravesical treatments
   a. Cystoscopy and hydrodistension
   b. DMSO
   c. Heparin
   d. Botulinum toxin A
      intravesical, intrasphincteric, levator antitrigger points
3. Acupuncture
4. Massage/physical therapy for pelvic floor trigger points
5. Posterior tibial nerve stimulation
6. Sacral nerve root stimulation

ENDOMETRIOSIS

Endometriosis is defined as the presence of endometrial stroma and glands outside the uterine cavity and uterine musculature. Endometrial tissues are dependent on ovarian steroids for biologic activity, which has important implications for treatment.

The prevalence of endometriosis is uncertain. Endometriosis is found in 12% to 32% of women of reproductive age undergoing laparoscopy to determine the cause of CPP, in 21% to 48% of women undergoing laparoscopy for infertility, and in 50% of teenagers with CPP.

The pathogenesis of endometriosis is not known. Genetic factors are important. A woman who has a first-degree relative with endometriosis is 7 times more likely to develop endometriosis than a woman with no family history of endometriosis.

Endometriosis most commonly presents as an asymptomatic, incidental finding at the time of other evaluation. For example, 6% to 43% of asymptomatic women undergoing elective laparoscopic sterilization are found to have endometriosis. Symptomatic endometriosis can present with the following symptoms: pelvic pain that can be unilateral, bilateral, low back, or diffuse; dysmenorrhea; dyspareunia; voiding dysfunction; abnormal menses; and infertility. Symptoms often increase perimenstrually.

Endometrial implants most commonly occur in the pelvis and less commonly in the abdomen. Rare cases of implantation have been reported in the breast, pancreas, liver, diaphragm, kidneys, vertebrae, peripheral nerves, and central nervous system.

An excellent history can be obtained through use of the International Pelvic Pain Society Questionnaire. This includes gynecologic, urologic, gastrointestinal, psychosocial, and musculoskeletal questions. It is available free of charge on the Internet, and only requires proper attribution for its use. Physical exam must include a pelvic examination. Diagnostic studies should include CBC, ESR, U/A, pregnancy test, cervical culture and sensitivity for chlamydia and gonorrhea, and pelvic ultrasound. The diagnosis of endometriosis should be confirmed by laparoscopy. The classification of endometriosis at laparoscopy is listed in Box 19-20. However, it is important to remember that there is no correlation between the stage of endometriosis observed and the presence or severity of symptoms. Infertility, however, is more likely to be associated with severe disease.

Treatment specific for endometriosis is outlined in Box 19-21. First-line treatment includes NSAIDs, COX-2s, oral contraceptives in monthly or 3 to 4 month cycles, and TCAs.

Box 19-20   Classification of Endometriosis at Laparoscopy

1. Minimal: isolated, superficial implants; no adhesions
2. Mild: superficial implants <5 cm aggregate; no adhesions
3. Moderate: multiple, superficial and invasive implants >5 cm aggregate; mild to moderate peritubal and/or ovarian adhesions
4. Severe: multiple implants, endometriomas; dense adhesions

Box 19-21   Specific Treatment of Endometriosis

1. First-line pharmacologic
   a. NSAIDs, COX-2s
   b. Oral contraceptives
   c. TCAs
2. Second-line pharmacologic
   a. Gonadotropin releasing hormone (GnRH) agonists
      (1) Lueprolide 3.75 mg IM q4 wks
      (2) Goserelin 3.6 mg s.c. q4 wks
      (3) Nafarelin 200 to 400 μg intranasal bid
      Treat for 2 months; resume therapy if symptoms recur
   b. Progestins
      (1) Medroxyprogesterone acetate 10 mg tid
      (2) Norethindrone acetate 5 mg qd
      Treat for 6 months
   c. Testosterone derivatives
      (1) Danazol 100 to 400 mg bid
      Titrate to amenorrhea
      Treat for 2 to 9 months
3. Surgery
   a. Laparoscopic endometrial ablation
   b. Hysterectomy
   c. Laparoscopic neural ablation

Second-line pharmacologic treatment is used only after failure of first-line treatment and is directed at the hormone responsiveness of endometrial tissue. Gonadotropin releasing hormone (GnRH) agonists are usually better tolerated than progestins or Danazol. "Add back" therapy with estrogen, progestins, bisphosphonates, parathyroid hormone, and calcitonin can be used to minimize the side effects of GnRH. Treatment is recommended for 2 months. If symptoms recur after discontinuation of therapy, resume the effective treatment regimen.

Surgery is indicated for the treatment of infertility due to endometriosis. Medical therapy is ineffective in restoring fertility. Other currently accepted indications for surgery are severe symptoms, the presence of endometriomas, and failure of medical management. There are no randomized, controlled studies that document the effectiveness of surgery at controlling symptoms. Laparoscopy with ablation of endometrial implants has been reported retrospectively to have up to 70% success at controlling symptoms; however, the recurrence rate can be as high as 40%. Hysterectomy has been reported to offer pain relief in 80% to 90% of women. Laparoscopic neural ablation of either uterosacral nerves or the presacral plexus has been reported, but their effectiveness is questionable.

Other general treatments for chronic pelvic pain due to endometriosis are the same as for chronic pelvic pain of any other etiology and are listed above and in Box 19-18.

SUGGESTED READING

Andren-Sandberg A, Hoem D, Gislason H: Pain management in chronic pancreatitis. European Journal of Gastroenterology & Hepatology 14:957-970, 2002.

Aronoff GM: Myofascial pain syndrome and fibromyalgia: a critical assessment and alternate view. Clinical Journal of Pain 14(1):74-85, 1998.

Bradley EL III, Bem J: Nerve blocks and neuroablative surgery for chronic pancreatitis. World Journal of Surgery 27:1241-1248, 2003.

Breitbart W, Dibiase L: Current perspectives on pain in AIDS. Oncology (Huntington) 16:818-829, 834-835, 2002.

Buskila D: Fibromyalgia, chronic fatigue syndrome, and myofascial pain syndrome. Current Opinion in Rheumatology 13(2):117-127, 2001.

Claster S, Vichinsky EP: Managing sickle cell disease. BMJ 327:1151-1155, 2003.

Davis CJ, McMillan L: Pain in endometriosis: effectiveness of medical and surgical management. Current Opinion in Obstetrics & Gynecology 15:507-512, 2003.

Kahl S, Zimmermann S, Malfertheiner P: Acute pancreatitis: treatment strategies. Digestive Diseases 21:30-37, 2003.

Nickel JC: Interstitial cystitis: a chronic pelvic pain syndrome. Medical Clinics of North America 88:467-481, 2004.

Okpala I. Tawil A. Management of pain in sickle cell disease. Journal of the Royal Society of Medicine 95:456-458, 2002.

Pardo C, McArthur J, Griffin J: HIV neuropathy: insights in the pathology of HIV peripheral nerve disease. J Periph Nerv Syst 6:21-27, 2001.

Sand PK: Chronic pain syndromes of gynecologic origin. Journal of Reproductive Medicine 49:230-234, 2004.

Sim J, Adams N: Systematic review of randomized controlled trials of non-pharmacological interventions for fibromyalgia. Academic Clinical Journal of Pain. 18(5):324-336, 2002.

Stinson J, Naser B: Pain management in children with sickle cell disease. Pediatric Drugs 5:229-241, 2003.

Strate T, Knoefel WT, Yekebas E, Izbicki JR: Chronic pancreatitis: etiology, pathogenesis, diagnosis, and treatment. International Journal of Colorectal Disease 18:97-106, 2003.

Weigent DA, Bradley LA, Blalock JE, Alarcon GS: Current concepts in the pathophysiology of abnormal pain perception in fibromyalgia. American Journal of the Medical Sciences 315(6):405-412, 1998.

Wolfe F, Smyth HA, Yunus MB, et al: The American College of Rheumatology 1990 criteria for the classification of fibromyalgia: report of the multicentre criteria committee. Arthrit Rheum 33:160-172, 1990.

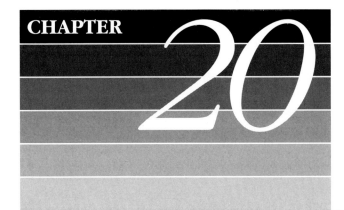

Cancer Pain

THERESE O'CONNOR

INTRODUCTION

The diagnosis of malignant disease carries with it many fears and anxieties. Apart from the fear of death, one of the most prevalent fears is that of pain. And indeed these fears may be justified. Cancer is the cause of 1 in every 10 deaths worldwide and 1 in 5 deaths in the United States. Analysis of published reviews reveals that more than two-thirds of patients with advanced cancer disease experience moderate to severe pain and pain is a major symptom in half of those undergoing active treatment. Pain may be severe or excruciating in 30% of cancer pain patients and moderate to severe in 50%.

The recent development of the specialties of pain medicine and of palliative care medicine has resulted in some progress in the relief of pain in cancer pain patients. However, significant limitations to the optimal management of pain remain and this results in less than optimal treatment, in part because of misconceptions about the administration of analgesic medication (especially narcotic drugs), but also because of lack of resources. Because of advancing disease, cancer pain often requires close titration of analgesics and frequent assessments to adequately manage even simple cancer pain problems, and this requires significant resources. For resistant or complex cancer pain, a multidisciplinary approach will optimize pain management. The oncologist, radiation therapist, anesthesiologist, neurosurgeon, and psychiatrist or psychologist should consult regularly and endeavor to pool their knowledge and experience to form pain management plans for such patients. Their aim should be to provide patients with maximum comfort while preserving organ function with minimal risk, cost, and discomfort.

Unrelieved pain can lead to a resignation to death as it is a constant reminder of the gravity of the disease and its progression. It is profoundly distressing to cancer patients and their loved ones; as pain physicians we must acquire the skills necessary to manage this symptom.

PATHOGENESIS OF CANCER PAIN

The pathogenesis of cancer pain among cancer patients involves multiple causes and mechanisms. Pain is not always the result of tumor progression, and it is essential that the precise cause be identified whenever possible, so that appropriate treatment can be initiated. Several common causes for cancer pain are listed in Box 20-1.

Types of Cancer Pain

Nociceptive or Somatic Pain

This type of pain results from activation of nociceptive afferent fibers as a result of tissue injury. It is usually well-localized and may be sharp and intense. Examples include musculoskeletal pain, bone metastases, and postoperative pain. Somatic pain usually responds to analgesic medications, such as opioids, nonsteroidal anti-inflammatory drugs (NSAIDs), local injection (e.g., joint injection with corticosteroid), somatic neurolytic nerve blocks, and radiation therapy.

Visceral Pain

Pain of visceral origin is common with intrathoracic, intra-abdominal, and pelvic tumors. The character of visceral pain can be described as deep, gnawing pain, experienced over a large area, being poorly localized. It is often referred to a cutaneous area (e.g., shoulder pain with liver metastases or hepatoma, back pain with endometrial or pancreatic carcinoma).

The likely mechanism of referred pain includes convergence in the spinal cord and the existence of branched afferent C-fibers that supply both visceral and somatic structures. Areas of referred pain may be tender to palpation. Visceral pain usually responds to opioid-based medications, although it is somewhat more opioid resistant than somatic pain. It is often possible to interrupt visceral pain using neurolytic blocks while preserving somatic motor and sensory function (Box 20-2).

Neuropathic Pain

While somatic and visceral pain occur in the presence of a normal functioning nervous system, injury to nerves by chemotherapy, radiation therapy, surgery, or tumor growth may produce neuropathic pain. This pain may be burning, shooting, or lancinating and may have associated neurological symptoms, allodynia, hyperpathia, or dysesthesia. Nerve injury can produce ectopic discharges, with paroxysms of stimuli, resulting in severe pain. This type of pain often responds poorly to opioids but may respond to drugs that modify nerve conduction (e.g., anticonvulsant, antidepressant, antiarrhythmic medications, and to interventions that decrease nerve ectopic activity, such as nerve blockade with added corticosteroid or neurolytic nerve blocks).

The pathogenesis of cancer pain may be complex in any individual and pain may be caused by a variable combination of all of the above. Comprehensive management requires careful assessment of the contribution of each type of pain and appropriate medications and/or interventions to address each.

Box 20-1   Common Causes of Pain in Cancer Patients

1. Tumor progression and related pathology
   Nerve compression, infiltration
   Bone pain
   Visceral pain
2. Operations or other investigative or therapeutic interventions
3. Treatment related pain
   Radiation neuropathy
   Chemotherapy-induced neuropathy
4. Infection
   Bacterial
   Herpes zoster
5. Muscle, joint, ligamentous pain from immobility, deconditioning
6. Common nonmalignant causes
   Arthritis
   Lumbar, cervical spine disease
   Headache
   Diabetic neuropathy

Box 20-2   Types of Visceral Pain

1. Distension of a hollow viscus
   Bowel obstruction
   Ureteral obstruction
2. Irritation of the mucosal and serosal surfaces
   NSAIDs
   Radiation therapy
   Chemotherapy
   Pancreatic enzymes
3. Mesenteric irritation, traction or torsion
4. Distension of the capsule of solid viscus
   Liver
   Spleen
   Kidney

Assessment of Cancer Pain

Studies of cancer pain management have demonstrated that poor pain assessment was the greatest barrier to effective pain control as careful evaluation is required when multiple causes of pain are possible. A comprehensive initial assessment followed by regular subsequent assessments is required to formulate a treatment plan and to evaluate the effectiveness of treatment. If the initial management does not address pain adequately, further assessment of causes related to cancer treatment, new metastatic lesions, or nonmalignant origins may be indicated. An outline of the assessment process is shown in Box 20-3.

Psychological Assessment

Patients who have pain with cancer have a greater risk of depression and other mood disturbances. As pain becomes more severe it increasingly intrudes on the patient's mood and quality of life and adequate pain relief reverses this effect. It is important to note that patients may be assumed to be depressed when the actual problem is undermedication of analgesic medication for severe pain. Patients may under-report pain for many reasons. They may fear that it will distract staff from curing their disease. They may assume that pain is a natural part of the illness or treatment. They may feel that staff will be less favorable to them if they continue to report unresolved pain problems. They may worry that potent analgesic medication will have side effects and cause addiction. All patients with cancer need to be assertive in reporting pain and communicating with staff

---

Box 20-3 Pain Assessment

History of pain
Onset and pattern
Quality
Location of each pain
Exacerbating and relieving factors
Intensity (Visual Analogue Scale or other scale)
Previous treatments and response
History of associated symptoms
    Nausea, anorexia, cachexia, constipation, dysphagia,
        dyspnea, urinary function
Physical examination
    General physical exam
Site of pain
    Tenderness, allodynia
Neurologic examination
Laboratory studies
Imaging studies
Psychological evaluation

---

when pain-relief measures are not working. Patients with pre-existing psychiatric disease need parallel management for both the psychiatric problem and the pain.

Diagnostic Evaluation

In order to optimize pain management and to reduce morbidity it is important that the pain physician be able to recognize the common pain syndromes that indicate disease recurrence or progression. Prompt recognition of these syndromes may also help to avoid or minimize neurological impairment when neurological structures are involved.

Bone Pain

While bone pain is common in primary bony cancers (e.g., sarcoma, myeloma), the incidence of those tumors is relatively low. Lung, breast, and prostate cancers are very prevalent and all have a high incidence of bone metastases. Renal and thyroid cancers also metastasize to bone, but are not nearly as prevalent. The vertebrae, pelvis, femur, and skull are the most common sites of metastasis to bone. Pain is usually well-localized and is dull and aching in character. Vertebral bony metastases may cause radiculopathic pain as a result of nerve root impingement. Complications include spinal-cord compression, hypercalcemia, and pathological fractures.

Bone metastases may be diagnosed by plain x-ray, where typical lytic, blastic, or mixed lesions are demonstrated and easily distinguished from other causes. Radioisotope bone scan is a sensitive diagnostic investigation for bone metastases and magnetic resonance imaging (MRI) may be helpful when bone has been previously irradiated and in cases of multiple myeloma.

Neuraxial Metastases

Epidural metastasis is a medical emergency and a common complication of prostate, breast, or lung cancer, melanoma, multiple myeloma, or renal cell carcinoma. Contiguous spread from vertebral metastases is the usual route of entry to the epidural space, although retroperitoneal spread, spread through intervertebral foramina, and bloodborne spread are possible. Pain is a reliable early sign and is usually midline or radiculopathic in the distribution of the affected nerve roots. Motor, sensory, autonomic, and bladder and bowel dysfunction may be evident. Diagnosis is by plain x-ray and MRI. A high index of suspicion will aid early diagnosis before neurologic signs develop and institution of appropriate treatment can avoid incontinence and paralysis. Treatment with corticosteroids or radiotherapy will often relieve spinal-cord compression, but surgical decompression is occasionally indicated.

Plexopathies

Brachial plexopathy is commonly caused by nerve infiltration by breast and lung cancer, by lymphoma and rarely, from metastasis to the brachial plexus. Like epidural metastasis, pain precedes neurological symptoms of sensory loss and weakness. Brachial plexus pain is experienced in the distribution of the involved roots and both upper and lower cords may be involved causing shoulder, forearm, elbow, and hand pain. Pancoast tumors of the superior pulmonary sulcus extend to the plexus in approximately 50% of cases.

Lumbar plexopathy is usually the result of direct compression by or invasion of the plexus as it passes through the psoas muscle, although metastatic spread is responsible for approximately 25% of lumbar plexopathies. The site of infiltration determines the distribution of pain, which is experienced in the lower abdomen, buttocks, and lower limbs. Pain precedes neurological symptoms and alerts one to the possibility of epidural spread causing spinal-cord compression and/or Cauda Equina syndrome. Pelvic CT scan, abdominal CT scan, and MRI are valuable diagnostic tools for prompt recognition of these syndromes.

Peripheral Neuropathy

Direct local compression or invasion of peripheral nerves by tumor may cause pain in the distribution of the affected nerve. Other factors, such as injury following radiation therapy, neurotoxic chemotherapy (e.g., vincristine, cisplatin, Taxol), or postoperative fibrosis of tissue can also cause peripheral neuropathic pain. Approximately 15% of patients with myeloma develop a progressive painful peripheral neuropathy associated with sensorimotor loss.

Herpes Zoster and Postherpetic Neuralgia

Suppression of the immune system in patients with cancer, especially in the elderly, leads to a higher incidence of varicella-zoster infection or reactivation and is twice as likely to occur in to occur in those with active disease as in those with remission. A high index of suspicion in cancer patients with unexplained pain particularly in the trunk or cranial nerve distributions with early institution of antiviral therapy and neuropathic pain medication (see below) can minimize discomfort and reduce nerve pain. Early initiation of epidural analgesia with local anesthetic or sympathetic blocks for trigeminal distribution herpes zoster has been shown to reduce the severity and duration of pain in the acute phase. However, there is little evidence that blocks reduce the incidence of postherpetic neuralgia.

Mucositis

Cytotoxic chemotherapy or radiation therapy to the head and neck may cause intense oral, pharyngeal, or esophageal pain with keratinization, sloughing, and ulceration of the involved mucosa. The pain intensity is related to the degree of damage to the mucosal tissue, is worse in the patient with concomitant periodontal disease, and may be complicated by superimposed infection. It is typically a burning pain that usually responds to local anesthetic mouthwash and systemic opioid administration.

PHARMACOLOGIC MANAGEMENT

Systemic analgesic pharmacotherapy is the mainstay of cancer pain management because it is effective, low risk, and usually of rapid onset. The guiding care principle is the individualization of therapy. Through a process of repeated assessments, drug selection, and administration is individualized so that a favorable balance between pain relief and adverse side effects is achieved and maintained through possible changing patterns of pain.

The World Health Organization (WHO) has proposed an "analgesic ladder," which is now widely used. This approach has been shown to be effective in 75% to 90% of patients with cancer pain. It is advised that the cause of pain should first be identified. Emphasizing that pain intensity should be the guiding principle it advocates the approach shown in Box 20-4.

Adjuvant drugs that treat other symptoms enhance analgesic efficacy or address specific types of pain independently (e.g., corticosteroids, anticonvulsants, antidepressants, antiarrhythmics) may be added at any step.

In order to maintain a constant serum level of drug, analgesia should be administered on a regular "by the clock" basis with breakthrough doses as appropriate. If

---

Box 20-4   World Health Organization Analgesic Ladder

Step 1: Patients with mild-moderate cancer pain should be treated with a nonopioid analgesic (e.g., acetaminophen, NSAIDs).

Step 2: Patients who fail to achieve adequate pain relief from a trial of nonopioid analgesics or are intolerant of side effects should be treated with an opioid for mild to moderate pain (e.g., codeine or hydrocodone as well as the nonopioid medication).

Step 3: If severe pain is present from the outset or there is failure to respond to Step 2, patients should be treated with opioid analgesic drugs of increasing strength until analgesia is achieved or unacceptable side effects occur.

Step 4: This is a modification to the WHO ladder and consists of invasive procedures, such as epidural or intrathecal drug administration.

the patient presents with moderate to severe pain step 2 or 3 are commenced from the outset.

Nonopioid Analgesics

Acetaminophen (Paracetamol)

The exact analgesic mechanism of acetaminophen is not clear. It may inhibit prostaglandin synthesis in some tissues but not in others and may be a weak inhibitor of cyclooxygenase (COX)-1 and COX-2 enzymes. COX-3, another enzyme isoform present in central nervous system tissue in some species, has been demonstrated to be more sensitive to acetaminophen than is COX-1 or COX-2. This drug is useful alone for mild to moderate pain and can provide additional analgesia when combined with an NSAID or opioid drug in the treatment of more severe pain. It is relatively free of upper gastrointestinal (GI) side effects and does not affect platelet function. However, it may in some circumstances reduce renal function. It may interact with anticoagulants, domperidone and metoclopramide, and anion-exchange resins. It is usually well-tolerated but may be hepatotoxic at higher doses of 10 to 15 g as a result of synthesis of toxic metabolites following dehydroxylation. In overdose depletion of glutathione may cause fatal hepatic necrosis. Paracetamol can also cause renal tubular necrosis and rarely, minor hypersensitivity reactions. It is safe in patients with bleeding diathesis as it has no effects on platelets.

Nonsteroidal Anti-Inflammatory Drugs and Cyclooxygenase-2 Inhibitors

NSAIDs are a chemically heterogeneous group of drugs that are unified by their common mode of action—inhibition of prostaglandin synthesis. Prostaglandins, biologically active lipids generated from arachidonic acid, contribute to the development of the inflammatory response and produce erythema, edema, and fever. They also produce sensitization of peripheral nociceptors and recent evidence suggests a central nervous system sensitizing effect for these agents in promoting the perception of pain. In addition to their role in mediating the inflammatory response, prostaglandins protect the gastric mucosa through the suppression of the release of gastric acid and increase in mucosal blood flow and mucus production. They are also involved in other important physiological processes including blood platelet aggregation, autoregulation in the kidney, and antiplatelet activity in the vascular endothelium.

NSAIDs provide analgesia primarily through peripheral inhibition of the enzyme COX, which is required for prostaglandin production. Consequent sensitization or activation of peripheral nociceptors is therefore inhibited, and it is possible that central mechanisms are also responsible for the analgesic effects.

It is now known that there are many different isoforms of the COX enzyme. The constitutive form, COX-1, is continually present in most cells in the body and is generally unregulated. It is responsible for the generation of prostaglandins that participate in many physiologic processes.

The COX-2 enzyme is normally absent in many tissues, or is expressed less prominently. However, following injury, such as trauma or infection it is rapidly induced, contributing to the inflammatory response. In general, COX-1 inhibition may produce unwanted side effects, such as gastritis and platelet dysfunction, whereas COX-2 inhibition produces anti-inflammatory, analgesia, and antipyretic properties.

Most of the standard drugs in the NSAID group are mixed COX-1 and COX-2 inhibitors. Over recent years specific COX-2 inhibitors have been developed, providing analgesia and anti-inflammatory effects with improved gastrointestinal tolerance. Serious gastrointestinal complications are still a risk with these drugs, but the incidence is roughly half that of mixed NSAIDs. Renal toxicity is a potential problem, and there is an increased incidence of ischemic cardiac events and stroke with some COX-2 antagonists.

NSAIDs are extensively bound to plasma proteins and therefore can displace or be displaced by other protein-bound drugs (e.g., digoxin, cyclosporin, methotrexate, Coumadin, and oral hypoglycemic drugs). Toxicity effects may therefore occur. Renal and hepatic dysfunction may occur, especially in patients who are elderly, those with pre-existing renal or hepatic function impairment, hypovolemia, and those who are treated with concomitant nephrotoxic drugs. COX-2 drugs are no less nephrotoxic than other NSAIDs.

Most COX inhibitors exacerbate ulcers and upper gastrointestinal symptoms, such as dyspepsia and epigastric pain and increase the risk of major GI toxic effects, such as hemorrhage, ulceration, or perforation. Despite improved GI tolerance, COX-2 inhibitors may delay healing of pre-existing GI ulceration. Because of their ability to increase bleeding time NSAIDs should be avoided if possible in patients who are thrombocytopenic or have clotting impairment. COX-2 inhibitors and the nonacetylated salicylates (salsalate and magnesium choline trisalicylate) have minimal effects on platelet function and are less likely to cause ulcers. They are safer in the coagulopathic patient, but are not risk-free.

A less common but potentially severe side effect is hypersensitivity reaction and skin rash, which can occur with all COX inhibitors. Therefore, careful monitoring for potential side effects should be carried out, especially in the elderly or in those with pre-existing GI, renal, or hepatic disease and those with decreased clotting ability (conditions present in many cancer patients).

Once an NSAID has been commenced the dose should be increased until adequate analgesia is achieved or the maximal recommended dose is reached. Because of a ceiling effect to their efficacy, if one from this group does not provide satisfactory pain relief, another should be tried before moving up the analgesic ladder.

Opioid Analgesics

Cancer pain of moderate to severe intensity should be managed with systemic administration of opioid analgesics. These drugs act on opioid receptors, which are seven-transmembrane receptors (the plasma membrane is crossed by the polypeptide chain three times) that are located in the central nervous system (CNS), mainly the spinal cord and brainstem, and in peripheral tissues. There are many types of opioid receptors, and the three main types are termed μ, κ, and δ receptors. μ-Agonist activation results in analgesia, euphoria, miosis, sedation, respiratory depression, cough suppression, decreased peristalsis with constipation, nausea and vomiting. In addition, δ and κ receptor activation also produces analgesia, although morphine-like drugs are more selective for μ receptors and therefore produces its well-known side effect profile as described above.

Opioid analgesics are a diverse group of drugs that may be structurally similar to morphine (e.g., codeine or hydromorphone) or may have a structure that is different from others in this group (e.g., buprenorphine, fentanyl, meperidine). Some are naturally occurring in opium (e.g., morphine) and others are synthetically manufactured (e.g., fentanyl, meperidine, and methadone). They are classified as full agonists, partial agonists, and mixed agonist/antagonists. Full agonists do not generally have a ceiling to their efficacy and have no antagonist action. Examples of full agonists include morphine, fentanyl, hydromorphone, oxycodone, codeine, and meperidine. Buprenorphine is an example of a partial agonist. There is a ceiling effect to its analgesic efficacy and it has relatively low intrinsic activity. The exact mechanism of action of tramadol is not known, but it does have a weak opioid effect. Pentazocine, nalbuphine, and nalorphine are examples of mixed agonists/antagonists. Because of the antagonist activity these agents should not be administered to patients who are receiving full opioid agonists as this may precipitate withdrawal syndrome and reverse pain relief.

While most opioids are μ-receptor agonists, there is considerable difference in their pharmacology, and failure to achieve adequate analgesia with one drug does not preclude success with another. In general, the dose of the selected drug is gradually increased until satisfactory analgesia is achieved or until unacceptable side effects occur. If side effects cannot be managed (e.g., analeptic drugs for somnolence, antiemetics for nausea), one should select another opioid. In general, it makes sense to select

a drug with higher efficacy or intrinsic activity. Intrinsic activity refers to the degree of receptor occupancy required to produce a given analgesic effect. A highly efficacious drug, such as sufentanil, will produce a given effect with occupation of a very low fraction of the available receptors, whereas low efficacy drugs, such as meperidine, require a much higher occupation to achieve the same effect. This becomes very important in tolerant patients or those with intense pain. In general, more potent drugs have a higher intrinsic activity, although this relationship is not always true. The relative efficacy of some commonly used drugs is shown in Box 20-5.

Methadone has a long duration of action as it is extensively bound to proteins and dissociates slowly, therefore producing less withdrawal symptoms. It is, however, as efficacious as morphine in its analgesic effect, but is less sedating in some patients, making it a useful drug for pain relief. It also has some N-methyl-D-aspartate (NMDA)-antagonist effect, which, at least theoretically, would provide some added benefit in neuropathic pain states.

Meperidine is now used uncommonly for cancer pain. It is a relatively weak (low efficacy) opioid that a toxic metabolite, nor-meperidine, which can produce CNS irritability, including seizures, when administered in high doses over prolonged periods.

Fentanyl has a high intrinsic activity and is often effective for patients who have not achieved pain relief with other opioids. Fortunately, it is available in a transdermal form for continuous administration and an oral transmucosal form for rapid administration for procedure or

---

Box 20-5 Potency, Intrinsic Activity, and Half-Lives of Common Opioids

Drug	Relative Potency*	Intrinsic Activity	Half-Life
Propoxyphene	0.5	Very low	6
Codeine	0.1	Very low	3
Buprenorphine	25	Low†	5‡
Meperidine	0.1	Low	3
Hydrocodone	3	Low-moderate	4
Morphine	1	Moderate	2
Oxycodone	3	Moderate	5
Methadone	1§	Moderate	30
Levorphanol	5§	Moderate	15
Hydromorphone	7	Moderate-high	3
Fentanyl	100	High	3
Sufentanil	500	Very high	2

*Estimated. Based on systemic equivalents for most drugs, oral equivalents for drugs available only as oral preparations (e.g., propoxyphene, oxycodone, hydrocodone).

†Partial agonist.

‡Long duration due to high receptor affinity.

§Applies to single IM or IV dose only. Accumulates with repeated doses.

breakthrough pain. Sufentanil has the highest efficacy of the available opioids. It is only available as an injectable, so it is administered as an intravenous infusion to highly tolerant patients who have failed other drugs.

All opioid analgesics exhibit tolerance (i.e., the need to increase dose over time to maintain the same degree of pain relief). However, increasing dose requirements usually indicate progression of the disease and in those patients where the disease is stable increasing doses is not usually required.

Physical dependence on opioids is exhibited when the drug is abruptly discontinued or an antagonist, such as naloxone is given. Withdrawal symptoms include nausea and vomiting, abdominal cramps, diarrhea, diaphoresis, irritability, joint pain, and lacrimation. Withdrawal symptoms occur sooner after discontinuation of opioids with short half-lives. The development of tolerance or physical dependence does not imply addiction or psychological dependence, which only rarely occur in this group of patients.

The optimal dose of opioids varies widely among patients and close titration of drug dose is required to give each analgesic a trial, before switching to a different drug. These drugs undergo extensive first-pass metabolism in the gut-wall and liver with oral administration. Therefore, other routes of administration (e.g., transdermal, sublingual, buccal, continuous subcutaneous, epidural, or intrathecal infusions may be considered if pain relief is inadequate).

Successful achievement of pain relief with opioid analgesics depends on:
1. Individualization of dose and route of administration
2. Regular administration (not on a prn basis)
3. Recognition and prompt appropriate treatment of side effects

Adjuvant Pharmacotherapy

Corticosteroids
Examples include dexamethasone, methylprednisolone, prednisolone, betamethasone, and triamcinolone. This group of drugs may be beneficial in the management of cancer as they are anti-inflammatory, antiemetic, stimulate appetite, elevate mood, and reduce peripheral edema. The anti-inflammatory effect is useful in the reduction of edema of the brain and spinal cord and helps reduce elevated intracranial pressure in brain metastases. Corticosteroids are a standard part of the treatment of spinal-cord compression and their direct inhibitory effect of spontaneous activity in excitable, damaged nerves also helps pain resulting from compression of peripheral nerves (e.g., brachial or lumbo-sacral plexopathy). Epidural corticosteroid may help pain from nerve root impingement by tumor or metastases.

Chronic use results in side effects that depend on the steroid given and both mineralocorticoid and glucocor-

ticoid side effects may occur. Hydrocortisone has a high mineralocorticoid effect and is therefore unsuitable for chronic pain. The risks are largely dose-dependant and the lowest effective dose for the shortest possible time should be used. Adverse side effects are usually reversible by dose reduction, but long-term effects may be permanent. Regular review is therefore indicated. It should be remembered that concomitant NSAID administration significantly increases the risk of peptic ulceration and prophylactic therapy should be added.

When pain relief is dependant on steroids the risk/benefit ratio for prolonged use should be carefully assessed and consideration should be given to alternative approaches to pain management.

Tricyclic Antidepressants
Examples include amitriptyline, doxepin, nortriptyline, imipramine, and desipramine. Through their action of blocking the reuptake of serotonin and norepinephrine at CNS synapses, tricyclic antidepressants (TCAs) are useful in the treatment of pain, particularly neuropathic pain. They may also help to improve analgesia by increasing plasma morphine levels. When administered at bedtime they improve sleep, and this can improve the ability to cope with chronic pain. Mood elevation may also help, although analgesic effect is observed at lower doses than the antidepressant effect.

There is more evidence that amitriptyline helps nerve pain although there are reports of beneficial effects with some other TCAs. Relative efficacy is unclear and amitriptyline is therefore the usual drug chosen in this group. The onset of pain relief occurs 1 to 2 weeks after commencement of therapy. It recommended that treatment be initiated with a small dose, titrating upwards to maximum dose slowly over a number of weeks to minimize sedative side effects in the elderly or debilitated patient. TCAs, especially amitriptyline and doxepin, have anticholinergic side effects and consequently dry mouth, constipation, and aggravation of prostatic symptoms may sometimes limit their usefulness. Of patients with neuropathic pain it is likely that approximately 30% of patients will obtain more than 50% pain relief. While minor side effects occur in 30% of patients on TCAs, major adverse effect necessitates discontinuation of the drug in only 4% of cases. Patients who experience intolerable sedation may be tried on desipramine, which is the least sedating of the class. Other antidepressants (e.g., 5HT reuptake antagonists) have fewer side effects but appear to be less effective in addressing neuropathic pain.

Anticonvulsants
Anticonvulsants have largely replaced the TCAs as first-line drugs for the treatment of neuropathic pain. The availability of a large number of new drugs with fewer side effects and drug interactions than carbamazepine,

valproic acid, and phenytoin and with a wide range of pharmacologic effects has greatly expanded their utility. Carbamazepine is still used extensively for classic trigeminal neuralgia, or tic douloureux, but is rarely the drug of choice for other neuropathies.

Gabapentin is the first-line drug for many neuropathic pain states. It has multiple mechanisms of action, including enhanced γ-aminobutyric acid (GABA) activity, reduction of voltage gated calcium currents, and some anti-inflammatory effects. It has few drug interactions and is usually well tolerated. It is started at doses of 100 to 300 mg tid and gradually increased to optimum effect, which usually occurs at doses of 600 to 900 mg tid to qid. Even higher doses are occasionally required. The dose is reduced if renal function is impaired.

Topiramate is also well-tolerated. It has multiple mechanisms of action, including GABA enhancement, sodium channel blockade, and block of some glutamate receptor subtypes. Topiramate and zonisamide both cause weight loss in some patients, limiting their utility in terminal cancer patients.

Lamotrigine blocks sodium channels and inhibits release of glutamate from primary afferent nerve terminals. Serious rashes, which can progress to Stevens-Johnson syndrome occur in up to 10% of patients.

Oxcarbazepine is an analog of carbamazepine, but has fewer serious side effects and fewer drug interactions. It has both sodium and calcium channel blocking properties.

Other drugs that have been used for neuropathic pain include levetiracetam, zonisamide, pregabalin, and tiagabine. There has been no clear rationale established for determining which drug to use when others have failed or produced intolerable side effects. A reasonable approach might be to select drugs with different mechanisms of action when rotating from one to another. Combinations of two anticonvulsants or of an anticonvulsant and a TCA may provide better pain control and fewer side effects than using a single drug alone.

NMDA Antagonists

NMDA antagonists have been shown to block or reverse central sensitization in animals following both inflammatory and neuropathic injury. They also reduce tolerance development to opioids and reduce the severity of opioid induced hyperalgesia. Ketamine has been used in intractable neuropathic pain states in subdissociative doses. It is effective orally at doses of 30 to 60 mg. For patients with excruciating pain that is unresponsive to high-dose opioids intravenous ketamine can be a useful rescue medication. Other available drugs with NMDA-antagonist effects include dextromethorphan, amantadine, memantine, propoxyphene, and methadone. NMDA-receptor antagonism may be a significant analgesic mechanism for amitriptyline as well.

Sodium Channel Blockers

Intravenous lidocaine is effective for a variety of painful neuropathic conditions. Unfortunately, its effect is short-lived, and oral administration can produce high levels of a toxic metabolite, monoethyl glycine xylidide (MEGX) through first-pass metabolism. Prolonged subcutaneous infusions have been used with some success, but there is a narrow therapeutic window for this drug.

Mexiletine, an antiarrhythmic drug, provides pain relief for some patients who are transiently responsive to lidocaine. Gastrointestinal side effects limit its utility. Patients with cardiac ventricular irritability may experience proarrhythmic effects.

Cannabinoids

δ-9-tetrahydrocannabinol has been demonstrated to have analgesic effects and reduce chemotherapy-induced nausea and vomiting. It is licensed for use in cancer pain in some countries. However, unacceptable side effects (e.g., drowsiness, dysphoria, hypotension, bradycardia) limit its routine use in chronic pain.

Bisphosphonates and Calcitonin

Bisphosphonates, such as pamidronate and clodronate, are highly effective for some cases of bone pain secondary to metastatic cancer. They inhibit tumor-induced bone resorption and reduce the incidence of pathological vertebral fractures and decrease radiation requirements for the treatment of metastatic disease of bone. They are orally absorbed, but are most effective when administered intravenously. Calcitonin, either injected subcutaneously or administered intranasally, has also been shown to be effective for treating pain from metastatic bone lesions. Both bisphosphonates and calcitonin have been reported to provide some relief for patients with complex regional pain syndrome (CRPS).

OTHER INTERVENTIONS

In general, the management of cancer pain should be approached by first-line treatment with NSAIDs, oral analgesics, and adjuvant drugs. Research has shown that a significant number of patients referred to pain clinics for neurolytic blocks or intraspinal narcotics respond promptly to adjustment of their oral medications. However, if there is unsatisfactory pain relief with oral drugs, many patients will benefit from techniques that modulate pain transmission and appreciation, without nerve destruction. In order to maximize pain relief to such patients, we need to fully understand the appropriate application of existing modalities for pain management. A combined approach encompassing oral medications, reduction in tumor size and spread, cognitive-behavioral therapy, physiotherapy, and non-neurolytic pain injection techniques should be explored prior to consideration of the drastic step of neuroablation and its often unacceptable side effects.

Transcutaneous Electrical Nerve Stimulation

Transcutaneous selective stimulation of large myelinated A-fibers by application of high-frequency, pulsed electrical current has been shown inhibit C-fiber activity and to reduce pain. Transcutaneous Electrical Nerve Stimulation (TENS) is thought to modify pain appreciation by stimulation of large fibers thereby blocking (or "closing the gate" to) the smaller C-fibers carrying nociceptive impulses to the spinal cord. There is also evidence that high-frequency stimulation of the skin decreases maximum firing rates and increases latency in small afferent fibers probably as a result of potassium efflux from the axon. This can produce conduction blockade in C-fibers as the current is increased. It is thought that the analgesia derived from the use of TENS is the result of a combination of these actions. High-intensity, low-frequency TENS may stimulate release of endogenous opioids.

Not all pain responds to TENS. If usual parameters do not produce pain relief, low-frequency, high-intensity stimulation may be tried at current amplitude level that produces mild discomfort and muscle stimulation. Burst stimulation may also relieve pain that is not responsive to conventional TENS where short bursts of high frequency stimulation are delivered at 1 to 2 Hz.

A TENS trial allows the patient to become familiar with the use of TENS and ensure that the pain is not aggravated by its use and should may be carried out prior to giving the unit to the patient to use at home. Length of application depends on the patient's response. Some patients will obtain several hours of relief following a 30-minute application, while others require constant use in order to obtain an effect. For full trial it is important to allow the patient to use the TENS at home for a period of at least 14 days.

Non-Neurolytic Nerve Blocks

Non-neurolytic nerve blocks may be helpful as an aid to diagnosis/prognosis but are also very useful in the management of intractable pain. In particular, neuropathic pain may respond dramatically to sympathetic nerve block or epidural or perineural steroid injections.

Non-neurolytic nerve blocks may also help to relieve severe acute pain (e.g., rib fracture) and provide temporary relief of incapacitating pain. As an aid to diagnosis, nerve blocks can differentiate between visceral and somatic pain, or between sympathetically-mediated and somatic pain, and they may be used to identify nerve distribution in neuropathic pain. They can help predict prognosis of neurodestructive procedures as well as helping the patient to experience possible side effects, such as anesthesia and motor blockade.

Complex regional pain syndrome is a syndrome that is characterized by pain, sensory distortion, autonomic instability in the affected area, and later in its course, dystrophic changes. Pain may be severe, usually burning in quality, and sensory changes (e.g., hyperaesthesia, hyperpathia, and allodynia) can be very distressing. In cancer patients, this type of pain may be triggered by radiation therapy, surgery, tumor spread, or pathologic fracture. Initial management usually involves local anesthetic sympathetic nerve block. The first block may produce analgesia that outlasts the duration of action of the local anesthetic drug. Several injections are usually required for permanent disappearance of symptoms. Extensive physiotherapy also helps achieve successful permanent relief. TCAs, gabapentin, and occasionally sympathetic blocking agents, such as prazosin or clonidine, may be helpful.

Plexus and Epidural Blocks

Research has shown that application of a targeted amount of steroid preparation to the site of injury of a nerve reduces the amount of ectopic firing in that nerve that may significantly ameliorate neuropathic pain. It is likely that nerve injury that is caused by tumor compression of that nerve is similar in pathology to that caused by nerve compression by other structures (e.g., lumbar radiculopathy from prolapsed lumber disc).

Perineural injections or epidural injections of a long-acting steroid preparation (e.g., triamcinolone diacetate or methylprednisolone acetate) will often result in improvement in symptoms over the following 2 weeks, and analgesia is usually effective for several weeks. The procedure may then be repeated to maintain pain control. Local anesthetic is injected with the steroid to signify correct placement of the preparation. Brachial plexopathy from Pancoast's tumor may respond to interscalene or subclavian brachial nerve block; pelvic floor tumors involving femoral plexus may respond to psoas compartment paravertebral nerve block.

It is important to warn patients undergoing such blocks that neurologic loss associated with the pain, such as numbness, may be unmasked by the block and pain relief, or the block itself may be blamed for the neurologic deficit.

Epidural steroid injection may be useful for the control of lumbar radiculopathy associated with epidural metastases or from noncancer origin.

Diagnostic and Prognostic Blocks

Local anesthetic blocks may be useful in determining whether a pain is of somatic or visceral origin or whether neuropathetic pain has a sympathetic component. Unfortunately, a positive response to local anesthetic sympathetic block does not necessarily predict long-term benefit from sympathectomy, although failure to relieve pain indicates that sympathectomy is unwarranted.

Local anesthetic blocks may be useful in predicting the efficacy of neuroablative procedures, such as gasserian ganglion ablation, surgical rhizotomy, and celiac plexus neurolysis. However, it is important to remember that pain may recur due to possible increased synaptic activity, development of aberrant connections from neuronal sprouts, and sensitization to neurotransmitters.

Regional Analgesic Infusions

Occasionally, cancer pain patients develop such severe pain that it cannot be controlled by oral analgesics with unacceptable side effects. In such patients continuous local anesthetic block, such as epidural infusion and brachial plexus infusion, may be very useful by providing complete analgesia and control of the crisis. Patients on long-term oral narcotics who have developed tolerance may benefit from a drug holiday that will increase the efficacy of their medications when recommenced after reduction.

Epidural analgesic infusions can be maintained for weeks or months in many patients. An epidural catheter can be tunneled subcutaneously to the flank to minimize displacement and allow the patient access to the exit site for ease of dressing changes. Combinations of low-dose bupivacaine plus an opioid, such as morphine, can be extremely effective. Portable infusion pumps that can be carried in a small shoulder bag or fanny pack reduce the inconvenience to the patient. If infusion therapy is unavailable or not supported by insurance, patients or family members can be instructed to do intermittent injections of opioids and local anesthetic.

For patients whose life expectancy is several months or more, implanted intrathecal drug infusion systems provide exceptional analgesia and are reasonably cost effective. For patients who have become extremely opioid tolerant, bupivacaine can be added to the intrathecal infusion. The advent of implanted pumps with high volume (40 ml) reservoirs allows for more effective daily doses of local anesthetic. Intrathecal baclofen, which is generally used for spasticity, has been shown to provide more effective analgesia than morphine for some patients, especially those with neuropathic pain or CRPS. Clonidine has also been used for patients who have become tolerant to opioids. Combining two or more of these agents may be required for optimum pain relief. Ziconotide, a conopeptide which acts as an antagonist to N-type voltage-gated calcium channels, is also effective for some patients who are refractory to opioids.

Myofascial Pain and Trigger-Point Injections

Cancer patients often develop myofascial pain, which is secondary to bony, neural, or visceral pain. Myofascial pain is characterized by tender spontaneously painful foci in muscles, known as trigger points. Injections of these trigger points with local anesthetic can bring about effective relief of pain and thus be an important aid to the patient's pain management. Repeat injections may be carried out for lasting relief. Physiotherapy interventions including gentle stretching of the affected muscle usually helps, too.

Neurolytic Blockade in Cancer Pain Management

Neurolytic blocks can be a useful tool for the anesthesiologist to utilize in relieving cancer pain. However, before proceeding to consideration of these techniques, other available modalities for the relief of pain should be fully explored including pharmacologic therapy, non-neurolytic nerve blocks and injections, tumor reduction therapy, and cognitive-behavioral therapy. Because cancer pain patients are living longer and nerve pain usually recurs after weeks or months at most, it is essential that we look critically at patient selection and timing and type of block before considering potentially hazardous neurolytic procedures. One possible exception is the use of visceral neurolytic blocks, such as celiac plexus or superior hypogastric plexus blocks. Early use of these techniques may spare patients several weeks to months of high-dose opioid use, providing a better quality of life and fewer side effects.

SUGGESTED READING

Abram SE: Cancer Pain. Boston, Kluwer Academic Publishers, 1989.

Elliot K, Portenoy R: Cancer pain. In Yaksh TL et al (eds): Anesthesia, Biological Foundations. Philadelphia, Lippincott-Raven, 1998, pp 803–819.

Lussier D, Huskey AG, Portenoy RK: Adjuvant analgesics in cancer pain management. Oncologist 9(5):571-591, 2004.

Management of Cancer Pain, Clinical Practice Guidelines No 9, U.S. Department of Health and Human Services.

Mantyh PW: A mechanism based understanding of cancer pain. Pain 96:1-2, 2002.

Mantyh PW, Hunt SP: Mechanisms that generate and maintain bone cancer pain. Novartis Foundation Symposium 260:221-240, 2004.

McNicol E, Strassels S, Goudas L, et al: Nonsteroidal anti-inflammatory drugs, alone or combined with opioids, for cancer pain: a systematic review. J Clin Oncol 22:1975-1992, 2004.

Mercadante S, Portenoy RK: Opioid poorly-responsive cancer pain. Part 3. Clinical strategies to improve opioid responsiveness. J Pain Symptom Manage 2:338-54, 2001.Yarwood R: Handbook of Pain Management. London, Haymarket Medical Imprint, 2004.

O'Connor TC, Abram SE: The Development and resolution of post-injury pain. In Yaksh TL, et al (eds): Anaesthesia, Biological Foundations. Philadelphia, Lippincott-Raven, 1998, pp 747-759.

Quigley C: Opioid switching to improve pain relief and drug tolerability. Cochrane Database of Systematic Reviews CD00484, 2004.

Smith HS: Drugs for Pain. Philadelphia, Hanley and Belfus, 2003.

CHAPTER 21

Neurolytic Blocks for Cancer Pain

STEPHEN E. ABRAM

INTRODUCTION

Destruction of nerve pathways with neurolytic agents has been a therapeutic option for the management of severe cancer pain for many decades. Its use has declined in recent years, partly because of rising medicolegal risks to the practitioner, but mainly because of improved treatment efficacy of radiation and chemotherapy, better pharmacologic options, and technical advances in neuraxial drug administration techniques.

Neurolytic blocks can be divided into three main categories: peripheral nerve blocks, neuraxial blocks, and visceral nerve blocks. The principle disadvantages to peripheral blocks are the risks of creating or increasing neuropathic pain, the risk of producing denervation dysesthesia, and the probability that pain will recur during and after nerve regrowth. Injection of superficial nerves can result in necrosis of the overlying skin. The technique should be avoided for mixed motor sensory nerves where motor blockade will produce significant functional loss. The risks of neuraxial blocks are mainly those of somatic motor loss and bowel and bladder dysfunction. For visceral blocks, the

main risks are for injury to adjacent somatic nerves and for injury to the blood supply of the spinal cord with resultant paraplegia.

PERIPHERAL NEUROLYSIS

In general, neurolytic blockade of peripheral nerves is not recommended. The risk of motor dysfunction, new-onset neuropathic pain, and denervation dysesthesia is fairly high. Intercostal blocks may be helpful for patients with very localized chest wall pain who are not expected to survive more than 2 to 3 months. Two ml 6% aqueous phenol is injected, usually at the lateral border of the paravertebral muscles, so that the lateral cutaneous branch is denervated. The most significant risk is for intraneural injection with subepineural spread of drug to the subarachnoid space. Cryoanalgesia and radiofrequency ablation are alternative procedures that do not share that risk.

Neurolytic blocks of the trigeminal nerve and its branches and the upper cervical nerve roots can provide significant relief for patients with head and neck cancers. There are significant risks of neurologic damage from intrathecal spread of the neurolytic agent, and in many centers neurolytic blocks have been largely supplanted by radiofrequency ablation techniques.

NEURAXIAL NEUROLYTIC BLOCKS

Intrathecal Neurolysis

For the most part, intrathecal neurolysis is used for pain in the thoracic dermatomes, where motor and sensory loss will not have devastating effects on upper or lower extremity function or on bowel or bladder function. Intrathecal injections are done with absolute alcohol or of 6% phenol dissolved in glycerin. With the alcohol injections, the posterolateral aspect of the affected cord segments is positioned uppermost. The alcohol is hypobaric and should bathe the dorsal roots with the patient so positioned. Phenol in glycerin is hyperbaric, so the dorsolateral aspect of the affected region is positioned downward. Drug volumes are usually limited to 1ml.

For patients with rectal pain who have undergone fecal and urinary diversion procedures, intrathecal saddle block with phenol in glycerin is an effective and relatively safe technique. A prognostic block with 3 to 4 mg hyperbaric bupivacaine should be done first and the effect of that block allowed to wear off. The patient is positioned in the sitting position and a dural puncture is done, preferably at L5-S1, using a 20 ga needle (phenol in glycerin is quite viscous and is difficult to inject through smaller gauge needles. The solution is injected in small (0.3 ml or less) increments at 5-minute intervals, evaluating pain relief and sensation after each injection. Generally, at least 1 ml is required, and the total volume should not exceed 2 ml. If the patient experiences numbness or paresthesias in the calf or foot no more should be injected. The patient should remain sitting for at least 45 minutes after the final increment.

Epidural Neurolysis

Aqueous phenol at a concentration of 6% is used for this procedure. An epidural catheter is placed using fluoroscopic guidance. If possible, the catheter is guided to the lateral epidural space on the affected side at the proper segmental level. A Racz type spring wire armored catheter can be modified by making a 10- to 20-degree bend near the tip, making the catheter steerable. Once the catheter is properly positioned, 1 ml radiopaque nonionic dye is injected "live" to ensure that the catheter is not intravascular, that the spread is epidural rather than intrathecal, and that the distribution is acceptable. A test dose of 2 ml 2% lidocaine is injected, again providing assurance that the catheter is not intrathecal, providing some prognostic information. After the local anesthetic effect dissipates, small incremental injections of 0.2 to 0.3 ml are begun, waiting 5 to 10 minutes between injections, with assessment of pain relief and sensory function before each subsequent increment. If pain is unilateral, it may be preferable to inject with the patient in the lateral position, with the affected side down. Total volume should not exceed 1 to 1.5 ml. The catheter is flushed with enough volume to clear the catheter and is secured. The patient is reassessed the following day. If there is residual pain, the procedure is repeated after again documenting catheter position and dye spread fluoroscopically. Two to three repetitions may be needed before adequate relief is achieved. If pain relief is inadequate,

the catheter can be left in place for the administration of local anesthetic and opioid infusions.

VISCERAL NEUROLYSIS

Visceral pain can often be interrupted by neurolytic blockade without appreciable loss of motor or sensory function. The pain of upper abdominal cancers (e.g., pancreatic, gastric, hepatic) can be relieved by celiac plexus or splanchnic nerve blocks, while pelvic pain can be relieved by superior hypogastric plexus blocks.

Celiac Plexus Block

The celiac plexus lies over the anterior surface of the aorta, surrounding the take-off of the celiac artery at the T12-L1 level. It contains vagal and sympathetic efferent fibers and visceral afferent fibers. It is the visceral afferents that are the target for nerve ablation. Destruction of autonomic fibers can produce changes in gastrointestinal motility, but these are rarely of serious consequence.

The patient should be assessed for coagulation defects and for atherosclerotic disease or aneurysm of the aorta, conditions that would cause serious consequences from aortic puncture. The patient is positioned prone. Opioid analgesia is usually required for the patient to tolerate this position. Sedation is acceptable, but should be light enough for the patient to provide feedback regarding changes in somatic sensory function and reduction in pain during the injection. A skin wheal is raised on each side, about 8 cm lateral to the midline. Under A-P fluoroscopic guidance, the 22 ga 6-inch needles (longer for obese patients) are advanced toward the anterolateral border of the L1 vertebral body. The needles should contact the upper one-third of the L1 body and should be directed to a position just past the anterolateral aspect. Switching to a lateral fluoroscopic view, the needles are advanced to a position 1 to 2 cm beyond the anterior border of L-1. The right needle will not usually enter a major vessel, but the left needle will usually enter the aorta. If it does, it should be advanced through the anterior aortic wall, at which point blood can no longer be aspirated. Two to 3 ml radiopaque dye is injected "live" through each needle to rule out intravascular injection and to determine the pattern of spread. The dye should spread in all directions, although the exact pattern will be dependent on the presence and extent of tumor in the region. Injection of 5 ml 1% lidocaine may be injected to determine if there is pain relief and no somatic blockade. A higher volume (10 to 12 ml each side) should be injected if alcohol is to be used, as the alcohol injection is quite painful. If phenol is to be used, local anesthetic is nor essential. The likelihood of spread dorsally to the nerve roots is very low.

If alcohol is used, up to 25 ml 50% alcohol or 12 to 15 ml absolute alcohol is injected through each needle. If phenol is used, 12 to 15 ml of 6% to 7% aqueous phenol is injected through each needle. Following alcohol injection, even if local anesthetic was injected previously, patients often have some burning pain, most commonly in the upper abdomen or shoulder. Shoulder pain is caused by irritation of the diaphragm. It usually subsides within 30 minutes.

The use of CT scan for needle placement allows for more accurate drug administration and, more importantly, for avoiding aortic puncture in patients at higher risk of bleeding or who have atherosclerotic disease of the aorta. The left-side needle can be passed lateral to the aorta to a position at its anterior border, and the right-side needle can be advanced between the aorta and the vena cava. Figure 21-1 shows needle placement and dye spread using CT guidance for such a technique as well as for the transaortic technique.

Splanchnic Block

This procedure is often referred to as retrocrural celiac plexus block, and the technique described above is called transcrural. The splanchnic nerves angle downward and forward over the lateral aspect of the lower thoracic vertebrae, traversing the diaphragm to partici-

pate in the formation of the celiac plexus. In order to block the splanchnic nerves, the needle tip is positioned posterior to the diaphragmatic crura. Using the approach described above, the needles are positioned at the anterolateral border of the upper one-third of the L1 vertebral body. They are not advanced beyond that site. Radiographic dye injected at these sites spreads along the anterolateral surface of the vertebrae. Five ml will generally spread upward to T10 to T11. If dye is seen to spread posteriorly to the region of the neural foramina, the technique should be abandoned in favor of a transcrural technique. The neurolytic agent will affect the visceral afferent and sympathetic efferent fibers in the splanchnic nerves. This technique is indicated when there is a very large tumor mass in the region of the celiac plexus that prevents the drug from reaching much of the plexus. Six to 8 ml of 6% to 7% aqueous phenol is injected on each side (see Figs. 21-2 and 21-3 for the relationship of needle position to the diaphragm).

Side Effects and Complications

The most common side effects of celiac and splanchnic nerve blocks are diarrhea and orthostatic hypotension. These are almost invariably transient, usually resolving within 72 hours. Diarrhea is related to loss of sympathetic

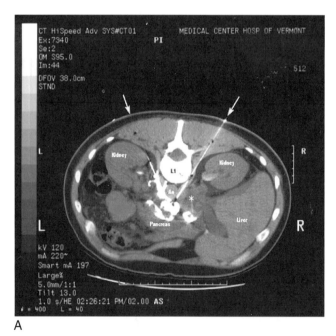

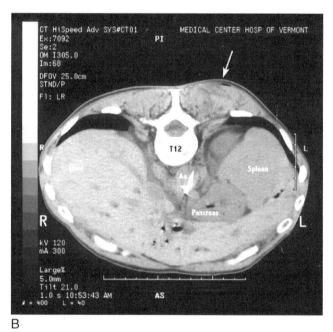

A   B

Figure 21-1   (A) Computed tomography after placement of two transcrural needles for neurolytic celiac plexus block. The arrows indicate the approximate needle trajectory on each side. Radiocontrast extends over the left anterolateral surface of the aorta and anteriorly along the posterior surface of the pancreas. There is a large soft tissue mass adjacent to the right-sided needle (asterisk) consistent with either metastatic tumor or adenopathy. Neurolytic solution has not yet been placed through the right-sided needle. (B) Computed tomography after placement of a single transaortic needle. The arrow indicates the approximate trajectory of the needle. The medial pleural reflection can be seen passing in close proximity to the needle path. (Reprinted from Rathmell JP, Gallant JM, Brown DL: Computed tomography and the anatomy of celiac plexus block. Reg Anesth Pain Med 25:411–416, 2000.)

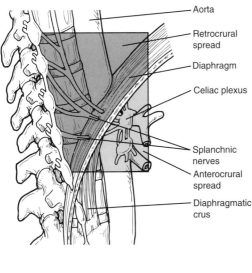

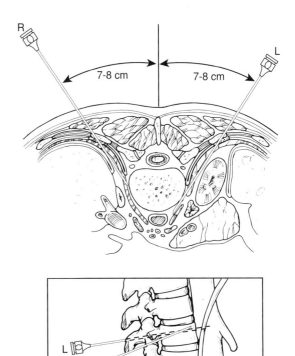

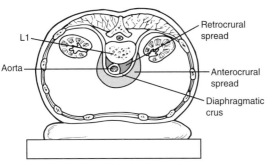

Figure 21-2   Celiac plexus block—retrocrural and anterocrural relationships.(Reprinted from Rathmell JP: Sympathetic blocks. In Rathmell JP, Neal JM, Viscomi CM (eds): Regional Anesthesia: The Requisites in Anesthesiology. Philadelphia, Mosby, 2004. Redrawn from Brown DL: Atlas of regional anesthesia, 2nd ed., Philadelphia, W.B. Saunders, 1999.)

Figure 21-3   Retrocrural and transcrural needle placement for celiac plexus block. Inset, the left needle (L) is retrocrural and results in spread of solution to block the splanchnic nerves. The right needle (R) is transcrural and blocks the celiac plexus directly. (Modified from Rathmell JP: Sympathetic blocks. In Rathmell JP, Neal JM, Viscomi CM (eds): Regional Anesthesia: The Requisites in Anesthesiology. Philadelphia, Mosby, 2004. Redrawn from Raj PP: Practical Management of Pain, 3rd ed. St. Louis, Mosby, 2000.)

innervation to the bowel with unopposed parasympathetic activity. It may also be related to opioid withdrawal.

More serious complications are listed in Box 21-1.

Hypogastric Plexus Block

Visceral pelvic pain can be treated by neurolytic blockade of the superior hypogastric plexus. This collection of nerves lies anterior to the L5 vertebral body, L5-S1 disc, and upper sacrum. It contains visceral afferent fibers that accompany sympathetic efferents from the lumbar and sacral portions of the sympathetic chain and those that travel with sacral parasympathetics to the midsacral foramina. The plexus is blocked at the anterior aspect of the lower end of the L5 vertebra.

Under fluoroscopic guidance, a 6-inch 22 ga block needle is introduced on each side, with an entry site 2 to 3 cm cephalad and 1 to 2 cm lateral to the tip of the L5 transverse process. This point is usually just medial to the upper edge of the iliac crest. The needle is angled mesiad and caudad passing just below the L5 transverse process and just lateral to the edge of the vertebral body. An L5

Box 21-1   Complications of Celiac and Splanchnic Neurolytic Blocks

Paraplegia
    Inadvertent epidural or intrathecal injection
    Injury or sclerosis of radicular artery
Radiculopathy
    Spread of drug to neural foramen
Pneumothorax
Chylothorax
Failure of ejaculation
Renal injury
Systemic toxicity (phenol)
    Seizures
    Cardiovascular collapse

paresthesia is often encountered as the needle is advanced, and the angle can be changed slightly in an effort to avoid the L5 nerve root. The needles are advanced just past the lateral edge of the vertebra in the AP view. On the lateral view, the needle tips should be .5 to 1 cm anterior to the anterior border of the L-5 vertebra or the L5-S1 disc. Injection of 2 to 3 ml radiographic dye is injected to rule out intravascular placement and to document proper spread. Ideally, the dye injections through the two needles should meet in the midline. Occasionally, tumor will prevent spread of the dye toward the midline, greatly reducing the chance of success. Each needle is injected with 6 ml 6% aqueous phenol. As with celiac plexus block, CT guidance should be used when it is critical to avoid injury to the major (in this case iliac) vessels. The technique of needle placement is shown in Figures 21-4 and 21-5.

Few complications have been reported with this technique. There is probably some risk of bowel or bladder dysfunction, spread of neurolytic agent to the L5 nerve root, and injury to the iliac vessels as well as systemic complication of intravascular injection.

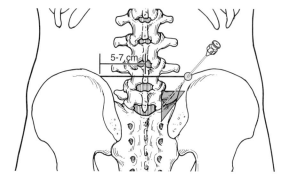

Figure 21-4   Posterior-anterior view showing the anatomic triangle through which the needle must pass for superior hypogastric plexus block. The triangle is bordered superiorly by the transverse process of L5, laterally by the iliac crest, and medially by the L5/S1 facet joint. (Reprinted from Rathmell JP: Sympathetic blocks. In Rathmell JP, Neal JM, Viscomi CM (eds): Regional Anesthesia: The Requisites in Anesthesiology. Philadelphia, Mosby, 2004.)

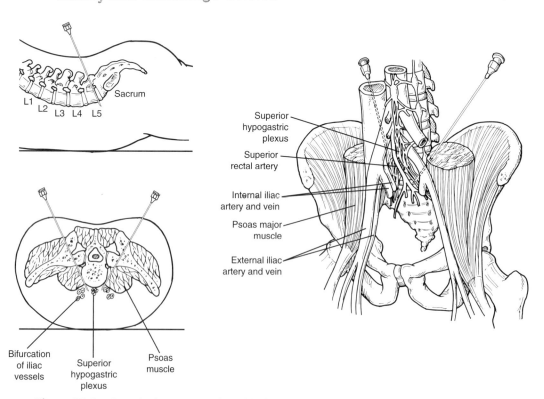

Figure 21-5   Superior hypogastric plexus block. (Reprinted from Rathmell JP: Sympathetic blocks. In Rathmell JP, Neal JM, Viscomi CM (eds): Regional Anesthesia: The Requisites in Anesthesiology. Philadelphia, Mosby, 2004.)

SUGGESTED READING

Abram SE, Boas RA: Sympathetic and visceral nerve blocks. In Benumof JL (ed): Clinical Procedures in Anesthesia and Intensive Care. Philadelphia, J.B. Lippincott, 1992, pp 787–806.

Patt, RA: Cancer Pain. Philadelphia, J.B. Lippincott, 1993.

Patt RA, Cousins MJ: Techniques of neurolytic neural blockade. In Cousins MJ, Bridenbaugh PO (eds): Neural Blockade, 3rd ed. Philadelphia, Lippincott–Raven, 1998, pp 1007–1062.

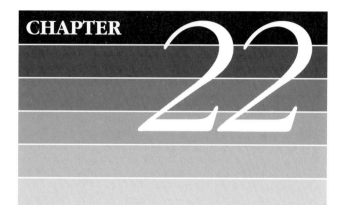

CHAPTER 22

Electrical Stimulation of the Nervous System

MIKHAIL FUKSHANSKY
PHILLIP PHAN
ARUN RAJAGOPAL

INTRODUCTION

Electrical stimulation of the nervous system describes the application of low-voltage electrical current to different neurologic areas to block the perception of pain. Although the underlying premise is the application of current to the affected area, different areas of the nervous system require wide variations in amplitude, pulse width, and frequency to cause pain relief. Thus, a wide variety of devices are available; some are external devices with power being applied transcutaneously, while others are fully implanted. Some devices combine both approaches with only the leads being implanted with an external power source.

In this chapter, the discussion will include five common modalities for electrical stimulation. These are spinal-cord stimulation (SCS), transcutaneous electric nerve stimulation (TENS), peripheral nerve stimulation (PNS), cortical brain stimulation, and deep brain stimulation (Box 22-1). Currently, SCS and TENS are the most widely used clinical applications of pulsed electrical energy. Both TENS and SCS were a direct clinical spin-off from the gate-control theory developed by Melzack and Wall in 1967. Cortical and deep brain stimulation techniques are gaining growing acceptance in the medical community and are being utilized with increasing frequency for treatment of intractable pain conditions.

HISTORIC PERSPECTIVE

Although a detailed historic overview of the variety of pain theories is outside the scope of this chapter, a brief mention of the subject is important in order to develop a better understanding of the history of evolution of the therapeutic techniques and current clinical applications of electrical stimulation. Our understanding of pain has changed over the past several thousands of years. Numerous texts from ancient Babylonia, Egypt, India, China, and Greece described a common experience of pain and its devastating consequences on the human condition. Many ancient civilizations believed the heart was a center of all sensation, especially of pain and pleasure.

In the Middle Ages, a concept of brain as a center of sensory perception, and also of pain, was introduced by Albertus Magnus and then modified and expanded by further research. Leonardo da Vinci thought of nerves as tubular structures. He also related pain sensation to touch sensation and associated the spinal cord as a conductor of sensation. Descartes described nerves as tubular structures containing microthreads that conducted sensation, including pain, via spinal cord to the brain.

Specificity and Intensive Theories

In the nineteenth century the specificity (sensory) and intensive (summation) theories were introduced. This was one of the earliest theories specifically attempting to explain basic pain pathways. The basic aspects of both of these theories, although seemingly mutually exclusive, helped to form a new understanding of the pathways conducting pain in the central nervous system.

Proposed by Schiff in 1858, the specificity theory described pain as a unique sensation conducted by a separate "pain pathway" different from touch (one to one conduction). Intensive theory, on the other hand, implied that pain resulted from overstimulation of touch receptors (central summation). Subsequent research led to further elaboration and refinement of both theories in later years.

Gate-Control Theory

The gate-control theory, proposed by Melzack and Wall in the 1950s, provided further insights into the nature of the mechanisms involved in the conduction of pain. This theory suggested that both specificity and intensive theories failed to account for the complexity of neurologic interaction involved in the conduction of pain.

Gate-control theory, as it was proposed in the original form, postulated that impulses generated at the periphery are transmitted to three distinct systems. Impulses are carried to the cells in the (a) substantia gelatinosa in the spinal gray matter, (b) dorsal columns, and (c) spinal-cord transmission cells that in turn conduct information to the brain. Transmission of stimuli is modulated by a *spinal gating mechanism* located in the dorsal horn. The spinal gate mechanism is controlled by the activity of the large-diameter (myelinated A) and small-diameter (unmyelinated C-fiber and lightly myelinated A-δ) fibers. Activity in the large-diameter fibers tends to *inhibit transmission* (closing the gate), whereas activity in C and A-δ fibers *facilitates transmission* (opening the gate). Thus, activation of A-β fibers can suppress conduction of painful stimuli carried by A-δ fibers and C fibers. In later years, Melzack and Casey modified the theory by incorporating new information derived from further related physiologic and behavioral research. By 1967, the gate-control theory was put to an early test by Shealy who utilized it for SCS first in the intrathecal space and finally in the epidural space.

Recent research also suggests that electrical stimulation of the nervous system might produce its beneficial effect through changes in the neurochemical environment at the dorsal horn and spinothalamic tract of the spinal cord. Studies have shown that levels of a number of neurotransmitters are altered in response to SCS.

SPINAL-CORD STIMULATION

Background

An SCS system consists of three basic components: a lead wire, which delivers electrical stimulation to the spinal cord, an extension wire, which connects the lead wires to a power source, and a power source, which generates the stimulatory signal. The power source may be fully implanted or deliver power via a radiofrequency signal transmitted to an implanted receiving coil (Figs. 22-1 and 22-2).

Patient Selection Criteria

Careful patient selection is an absolute requirement for a successful outcome of SCS. In general, SCS is indicated for chronic intractable pain of the limbs. Patient selection criteria are shown in Box 22-2.

Techniques of Implantation

Implantation of the spinal column stimulator is a technically complex interventional pain procedure. Assuming the patient has generally met the selection criteria shown in Box 22-2, the initial phase involves a trial. The trial allows both the patient and the physician to gauge the benefits prior to implantation of a permanent device.

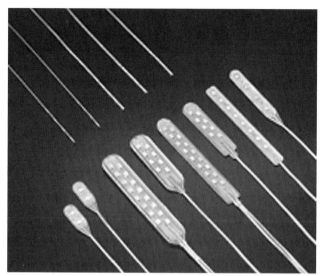

Figure 22-1   An assortment of electrodes is shown. Percutaneous leads are in the upper left and surgical leads have a "paddle" shape and are placed via a laminotomy incision. (Courtesy of Advanced Neuromodulation Systems, Inc., Plano, Texas).

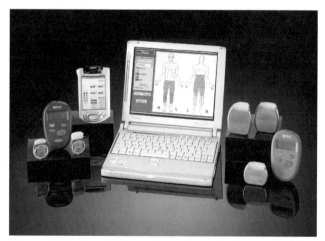

Figure 22-2   In addition to the implanted leads, spinal-cord stimulation includes the implanted generator, screener, and programmer. (Courtesy of Advanced Neuromodulation Systems, Inc., Plano, Texas.)

In the majority of patients, the initial spinal-cord stimulator trial can be performed with low morbidity and emulate the permanent procedure to a large degree.

Trial Phase

The following is a description of the implantation technique applied at our institution. In order to maintain strict aseptic technique, all trials and permanent implantation are performed in the operating room. The patient is placed in the prone position with adequate padding under the abdomen to slightly flex the lumbar spine. Light sedation is provided. After the back is prepared and draped in sterile fashion, under fluoroscopic guidance,

---

Box 22-2   Patient Selection Criteria for Spinal-Cord Stimulation

- More conservative therapies have failed.
- A pathology is the basis for the pain complaint.
- Further surgical intervention is not indicated.
- No serious untreated drug habituation problem exists.
- Psychological clearance has been obtained.
- No contraindications to implantation are present.
- Trial screening has been successful.
- Patient is able and willing to use the therapy.
- Patient understands the limits and risks of the therapy.

Provided courtesy of Medtronic, Inc. Spinal Cord Stimulation Patient Management Guidelines for Clinicians, p 12.

the appropriate landmarks are identified. For pain in the lower extremities, the entry point is at the level of L1-L3. For pain in the upper extremities, the entry point is approximately T12-L1 and for the cervical area, entry may be achieved at C7 to T1.

After adequate local anesthetic is infiltrated, the supplied 15 ga. A Tuohy needle is used to enter the epidural space. The angle of entry is as shallow as possible and as such, only a paramedian approach is generally used. The paramedian approach allows the angle of entry to be shallow; this is important to prevent the lead from migrating to the anterior epidural space. Once the epidural space is entered, the supplied guide wire may be used independently to gently probe the epidural space for ease of entry of the lead wire. The lead wire is slightly bent at the tip to facilitate "steering" in the epidural space (Figs. 22-3 and 22-4). Note that the specially designed Tuohy needle allows withdrawal of the lead through the needle without

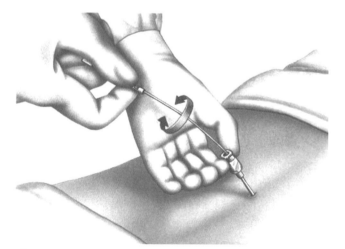

Figure 22-3   With the Tuohy needle in the epidural space, the lead wire is turned gently to steer the lead to the correct place. (Courtesy of Medtronic, Inc.)

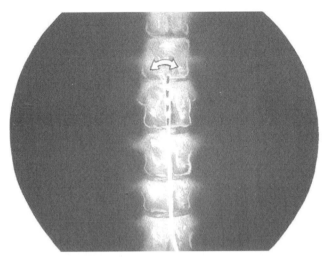

Figure 22-4   The tip of the lead wire is slightly bent, allowing it to be steered slightly to the left or right. (Courtesy of Medtronic, Inc.)

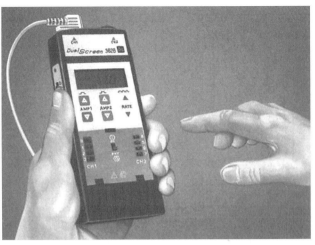

Figure 22-6   The lead wire is connected to the screener via the extension wire. Various parameters are tried to optimize analgesia. (Courtesy of Medtronic, Inc.)

shearing (Fig. 22-5). However, if resistance is encountered during withdrawal of the lead wire, both needle and lead should be withdrawn *en bloc* and the needle should be reinserted by itself.

The patient should be awakened and the lead wire should be carefully advanced under fluoroscopic guidance while steering the lead wire by applying gentle rotational pressure to the lead wire at the needle hub. The lead wire should be positioned as close to midline as possible and when it is at the desired level, steered to the left or right side as indicated. A lateral radiograph at this point will confirm placement in the posterior epidural space. The supplied sterile extension cord is then attached to the lead wire and the other end is passed over the drape to the assistant, who will connect the lead wire to the trial programmer or screener (Fig. 22-6).

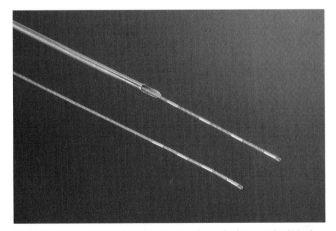

Figure 22-5   Electrode leads shown through the supplied Tuohy needle. The proximal edge of the opening in the Tuohy needle is blunt, allowing gentle withdrawal of the leads without shearing. (Courtesy of Advanced Neuromodulation Systems, Inc., Plano, Texas.)

Once the lead wire is connected, various stimulation parameters are tried until optimal coverage is achieved over the affected area (see Programming section below). During this phase, the patient is actively involved in reporting the area and strength of coverage. It is not unusual for lead wires to need repositioning and coverage parameters adjusted until the patient reports a satisfactory result. Once optimal coverage is achieved, the needles are withdrawn, the lead wires are secured to the skin using a nondissolving suture looped around the lead wire, and a final radiograph is taken to ascertain position of the leads. A sterile dressing is applied and the lead wires are connected to a programmer the patient can keep for 3 to 5 days.

During these 3 to 5 days, the patient is encouraged to continue with usual activities although allowing the lead placement area to become wet is discouraged. The patient may keep a log of pain scores and degree of improvement from baseline. After 3 to 5 days, the patient returns to clinic and reports on the outcome of the trial. Whether successful or not, the trial lead is removed to minimize the risk of infection in the epidural space. The single suture is clipped and the lead is easily withdrawn. If the trial is successful and the patient reports satisfactory improvement in pain scores, a permanently implanted system may be considered.

Programming

The underlying principles of programming are very complex and are beyond the scope of this chapter. However, a brief overview of these principles will allow the reader a greater depth of understanding of how these devices work. In general, in order to stimulate specific nerves, a flow of energy has to be delivered to the nerve. This energy is delivered by a flow of electrons (a "current") from the negative (−) to the positive (+)

terminal of a closed circuit. In this case, the circuit is the lead wire. Since the lead wire has multiple contact points or electrodes, each can be programmed independently to serve as the cathode or anode. Once this is done, a circuit is established and current flows in a local area around the electrodes. (In some instances, the lead wire can serve as the negative lead and the implanted generator chassis can serve as the positive lead.)

The choice of which electrode to set as the anode or cathode is empiric. In general, a broad area of coverage is applied and is then made smaller by using the middle electrodes in each lead wire. This allows for readjustment if the lead migrates in a cephalo-caudal direction. During programming, electrode settings are first adjusted to achieve anatomic coverage. Then the pulse width and pulse rate are adjusted to achieve the individual patient's maximum comfort. The patient can further adjust the voltage up and down to fine-tune individual comfort level. The lowest acceptable settings on all four parameters should be used to conserve battery life of the pulse generator. The patient's pain level can change over time, and the stimulator is reprogrammed to adjust to the patient's need.

Once the circuit is established, the pattern of energy flow has to be adjusted to match the stimulatory requirements of the specific nerves (Box 22-3). This is done by adjusting the pulse width and frequency of the current flow. For spinal-cord nervous tissue, the usual values are a pulse width of approximately 210 microseconds and frequency of 30 to 80 Hz. At a lower frequency, the patient experiences a "thumping" sensation over the painful site. At a higher frequency, the patient feels a "buzzing" sensation. A final parameter, the amplitude, determines the strength of the incoming current and is adjusted up or down based on patient comfort. This is usually in the range of 0 to 10 volts.

Implantation Phase

If the trial is successful, the patient may elect to have a permanently implanted system. In the operating room, another lead wire is placed as described above during the trial phase. After the lead wire is placed successfully, a 3-cm incision is made around the needle in a cephalo-caudal direction. The depth of the incision should be to the supraspinous ligament. The lead wire should be secured to the supraspinous ligament using one of the

supplied anchors. Using the supplied connectors, the lead wire is attached to the extension wire.

A suitable site is chosen for the implantable generator. The generator is about the same size as an implanted pacemaker although the units with an extended battery life are slightly larger (Fig. 22-7). Common areas are the lower abdominal wall and superior gluteal area for lower extremity stimulators. The selected site should be the area where the patient can feel comfortable accessing the area with their dominant hand for adjustment of the lead settings with the remote control unit. The upper anterior chest wall is used for cervical stimulators. A small horizontal incision, equal to the diameter of the generator, is made to a depth just deep to the subcutaneous tissue. Using gentle blunt dissection, a pocket is made approximately the size of the generator. Care should be taken not to make the pocket too big because a loose-fitting generator can sometimes turn in the pocket and dislodge the lead wires or a seroma may form in the space between generator and pocket.

The pocket should be checked for hemostasis and gentle electrocautery may be used. Excessive electrocautery use may lead to excessive amounts of necrotic and burned tissue. This is conducive to formation of an inflammatory reaction and may contribute to the formation of a seroma. The pocket should also be irrigated with antibiotic irrigation solution. Once the pocket is ready, the supplied tunneling rod should be used to connect the back incision (with lead wire) to the front incision (pocket for the generator). The extension wire is then passed through the tunneler and connected to the generator. Prior to final closure, the stimulatory parameters should be checked again to ascertain the lead wires have not moved from their original location. The incisions are closed with dissolving suture in the deeper tissues with nondissolving sutures or staples at the skin.

Box 22-3   Adjustable Parameters for Spinal-Cord Stimulation

Amplitude (volts or V)
Pulse width (microseconds or μs)
Frequency (hertz or Hz)
Electrode selection

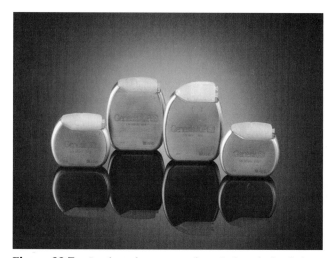

Figure 22-7   Implanted generators for spinal-cord stimulation, peripheral nerve stimulation, and deep brain/cortical stimulation. (Courtesy of Advanced Neuromodulation Systems, Inc., Plano, Texas.)

Complications

Complications with SCS are variable, ranging from failure of paresthesia coverage to more serious consequences of paralysis, nerve injury, and death. Prior to proceeding with SCS trial, extensive educational discussions with the patient and the family members should be carried out to include explanations of possible complications and risks.

In general, complication can be classified into perioperative surgical complications and complications with the implanted stimulator itself. Surgical complications include bleeding, subcutaneous infection, cerebrospinal fluid (CSF) leak, epidural abscess, stimulator pocket hematoma, or seroma. Bleeding at the surgery site itself is usually minimal because the lumbar area, the anterior abdominal wall, and the superior gluteal region are not heavily vascularized. Pressure tamponade with gauze and selective use of electrocautery will stop any significant bleeding at incisional sites.

Although most complications are minor, two potentially devastating complications are an epidural abscess or epidural hematoma. An epidural hematoma is extremely rare but has been reported in the literature with devastating consequences including paralysis and death. At our institution, patients are kept overnight for observation and sequential neurologic exams are performed postoperatively. Most infections are minor and involve only the superficial wound area. These may be managed conservatively with antibiotics. However, if the hardware is infected or an epidural abscess is suspected, it may be necessary to explain the entire system. An epidural abscess can progressively lead to paralysis and death if not recognized quickly and treated aggressively. Close monitoring of the infected patient for clinical signs and symptoms of neurologic deterioration is recommended. Emergent CT scan imaging and neurosurgical consultation may be warranted if the patient shows neurologic compromise. At our institution, in addition to performing these procedures in the operating room, the standard of care has been to use antibiotic irrigation in all wounds, perioperative systemic antibiotics, and close observation for the first 24 hours postoperatively. In general, the reported rate of localized infections has been 4% to 5%.

Another complication of stimulator implantation involves formation of a hematoma or seroma at the incisional site or in the pocket. Hematoma formation can be prevented by careful hemostasis of wound sites and generator pocket prior to closing. Seroma formation results from collection of body fluid at the wound site due to localized inflammation or from breakdown of an old hematoma. As discussed in the Technique section, we try to minimize tissue trauma or excessive use of electrocautery during the implantation procedure to prevent an inflammatory reaction at the wound sites.

If a seroma or hematoma does occur, the collection of fluid or blood may be bothersome to the patient but this is generally benign, resolving spontaneously and requiring no intervention. Aspiration of the fluid collection should be minimized because this puts the patient at increased risk of infection. If necessary, surgical revision can be performed under sterile conditions in the operating room. Use of an abdominal binder is sometimes helpful to increase pressure in the fluid pocket and prevent fluid accumulation.

CSF leaks can sometimes occur during the procedure, with inadvertent placement of the epidural needle in the intrathecal space. If this occurs, the needle should be reinserted at a different level. If patient develops a postdural puncture headache, conservative measures, such as nonsteroidal anti-inflammatory drugs (NSAIDs), hydration, and IV caffeine are recommended. As a last resort, epidural blood patch can be performed under fluoroscopic guidance. This should be done carefully because of the increased risk of lead migration or breakage.

A second category of complications involves problems with the implanted stimulator system itself. By far, the predominant complications consist of lead migration and lead fracture or breakage. The rate of lead migration has been reported at about 20%. Lead migration results in undesired change in paresthesia coverage of the painful area. It is commonly observed immediately after surgery or later as a result of trauma, such as a fall. Most lead migration is seen in the horizontal plane, across midline, or to the anterior epidural space. Patients with lead migration will often describe a change in paresthesia coverage or a new area of stimulation. Anteroposterior and lateral radiographs of the spine confirm lead migration. Most patients with lead migration will require surgical revision of the leads. We recommend totally exchanging the existing migrated lead with a new percutaneous lead. Lead fracture or breakage will also require surgical replacement of the broken implanted lead.

Outcomes

In the United States, the number one indication for SCS is failed back syndrome. The use of SCS for failed back surgery syndrome has been reported since 1991 with several studies reporting favorable outcomes. In Europe, however, the most common use for spinal-cord stimulator is for peripheral vascular disease. In general, approximately 59% of patients reported long-term relief of at least 50% reduction in pain from SCS. SCS has also been reported to be superior to reoperation in patients with failed back surgery syndrome. Finally, SCS has been reported as cost-effective as compared to chronic medication use.

Over the past two decades, our understanding of neuromodulation and spinal-cord stimulator implantation techniques has improved dramatically. Such continuing improvements contribute to decreased morbidity and greater efficacy of use of SCS. Use of SCS in the United States is likely to expand beyond treatment of chronic back pain to include other pain conditions.

TRANSCUTANEOUS ELECTRICAL NERVE STIMULATION

Background

TENS is the process of applying low-voltage electrical impulses to the skin to affect conduction in the underlying nerves. The electrical impulses are applied through pads adherent to the skin over painful areas. The underlying mechanism explaining the efficacy of TENS is based on the gate-control theory. It is felt that stimulating the larger A-β fibers by selective application of electricity may inhibit nociceptive conduction by the smaller A-δ and C fibers. Another possible mechanism may involve the release of endorphin-like substances from nerve endings, triggered by the electrical impulses.

Mechanism of Action

TENS controls pain by applying electrical impulses to the skin. Traditionally, TENS exists in two forms: high-frequency, low-intensity TENS (conventional TENS) and low-frequency, high-intensity TENS (electroacupuncture), although recently several new modes of action have been described.

It is thought that conventional TENS works by the mechanism postulated in the gate-control theory (see above). It is postulated that stimulation of the large myelinated fibers blocks nociceptive transmission at the level of the spinothalamic tract. Presumably, TENS can produce neuromodulation by three different routes:

1. Presynaptic inhibition of the spinal cord;
2. Direct inhibition of an excited, abnormally firing nerve; or
3. Restoration of afferent input. TENS at rates of 50 to 100 Hz produce analgesia that is not reversible with naloxone.

The second type of TENS, or electroacupuncture, uses high-intensity stimulation, which has been shown to increase endogenous opioid production in the brain. This form of TENS has proved to be most successful when used prior to flexibility exercises. This form of stimulation might provide better results than stretching alone. The effects of this type of TENS stimulation has been shown to be reversible with naloxone, suggesting the effects are mediated through endogenous opioid receptor activity.

As mentioned earlier, delivery of TENS energy comes in several varieties; however, there is no current research to support one form of stimulation over the other (Table 22-1). Recent research also suggests that the mechanism of action of TENS is multifactorial. It has been reported that TENS reduces the mean axon terminal content of glutamate, aspartate, and glycine in the neuropathic pain rat model.

Patient Selection

TENS is used frequently for the treatment of various painful conditions. TENS is a safe, nonpharmacologic, nonaddictive mechanism for pain relief. Since TENS only interferes with nociceptive transmission and does not affect the underlying painful condition, it is most useful as an adjunct with other modalities.

In cases of cervical stenosis, early application of TENS is recommended among other modalities for treatment of radicular pain. Patients who experience severe pain secondary to peripheral neuropathy should have a trial of TENS unless otherwise indicated. TENS is also recommended for treatment of phantom limb pain. Application of a TENS unit has been found to produce benefits in a variety of neuropathic conditions including thoracic radiculopathy, femoral neuropathy, and radial neuropathy. In non-neuropathic conditions TENS has been used with variable success in treatment of osteoarthritis, piriformis syndrome, labor pain, and pain associated with stroke (Box 22-4).

Equipment

The most commonly available commercial TENS unit consists of a small, battery-operated device that may be easily attached to clothing. Two output channels, each allowing dual lead attachment, are present. The clinician may program the stimulation modes and other parame-

Table 22-1 TENS Parameter Settings

	Parameter		
TENS Mode	Pulse width (μs)	Amplitude (mA)	Frequency (Hz)
Conventional (high-frequency, low-intensity)	50 to 100	10 to 30	60 to 100
Electroacupuncture (low-frequency, high-intensity)	200 to 300	20 to 50	5 to 10 100–Hz pulses at 1 to 2 Hz

Box 22-4   Indications for TENS

Myofascial pain syndromes
Neuropathic pain
Pain from vascular insufficiency
Acute pain (postoperative pain)
Multiple sclerosis
Focal pain from malignancies
Labor pain

ters. The patient is allowed to control the intensity of stimulation independently for each output channel. Adhesive electrodes are applied to the affected area and connected to the jacks (Fig. 22-8).

Prior to application, the skin is cleaned gently with mild soap. Although excess hair may be trimmed off, shaving immediately prior to application of electrodes is not recommended. If the affected area needs to be shaved, it should be done 24 hours in advance to minimize skin irritation during electrode application.

Complications and Precautions

The most common problem with TENS units is skin irritation from the electrodes. These can be treated by changing the type of electrode, using a different type of gel, or perhaps applying a small amount of over-the-counter steroid ointment before applying the electrodes. Since TENS uses electrical impulses for stimulation, there is a risk of interference with similar devices. Thus, application of a TENS unit is contraindicated in patients with cardiac pacemakers. If the TENS leads are placed across the heart, there is a theoretic risk

of interference with myocardial electrical conduction although this is a very slight risk given the low current in a TENS unit. The TENS unit should not be placed over the carotid arteries because of the risk of hypotension or bradycardia from stimulation of the carotid sinus. Overall, TENS is a very safe device largely free of serious side effects.

PERIPHERAL NERVE STIMULATION

Background

PNS, a technique for providing pain relief, started in 1967 as a direct result of Wall and Sweet's work to demonstrate the gate-control theory. Although satisfactory analgesia was produced, there was a lack of commercially available equipment and interest waned until the 1980s. In the 1980s, the introduction of commercially available equipment, specifically the introduction of the flat Resume electrode by Medtronic, rekindled interest in PNS. Today, with careful patient selection, PNS offers a method of nerve stimulation without the disadvantages of SCS (Table 22-2).

Mechanism of Action

Historically, four methods of stimulation have been described. The first one utilizes metal electrodes placed over peripheral nerves (this became a prototype for TENS). In the second method, percutaneous electrodes were placed near the affected nerves. These electrodes produced a tingling sensation in the distribution of the nerve. In the third method, silicone cuff electrodes were

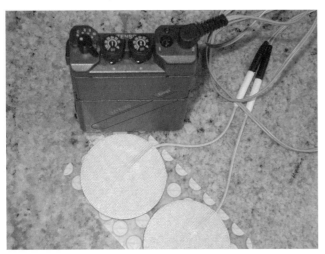

Figure 22-8   Commercially available TENS unit with adhesive electrodes, attached to output channel 2. Note that two additional electrodes may be attached to output channel 1.

Table 22-2   Comparison of Peripheral Nerve Stimulation with Spinal-Cord Stimulation

PNS	SCS
No involvement of the central nervous system	Higher likelihood of central nervous system problems
Less likelihood of lead migration	Epidurally-placed leads may migrate
Unilateral stimulation	Higher likelihood of unwanted bilateral stimulation
Mixed nerve stimulation can lead to involuntary movement with paresthesias	Dorsally-located epidural leads unlikely to result in involuntary movement
Scarring can occur around nerve	Scarring possible around catheter, less likely to involve nerves
Initial placement more invasive	Initial placement less invasive with percutaneous approach

placed around affected nerves and attached subcutaneously to the rheumatoid factor unit (modern PNS evolved from this technique). The fourth method, which gave rise to present SCS, involved placement of flexible electrodes into the epidural space and stimulation of the dorsal columns.

Implantation Technique

The equipment used for PNS is the same as that used for SCS. Like SCS, PNS requires a trial period. However, even the trial electrode is placed surgically and under aseptic conditions. A small incision, usually about 5 cm, is made directly over the nerve and the underlying tissue is carefully dissected. A small fascial flap, about 1 × 5 cm, is placed over the nerve and attached with interrupted sutures. The electrode is placed over the fascial flap to prevent direct contact with the nerve. This is analogous to the dura mater in SCS, which is positioned between the electrode and the nervous tissue. With the cuff electrode, which wraps around the nerve, no fascial flap is required. However, the cuff is not sewn directly to the nerve. A second incision is made proximal to the first to allow room for the percutaneous wires to be connected to the leads. If the trial is successful, the electrode is left in place and only the percutaneous extension wire is removed. The electrode is then connected to the implanted generator which is usually implanted in the infraclavicular region (for upper extremities) or in the lower abdominal wall (for lower extremities).

Patient Selection

PNS has been utilized with variable success in treatment of sympathetically-mediated post-traumatic causalgia (CRPS II). Some investigators reported significant success rates in patients with peripheral nerve injuries, up to 61%. PNS can be utilized for treatment of causalgia in the distribution of ulnar, median, radial, tibial, common peroneal, brachial plexus, or saphenous nerves.

The criteria for patient selection are similar to those of SCS. Prior to implantation, a definite cause should be well-established. Patients considered for possible PNS should demonstrate prior failure of conservative therapy and/or surgery. Habituation problems should be ruled out. Some practitioners advocate use of psychological testing prior to implantation to rule out any underlying psychological problems.

Complications and Precautions

A number of studies in the literature have reported complication rates of between 5% and 43% with a mean complication rate of 18%. Most complications are minor,

including revisions for repositioning of electrodes, or superficial infections. Some complications are more serious, including injury to the nerve during implantation, ischemia from wrap-around electrodes that may have been too tight or foreign-body reactions to the implanted material.

CORTICAL AND DEEP BRAIN STIMULATION

Background

The placement of electrodes in the intracranial space began in the late 1970s as an option for patients who had exhausted all other modalities. Although initial studies were promising, follow-up studies were less so and this procedure has been relatively underutilized since then. Some of the difficulties with this procedure may be due to the difficulty mapping the exact location to stimulate. Studies have shown that different types of pain respond differently to stimulation at different regions of the brain. Stimulation of the brain has involved two areas, the so-called *deep brain stimulation* for deafferentation pain and nociceptive pain and *motor cortex stimulation* for poststroke pain.

For deep brain stimulation, the two major areas for stimulation in the brain are the sensory thalamic nuclei and the periaqueductal/periventricular (PAG/PVG) gray area. Deafferentation (or neuropathic) pain responds much better to stimulation of the sensory thalamus and nociceptive pain responds better to PAG/PVG stimulation. Although some forms of deafferentation pain may respond well to SCS (which is also indicated for neuropathic pain), for certain types of injuries, SCS may not be an option. These include pain after spinal-cord injury, possibly postherpetic neuralgia, trigeminal neuropathic pain, and phantom limb pain.

More recently, stimulation of certain areas of the motor cortex has shown some promise for poststroke pain and perhaps for trigeminal neuralgia. Although the mechanism for pain relief is not precisely known, the prevailing theory is that stimulation of the motor cortex may inhibit spinothalamic neurons to a certain degree. There are no reliable predictors for success with this procedure and this should only be attempted after all other modalities have failed. Based on the available data from the literature, this procedure has shown some promise in poststroke pain and trigeminal neuralgia.

Implantation of the electrodes is usually accomplished through a small craniotomy, performed near the motor cortex. The locations in the brain are confirmed by changes in the operative somatosensory evoked potentials. The location in the brain from which a good muscle contraction occurs must be mapped as carefully as possible. If successful, the generator is implanted in the infraclavicular area (Fig. 22-9). The experimental evidence is limited. Available information describes approximately 50% of patients who achieved satisfactory or excellent pain control over 2-year period.

Stimulation Parameters

Patients receiving deep brain or cortical stimulation should undergo a trial of 1 to 2 weeks. The infection rate with an external system like this is very low and prophylactic antibiotics are recommended. A lengthy trial period of 1 to 2 weeks will allow the clinician to gauge the effectiveness of the placement, the degree of any discomfort from the actual stimulation, and possibly minimize the placebo effect. In general, the degree of pain reduction should be at least 50% to proceed to permanent implantation.

For thalamic stimulation, the period of stimulation should be about 15 to 30 minutes. The frequency is set between 40 to 70 Hz, based on patient comfort. The pulse width is usually about 200 μs and this regimen may provide several hours' pain relief. Patients are instructed to use the stimulator no more than 3 to 4 times in 24 hours.

For motor cortical stimulation, pain relief has been reported after 10 to 15 minutes of stimulation with a post-stimulation effect lasting several hours. The stimulation intensity is widely variable and is set at approximately 80%

of the intensity needed to induce muscle contractions. The frequency and pulse width are also widely variable at 40 to 130 Hz and 60 to 350 μs, respectively.

Complications

In general, there have been very few complications from these procedures with a reported complication rate of about 3%. These complications include hemorrhages at the local site, superficial infections, transient diplopia (during stimulation of the PAG/PVG), or stimulation-induced pain.

CONCLUSION

Electrical stimulation of the nervous system by one, or more, of the methods discussed in this chapter is a useful adjunct in pain management. It is important to discuss these procedures extensively with patients and attempt to match the patient's expectations with what these procedures can reasonably accomplish. TENS is a useful, noninvasive, and safe modality for many types of pain and its favorable risk-benefit ratio makes it a worthwhile adjunct to consider. SCS continues to enjoy an expanded role for chronic pain, cancer-related pain, and for vascular problems. The advantages of PNS make it a worthwhile adjunct to consider, although the placement of electrodes is considerably more invasive, even in the trial phase. Deep brain and cortical stimulation are generally underutilized because of their invasiveness but both have demonstrated promise in many pain syndromes that are refractory to other means. Electrical stimulation of the nervous system should continue to expand as new clinical applications are discovered.

SUGGESTED READING

Benzon H: Essentials of Pain Medicine and Regional Anesthesia. Philadelphia, Churchill Livinstone (Elsevier), 1999, pp 111–114, 395–398.

Burchiel KJ: Surgical Management of Pain, Part IV. New York: Thieme Publishing, 2002, pp 498–576.

Kanner R: Pain Management Secrets: 2nd ed. Philadelphia, Hanley & Belfus (Elsevier), 2002.

Loeser JD (ed): Bonica's Management of Pain, 3rd ed. Philadelphia, Lippincott Williams & Wilkins, 2001, pp 1849–1890.

Raj PP: Pain Medicine: A Comprehensive Review, 2nd ed. Philadelphia, Mosby Publishing, 2003.

Rajagopal A, Abram SE: Electrical stimulation of the nervous system. In Abram SE, Haddox JD (eds): The Pain Clinic Manual. Philadelphia, Lippincott Williams & Wilkins, 2000, pp 109-115.

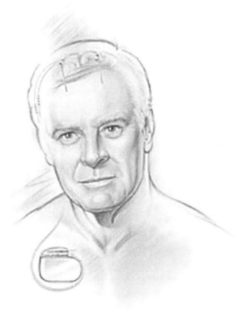

Figure 22-9   Position of deep brain stimulation leads and implanted generator in the infraclavicular space. (Courtesy of Medtronic, Inc.)

Index